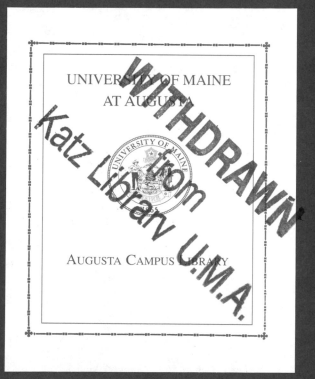

CALIFORNIA/MILBANK BOOKS ON HEALTH AND THE PUBLIC

Big Doctoring in America

Big Doctoring in America

Profiles in Primary Care

Fitzhugh Mullan, M.D.

Photographs by John Moses

UNIVERSITY OF CALIFORNIA PRESS
Berkeley · Los Angeles · London

THE MILBANK MEMORIAL FUND
New York

The Milbank Memorial Fund is an endowed national foundation that engages in nonpartisan analysis, study, research, and communication on significant issues in health policy. In the Fund's own publications, in reports or books it publishes with other organizations, and in articles it commissions for publication by other organizations, the Fund endeavors to maintain the highest standards for accuracy and fairness. Statements by individual authors, however, do not necessarily reflect opinions or factual determinations of the Fund.

University of California Press
Berkeley and Los Angeles, California

University of California Press, Ltd.
London, England

Library of Congress Cataloging-in-Publication Data

Mullan, Fitzhugh.
    Big doctoring in America: profiles in primary care /
by Fitzhugh Mullan.
        p.   cm. (California/Milbank books on health and the
public ;5)
    Includes bibliographical references and index.
    ISBN 0–520–22670–4 (cloth : alk. paper)
    1. Primary care (Medicine)—United States.
    [DNLM: 1. Primary Health Care—trends—United
States—Personal Narratives.   2. Family Practice—trends—
United States—Personal Narratives.   W 84.6 M958b
2002]   I. Title.   II. Series.

R729.5.G4 .M85   2002
362.1'0973—dc21   2001005492

Manufactured in the United States of America
10   09   08   07   06   05   04   03   02   01
10   9   8   7   6   5   4   3   2   1

For Caroline

Contents

Foreword

The Milbank Memorial Fund is an endowed national foundation that engages in nonpartisan analysis, study, research and communication on significant issues in health policy. The Fund makes available the results of its work in meetings with decision-makers, reports, articles, and books.

This is the fifth of the California/Milbank Books on Health and the Public. The publishing partnership between the Fund and the Press seeks to encourage the synthesis and communication of findings from research that could contribute to more effective health policy.

Fitzhugh Mullan uses the methods of oral history and personal journalism to humanize the phrases "primary care" and "medical generalism." Mullan traveled the country to interview 74 primary care practitioners, the "big doctors" of his title (in contrast to specialists, whose knowledge is narrower and often focused on technology rather than patients). Most of these big doctors are family physicians, internists, or pediatricians. But Mullan also interviewed nurse practitioners and physician assistants. He transformed interviews with fifteen practitioners into first-person stories about their professional lives. Next he set these stories in context by adding opening and closing chapters and introducing each story. John Moses, a professional photographer as well as a primary care physician (as is Mullan), visited each of the practitioners to take the photographs in the book.

In the final chapter, "Building a Better Future: The Case for Primary Care," Mullan describes policy that could enable more Americans to benefit from access to health care generalists. He believes that a fundamental challenge for the politics of health policy is whether "to give all of our citizens affordable humanistic care" or instead "emphasize the right of the individual to seek technological solutions regardless of the consequences for society as a whole."

Daniel M. Fox   Samuel L. Milbank
President   *Chairman*

Introduction

Big Doctoring is a book about the generalist in America, the practitioner of primary care medicine in the United States at the opening of the twenty-first century. Big doctoring is what the generalist does: doctoring that embraces the whole person, that values comprehensiveness and continuity, that welcomes the richness and the complexity of the complete human being. I set about writing this book because I am a primary care physician, a pediatrician, and I am, by turns, puzzled, fascinated, and troubled by what is happening to health care in this country.

I chose medicine as a career because, I realize now, I was drawn to big doctoring (though I would hardly have called it that in 1964 when I started medical school) by my father and grandfather. My father was a psychiatrist and a group therapist who invited me from an early age to sit in with him occasionally on counseling and therapy sessions with groups and even individuals. Though he was not a literal layer-on of hands, I was fascinated by the breadth and intimacy of his work with people, by the privilege and the license that allowed him to explore and advise on all aspects of his patients' lives. He got to know his patients well, and I remember vividly how he came home, for better or for worse, full of their troubles. He worried about them as people, as complete, struggling human beings. My grandfather trained in medicine in the first years of the twentieth century and then spent thirty-five years as a Commissioned Officer in the United States Public Health Service. Although he worked in many parts of the United States, in Canada, and in Europe, his assignments kept bringing him back—five times in all—to Ellis Island in New York harbor. As an examining physician, he had a responsibility to both the immigrants he screened and the nation they were joining. His message to me was, likewise, that doctoring was a broad, multifaceted undertaking. It was a big enterprise that involved the whole person and the society as well.

My instincts in medical school all ran toward big doctoring. The mid-sixties, however, was a time when medical education was moving briskly away from the generalist ideal based on the virtually unchallenged premise that the growing volume of science available to medicine meant that the future of medical practice was the specialist. The job of training programs was to produce specialists in increasing numbers and varieties. General practice as a calling was dying—faculty openly told us "no one from a decent medical school ever becomes a GP any more"—and the new model of family medicine had not yet been launched. So I chose pediatrics as my version of big doctoring, a discipline where I hoped that making a difference for a little person would over many years make a big difference. Pediatrics also meant engaging parents and families as well as the child, and had a rich tradition of work in schools and communities. After four years of residency at city hospitals in New York, I joined the National Health Service Corps—a brand-new program of the United States Public Health Service that sent doctors to poor and rural areas to work with people in need. I was assigned to a clinic in New Mexico, where for three years I practiced a mixture of pediatrics and, of necessity, family medicine. Although the time and the place were different, I did have a sense of following in my grandfather's footsteps, and I certainly had found my way to big doctoring.

In the mid-1970s, I moved to Washington and from 1977 to 1981 served as director of the National Health Service Corps, running, in essence, a 2,000-person national primary care practice. This was big doctoring heaven. By the early 1980s I was firmly committed to the Public Health Service and remained as a Commissioned Officer until 1995, managing a number of programs supportive of primary care education, research, and practice. From 1992 to 1994, I served on the Task Force on Health Care Reform and worked on the resultant Health Security Act that envisioned primary care as a central feature of a reformed system. But legislated health care reform did not come to pass. Instead, market-driven managed care swept across the country, rearranging the lives of doctors, patients, and hospitals. Most forms of managed care called on primary care physicians to serve as gatekeepers—a pivotal and controversial role that asked them to see all patients, render appropriate care, and determine when specialty referrals were warranted. Controversial or not, the prominence of primary care was sudden, and the demand for the services of generalists rose perceptibly.

In 1996, after more than twenty years in the United States Public Health Service, I left federal service intent on resuming my identity as a primary care doctor. I spent time retraining in pediatrics and went to work at a community health center in inner-city Washington, D.C. More than this, though, I wanted to explore the evolving role of medical generalism in the United States. I wanted to bear witness to it, to understand its potentials and its debilities, and to provide testimony for it. Advocate I certainly was—and am—but I was acutely aware that this would be a tough task in contemporary America, a wealthy nation endowed with a powerful tradition of individualism and a strong sense of entitlement. These cultural realities, combined with the steady advances in clinical science, were serving to promote ever-higher popular expectations of the medical system and the common belief that pinpoint specialized interventions were the way of the future. In this environment, rich in transplant thinking and awash with anticipatory excitement about the Human Genome Project, primary care was seen by many as irrelevant or a remnant of the past.

AMERICAN MEDICAL QUANDARIES

The United States is mired in a profound, expensive, divisive, paradoxical medical swamp—and has been, with increasing malign consequences, for at least fifty years. Despite spending an average of $4,270 on medical care for every man, woman, and child in the United States each year—55 percent more than the next most munificent nation (Switzerland) and a full 3.4 percent more of our gross national product than the next most medically committed nation (Germany)[1]—we get undistinguished (some would argue terrible) results for our investment. A recent global comparison of health systems conducted by the World Health Organization rated the United States as number 37 overall, behind virtually all Western European nations, Canada, Colombia, and Morocco.[2] The U.S. system's levels of responsiveness as scored by the WHO did not offset its very low ratings on costs and fairness, confirming many transnational and domestic studies that document high degrees of frustration with the medical care in this country. Most troubling, the United States does not receive good outcomes for its prodigious expenditures, ranking twenty-fourth in the world in life expectancy, below countries such as Japan, Greece, and Iceland.

The WHO document analyzes global data, but its findings are in no way contrary to multiple surveys, studies, and consensus documents published over the years in this country. Fifteen percent of our population has no health insurance. Infant mortality and longevity figures lag well behind countries that spend much less on health care but enjoy more comprehensive systems. In a business-driven campaign to control medical costs, many whose insurance is provided through employers have been moved into systems of managed care, which many think limit patient choice and compromise quality. Despite this widespread phenomenon, medical costs are again rising, led by pharmaceuticals, which are now aggressively marketed to the public as well as to physicians. Medicare (government-mediated health insurance for the elderly) remains an extremely popular but expensive program that, despite its lack of coverage for drugs and nursing homes, is headed for insolvency in the future. Medical information is everywhere—in newspapers and magazines, and now on the Web—but the consumer, newly rich in data and opinion, has a new problem of sifting and evaluating this proliferation of advice. Despite the resplendency of our medical technology and the monumental outlay that we make for health care, we are not doing well in outcomes, satisfaction, or fairness.

A national primary care system of robust quality is a necessary prerequisite to draining our national health care swamp. This generalist ideal is a concept that flourished in earlier times, when, to be sure, medical knowledge was far more limited and an individual doctor could "own" a significant portion of it. The proliferation of knowledge in the twentieth century spawned and promoted specialism, but has led to the current situation in which specialty physicians in the United States outnumber generalists two to one, are paid at substantially higher rates, and enjoy far more prestige than their generalist colleagues. These circumstances and the general gusto with which American medicine has adopted the specialty ideal are at the heart of the quandary in which we find ourselves. Not coincidentally, primary care physicians play more central roles in virtually all of the national systems that rate ahead of the United States in satisfaction and quality. Quantities of evidence demonstrate the ability of generalist physicians to manage medical care more cost-effectively than highly compartmentalized specialists. Primary care must be the basis of any future strategy to extend care to all of the American population as well as all of the current "safety net" efforts to provide care to the uninsured. New patterns of training in areas such as the primary care disciplines, combined with powerful and portable new information technologies, will make the generalist of the future a far more effective manager of information than those of the past. The skilled generalist working in partnership with patients is the antidote to the complexity, inconsistency, and anomie that we all experience in our ever more complicated system. The complete generalist is a clinician, a navigator, and a personal coach—the medical friend whom we all need.

Many questions came immediately to mind when I considered the status of big doctoring at the end of the twentieth century. The physician with a horse and buggy faithfully traveling the countryside to treat patients at all hours and in all seasons is a powerful but dated American image. The house call and the cradle-to-grave care are important national lore but these images, too, tend to come from the past. Marcus Welby was celebrated on TV, but that was forty years ago. Who are the generalists of today, women and men, rural and urban, physicians and, in fact, nonphysicians? How are they trained? What are their practices like? How do they balance their work and their personal lives? How do they see the changing medical world in which they live? How do patients regard them, given the specialist bent of our society? What do they think about managed care and their prominent role in it? How do they feel about keeping current given the continued growth of clinical science? What about the tedium of routine care and the hassle factor of dealing with a dizzying array of billing codes and insurance forms . . . and the future?

ORAL HISTORY

I needed a better understanding of the present and past before taking on the future. I wanted to understand how primary care practitioners viewed this tradition of doctoring, what these clinicians thought about their lives in medicine and their lives in general. So I set about talking to them, traveling the country and recording the oral histories of some seventy-four generalist practitioners—sixty-three primary care physicians, eight nurse practitioners, and three physician assistants. I identified and selected candidates for interview by a simple process of networking, starting with individuals I knew in various parts of the country and asking them who came to mind in response to the words "primary care," "experienced," "thoughtful," "articulate," and "colorful." From there I followed my leads, trying to keep a balance with regard to geography, gender, urban and rural practices, ethnicity, and discipline as I went.

The path was rarely straight but always interesting. I had one New England candidate lined up for interviewing at a time when he was scheduled to go fishing and, he told me firmly, "Nothing interferes with my fishing." When I asked him whom he might recommend, he thought for a moment and said, "I got it. Another old gopher just like me. I'm sure he'll have the time." He did, and he had a wonderful story to tell. In another instance, I sat down to interview an internist recommended by a friend of a friend and discovered, part way through the session, that he and I had spent a week together in 1965 being trained in first aid and nonviolence by the Medical Committee for Human Rights before traveling to Mississippi as civil rights workers. My subjects (the word is unfairly and inaccurately impersonal) were extremely generous of their time and attentiveness, sometimes feeding me, housing me, and, on one occasion, flying me to my next interview. People told me their stories on rustic porches overlooking the Gastineau Channel in southern Alaska and on Maine's Penobscot Bay, in corporate boardrooms in Miami and Albuquerque, in a battered community health center in Washington, D.C., and in the magnificent National Academy of Sciences building a mile or two away in the same city. One interview had a forty-five-minute obstetrical delay while my subject plied her trade in a delivery room down the hall before she returned to telling me her story.

Oral history has been with us since humans began contemplating themselves and their origins. Tribal legend and family lore are special and common forms of oral history. More recently, and with the advent of recording equipment, oral history has become a form of documentation used by scholars to chronicle the perspectives of participants in epochal events— warriors, politicians, scientists. Social scientists and, increasingly, family members have used oral history to collect the stories and insights of citizens, community members, parents, and grandparents in an effort to capture and understand the immediate past.

I chose the oral history format because the intent of my interviews was to try to understand my subjects not just as physicians in the 1990s but as individuals who had grown up in the midst of the twentieth century, buffeted by the many winds blowing through American life and medical practice. I was especially interested in their values and the decisions that had drawn them into primary care. Where had those values come from, and how had they been formed, nurtured, rewarded, or disappointed? These questions have a relevance not only for understanding ourselves and our past but also for envisioning the future. The generalist of the new century will surely continue to provide day-to-day personal and preventive care. While medical science and new therapies may well alleviate or eliminate certain diseases, many of the imponderables of medical life—clinical uncertainty, patient debility, emotional pain, family disruption, and Solomonian medical choices—will remain central to the work of generalists. What do the lives and the experiences of current generalists tell us about recruiting, educating, and supporting future generations of generalists?

Oral history is not just an open mike. The historian structures the conversation with the flow of questions and nudges the subject to get at frustrations and disappointments, which are generally much harder to learn about than passions and achievements. My interviews were as varied as the people were, but I always asked about the youth and background of the individual, especially about the decision to become a clinician and what prompted the choice of a career in primary care. We usually talked about the person's practice, social and community experience, and view of the present and future of health care. In the interviews I labored to get at what motivates these individuals, what they love and what troubles them about their life and their work. Most were marvelously open, talking to me with candor about their professional and at times their personal lives, sharing recollections, stories of youth, moments of pride, disappointments, hopes.

ORGANIZATION

Each oral history was transcribed, returned to the individual for editing, and revised accordingly. All of the transcripts were then deposited as the Primary Care Oral History Collection at the National Library of Medicine in Bethesda, Maryland, for the use of future scholars as well as anyone interested in the history of medicine at the end of the twentieth century. In 1998 and 1999, the *Journal of the American Medical Association (JAMA)* published five pieces drawn from the oral history collection under the heading "Profiles in Primary Care." For this series, I edited and condensed each profile so that it read as a mini-autobiography, with the practitioner telling the story in his or her own voice. The core of *Big Doctoring* is the five *JAMA* profiles and ten more edited in a similar fashion to create a mosaic representation of the lives of generalist practitioners.

Each of the profiles is accompanied by a photographic portrait depicting the protagonist of that particular profile. These pictures were taken by John Moses, M.D., an accomplished documentary photographer and, as it happens, primary care pediatrician who is on the faculty of Duke University School of Medicine. Dr. Moses spent time with each of the individuals, learning about their work and taking photographs in settings that would capture their practices and personalities.

In rereading and selecting among the rich cache of human stories that I had collected, I discovered two unexpected characteristics of my "data." The first was that my subjects were virtually all born before 1960 and most before 1950, meaning that I had not spent time with generalists in training or in their early years of practice. This bias came about because in my oral history mode I was looking for experience and perspective, which usually came from subjects who had been around for a while. The profiles in *Big Doctoring,* therefore, represent the end-of-the century generation of generalists, men and women who for the most part were trained in the 1960s and 1970s and who have been practicing since then—well versed in issues such as the escalation of medical costs, the uninsured, technological acceleration, and managed care. These are seasoned and opinionated commentators—veterans.

My second discovery, linked to the first, was that in my effort to find subjects with colorful stories to tell, I had managed to identify an extraordinary group of people who probably have more clinical, community, and professional involvements than the average generalist practitioner. These are unusually committed people whose stories go well beyond the typical and common issues of clinical medicine and practice management. They demonstrate an abundance of idealism, activism, and a willingness to deal with risk, adversity, diversity, and uncertainty. Their commitment to purpose and the vitality with which they approach their clinical and personal lives are evident. While it could be argued that the cast of *Big Doctoring* is not "typical," these people represent the best values and instincts of clinicians drawn to big doctoring and the primary care movement.

While these fifteen lives make strong statements about primary care today, they are all set on the larger stage of the evolving history of medical care in America. To put them in context, it is important to understand the legacy of medical generalism as well as the particular organizational, economic, and policy issues that bear on primary care today. *Big Doctoring* opens with a chapter titled "Primary Care Roots" which discusses the values, mind set, and definition of primary care. It traces the history and emerging philosophy of medical generalism in twentieth-century America and brings the story to the present with the challenges and opportunities of today's complicated medical marketplace.

The profiles themselves raise questions about the future, with many of the subjects reporting current dilemmas as well as explicit and implicit challenges that they see down the road. The policy debates of the present—the intellectual and political struggles over issues such as system reform, compensation, educational strategies, the coverage of the uninsured—will determine a great deal about the future of big doctoring in this country. What the public understands and what the public thinks about primary care is essential to how the system of the future will be structured—and what role primary care plays in it. The last chapter in *Big Doctoring* is devoted to the future. It moves from the biographical to the political. If the patients of America are going to continue to benefit from practitioners like those whose lives are chronicled here, what has to happen in the realms of public opinion, public policy, health policy, and educational strategy?

LANGUAGE

Throughout *Big Doctoring,* I use the terms "generalist" or "generalist physician" and "primary care," "primary care provider," or "primary care clinician" more or less interchangeably. I do this knowing that I am blurring certain professional lines of demarcation. There certainly are distinctions that can be drawn between these terms, and there are activities or clinicians that are typically designated by one or another of the labels. Generalism as a term has broad implications and links to concepts well beyond medicine and, as such, has particular importance to certain discussions, whereas primary care has a more specific applicability to health care and, therefore, a special role in other discussions. Yet the commonality of the work of generalist practitioners substantially outweighs the differences in nomenclature that complicate the domain of primary care, and the message of *Big Doctoring* is one of ecumenicism, not of schism. Therefore, at each opportunity I have attempted to choose the term that makes most substantive sense and avoids semantic awkwardness.

These linguistic issues are enriched and complicated by the arrival of clinicians from backgrounds other than medicine in the primary care sector—specifically, nurse practitioners and physician assistants. Nurses, in particular, have well-developed identities and a long tradition of nursing practice, so that their new presence in the realm of "medical practice" has created multiple challenges of language. Words such as "provider" and "clinician" have to some extent taken the place of "doctor" or "physician." In some circles the very word "medical" is considered both exclusionary and passé, and the term "health care" has supplanted "medical care." These conflicts can be more than struggles over vocabulary. At times, they are actual contests for professional identity and position, with certain professional groups pressing hard for new linguistic rules that will promote their view of the professional world.

In choosing the title *Big Doctoring*, I concede from the start that I am not going to try to force my view and experience with the world of primary care into a language that might be topical but does not talk to the public as a whole. The title "Big Providing," for instance, simply didn't work. Throughout the book I have followed this same convention. I consider nurse practitioners and physician assistants core members of the primary care family, and my interviews and writings include them in significant numbers. But the work that they do falls under the banner of what for centuries society has considered to be doctoring. I have tended to use language that welcomes them to that role, in the spirit of collegial embrace and in the hopes of an increasingly unified world of big doctoring.

Some readers will undoubtedly raise questions about my selection of primary care disciplines. The boundaries of primary care are not uniformly defined, and there are many professional disciplines within health care that regularly or, on occasion, identify themselves as primary care providers. Common examples include obstetrician/gynecologists, dentists, and podiatrists. Others lay claim to practicing primary care under certain circumstances, such as oncologists who sometimes treat non-cancerous conditions of cancer patients. While the contributions of these clinicians to the delivery of primary care is important, in *Big Doctoring* I chose to limit my interviews to five categories of health professionals whose educational programs are designed to prepare them to care for most of the problems that trouble most people most of the time and whose practices reflect that training. These are family physicians, general internists, general pediatricians, nurse practitioners, and physician assistants.

It is my hope that *Big Doctoring* will help make the work of primary care more discernible to the public as a whole as well as to practitioners and students of medicine and the health professions. These lives tell a great deal about healers whose specialty is knowing and treating people over time and helping them navigate the opportunities and the hazards of an ever more complex health care system. Taken together, they make an eloquent case that primary care is a fascinating, important, and precious calling.

CHAPTER ONE

Primary Care Roots

Big Doctoring is about a way of medical life, an approach to health care
and healing, a skill set, and a mind set that is called primary care. It is
about doctoring that is humanist, comprehensive, efficient, and flexible,
doctoring that builds on the legacy of the past and the rich tradition of
care in medicine and nursing. To that it adds the science and technology
of the contemporary world, applied in a measured, evidence-based, and
coordinated fashion. In our current culture of medical care—noteworthy
for its sophistication of technology, its inexorable cost increases, the absence of uniform access to its benefits, a high rate of medical errors, and
the uncertainty of many outcomes—primary care provides a foundation
for health care that blends good science with good judgment.

Yet primary care is not a philosophy or a vocational inclination shared
by everybody in the healing sciences. In fact, for decades a tug-of-war
has been taking place between advocates of generalist approaches to medical care and proponents of narrower, specialty-based philosophies. The
fifteen primary care clinicians profiled here are men and women whose
work is characterized by a broad approach to patient care and the community: they are practitioners of applied generalism, dedicated holists.
Their work, however, takes place in the larger setting of the economics
and politics of health care in the United States, and an understanding of
this larger context is essential to any discussion of the present and future of primary care in the United States. The definition of primary care,
its values, the role of generalism in contemporary life, and a review of

the history of primary care in the United States are all elements of that understanding.

WHAT IS PRIMARY CARE?

Like the Mona Lisa's enigmatic smile in Leonardo da Vinci's masterpiece, primary care means different things to different people. Unlike many elements of health care today, primary care is not defined by an organ system (cardiology), a place (the outpatient department), or a financial precept (capitation payment). It is an idea that, by turns, describes a type of practitioner, a domain of service, or a philosophy of care. This definitional ambiguity means that many roles can be ascribed to primary care, but it also can be an area of troublesome imprecision and confusion.

To clinicians primary care is a label that describes certain types of practitioners—even though no one is actually schooled or board-certified in a discipline called "primary care." Family physician, pediatrician, internist, physician assistant, and nurse practitioner are the professions most often grouped under the heading of primary care, but on occasion many other medical and nonmedical specialties claim primary care status. To patients primary care can mean the provider (a word that is itself greeted with ambivalence) who knows them best, giving comprehensive, "high touch" care over the years. Or it can mean the designated medical grinch who bars their access to coveted specialty services. Payers and policymakers see primary care as a set of attributes and a level of care that promote the rational and cost-effective delivery of medical services in a culture much given to unwarranted subspecialty care and the use of the hospital.

These definitions are further complicated by an important but largely unarticulated divergence of opinion about the ethos of primary care, about why primary care matters. Beyond its functional role, what is the moral role of primary care in society? Many proponents have seen the primary care movement as a battle for the soul of medicine. This struggle has been especially apparent in poor and rural communities that have been largely abandoned or neglected by contemporary medical practitioners and where primary care is viewed as a special mission to serve the underserved. In both mainstream and marginalized communities the role of primary care is seen as bringing competent, comprehensive doctoring to bear, healing in an omnibus sense. In this view, biopsychosocial skills are important, as are capabilities in areas as diverse as epidemiology, Spanish, community organizing, and short-term psychotherapy. This might be called the "social justice" view of primary care.

Set against this is the "industrial efficiency" view that sees primary care as the foundation of all systems of health care. From this perspective, the primary care provider is simply the "field captain" best qualified to make sense of a complicated and often inefficient system. Not only can the primary care clinician treat the majority of the problems that patients bring to the medical system, but he can carry out well-informed triage for hospital and specialty referrals. It is this latter gatekeeping capability that has special appeal to the business-oriented values of health systems planners and insurers.[1]

Working in the midst of these competing and sometimes conflicting definitions, the Institute of Medicine of the National Academy of Sciences convened a panel in 1994 to deliberate on the future of primary care. That panel produced a working definition of primary care that has stood up well in the ensuing years and certainly captures the essence of primary care as it is being lived by the practitioners whose lives are documented here: "Primary care is the provision of integrated, accessible health care services by clinicians who are accountable for addressing a large majority of personal health care needs, developing a sustained partnership with patients and practicing in the context of family and community."[2] Here I have limited my discussion of primary care to clinicians whose training and practice conforms most closely to this definition: general internists, general pediatricians, family physicians, physician assistants, and nurse practitioners.

VALUES

The values of primary care have always been present in the medical care system under one label or another. These are the values of medical generalism (a term I use interchangeably with primary care), and they center on the treatment of the whole person with attention to his or her biology, psychology, and social and community situation. Primary care encompasses mental health, public health, and community health as well as personal health care. It involves both first-contact care and care that is given over time. Comprehensiveness, continuity, and coordination have always been associated with primary care practice, as have accessibility and accountability.[3] The proverbial horse and buggy, the home visit, the doctor who delivered the baby and treated grandma in her final illness, affordable care, and general practice are traditional ideas that have given expression to the values of primary care. To these concepts have recently been added family medicine, health promotion and disease prevention, a "medical home," the general internist and pediatrician, geriatric care, patient and community education, and the new disciplines of the nurse practitioner and the physician assistant.

The generalist approach to medical care is more than a tradition or a stylistic preference. Primary care brings benefit to both the care of the individual and to the health care system as a whole. From a personal perspective, "knowing a doctor who knows you" is a widely held value but one that can be hard to fulfill in a system dominated by specialists skilled in one organ system or another but who disavow responsibility beyond their own area of expertise. A friend recently discharged from a hospital stay captured this sentiment poignantly: "It would have been fine if I could have dropped my body off the way I do my car at the repair shop, and picked it up a week later. The problem was that I had to stay with my body, and that was awful. Nobody really took charge. Everybody took care of their own thing, and I was left ultimately to fend for myself. Whatever happened to doctoring?" A skilled clinician who values discussion, education, and prevention, and who can make referrals and provide insider advice on the system, is an asset to individuals and families. Finding and retaining a clinician with these qualities is not always easy, but few among us would question the value of having a proficient generalist as a personal physician.

Studies have documented time and again that systems of care based on the generalist model cost less, provide excellent quality, and have high levels of patient satisfaction.[4] In nations such as Canada and Great Britain, which have built their medical care systems on an explicit primary care model, health care systems enjoy higher levels of citizen satisfaction despite considerably smaller expenditures than in the United States.[5] Similarly, the health maintenance organization (HMO) movement, from its earliest manifestations in the 1930s to the present, has always held that strong primary care must be the basis of any sensible system of quality care.

Primary care has its detractors who argue that it is a bad idea or, at the most, a nice idea from the past that has diminishing relevance in the present and the future. This argument stems from the premise that doctoring today has emerged from centuries of practice that were based largely on tradition, personal belief, and hokum. Today's medicine is increasingly evidence-based and scientifically complex. This being the case, the argument goes, specialism, reductionism (focusing on the parts rather than the whole), and the division of knowledge and practice into ever-smaller units are natural and necessary developments. Because no practitioner can possibly stay abreast of the exploding world of clinical information, specialization and subspecialization are requirements of competency. And because the growth of knowledge is accelerating, the current arguments for clinical reductionism will be even more compelling in the future. The idea of the general practitioner is hopelessly ill-suited to the epoch of the heart transplant and laser surgery.

This view is not wrong in its assessment of science or the challenges facing clinical medicine. Rather it is wrong in its assumptions about the human being. Despite the magnificent march of science, the human being remains a complex animal whose body and mind, self and family, person and community are linked in ways that will resist the effort to compartmentalize every pain or blemish as the domain of an expert but narrow specialist. Doctoring as serial specialty visits has not worked well in the past and, despite the onrush of specialized knowledge, will not work well in the future. The late Avedis Donabedian, the leading American scholar and proponent of quality measurement in health care, reflected this in a commentary about his final illness. Dr. Donabedian noted the irony in his need to coordinate much of his own care, observing that quality seemed to mean only "technical competence and, more recently, superficial attention to the interpersonal process. Keep the patient happy, be nice to the patient, call him Mr. or Mrs., remember his name. . . . Today people talk about patient autonomy but often it gets translated into patient abandonment."[6] The increasing complexity of medical science, in fact, will create the need for more—not less—integrative medical care. To the traditional generalist values of comprehensiveness, continuity, and coordination will be added imperatives from the emerging system: interpretation, integration, and navigation.

GENERALISM IN HUMAN ENTERPRISE

Generalism as a phenomenon is not limited to medicine. To some extent, there is a competition in all human endeavor between the instinct to keep things whole, complete, and general, and the tendency to distinguish, sort, and reduce. The famous distinction between "lumpers" (those who prefer pulling things together) and "splitters" (those given to dividing things wherever possible) is evident in our daily lives. The way we organize our desks or our refrigerators, for instance, is subject to lumping and splitting preferences, as are our patterns of friendship and our choice of jobs. Virtually any task can be approached holistically or in a reductionist manner though some clearly commend themselves more to one approach than the other.

Generalism in human terms can be defined as a tendency to remain broadly focused, protean, and varied in worldview and activity. The generalist is interested in the big picture with all of its nuances, connections, and complexities. Generalism requires a willingness to think broadly and to maintain sets of knowledge and ideas that are disparate and often not mutually reinforcing. Since the generalist's domain is typically large and complex, it often lacks the certainty and predictability that typifies the world of the specialist. The generalist needs to have a reasonable tolerance for living with uncertainty.

Generalism in human enterprise and as an approach to professional life is vitally important to society as a whole. The generalist labors in broad areas of human endeavor that call for an integrator and a coordinator, someone who can see the big picture and work accordingly. In earlier times the generalist was the norm. The family farmer, the local school teacher, the owner of the general store, the lawyer, and the banker were all general practitioners. Over the past century, however, developments in transportation, communications, and information management have created an environment where vocational specialization is possible, useful, and encouraged. Consequently, most professions have shifted toward more specialized training and practice. The benefits of reductionism are apparent in the growing variety and sophistication of educational opportunities, choice of foods, and telephone service. The specialization of knowledge and the expansion of consumer services seem to go hand in hand and suggest an inevitability to the march of specialization.

The development of specialism is favored not only by the growth of technology but also by the universal desire for personal mastery. One is more likely to achieve proficiency and excellence if one can reduce one's task to the smallest and most specific elements possible. Labor efficiency likewise favors dividing tasks in such a way as to assure a high level of worker competence in a focused and repetitive area. Specialized training and experience tend to reinforce each other and assure efficient production from a compartmentalized work force. In short, reducing knowledge, information, and tasks to units that are as small and as specialized as possible addresses important needs of individuals and societies.

The very word "specialist" implies a superiority over the nonspecialist in the hierarchy of knowledge. The specialist, indeed, has often earned that title through advanced training that has upgraded her skills in a specified area and, in the process, narrowed her field of endeavor. The result is a presumption of advanced practice and high technical competence that society tends to reward with increased prestige and compensation. Implicit also in the hierarchical idea of competency is the assumption that specialist work is more difficult and more taxing than generalist work; that teaching everything to the third grade is easier than teaching calculus to high school seniors; that doing mental health intake at a community health center demands less expertise than practicing analytic psychotherapy; that being a family physician is less challenging than being an anesthesiologist.

And yet what is the evidence that specialty work is harder than generalist work? The specialist deals in a definitionally limited range of challenges. Teaching calculus involves a much narrower curriculum and a far more restricted set of issues than teaching arithmetic, social studies, science, and reading to eight-year-olds while simultaneously coping with classroom discipline and inquiring parents. The specialist in any field may deal with severe manifestations of problems, but the problems will have predictability and repetitiousness. If a problem falls outside the specialist's zone of competence, he refers it on. The generalist does not have that luxury; she starts with ownership of all of the problems that patients bring. Triage and referral are important roles for the generalist, but diagnosis and treatment come first. The elementary school teacher, the general dentist, the parish priest, the neighborhood police officer are examples of practicing generalists all of whom have training and capabilities that provide the basic foundation of much of societal life. Generalist practice is multifaceted, unpredictable, and often complicated, calling on skills drawn from various disciplines. Sorting and weighing problems, deciding on programs of action, and knowing when and how to refer (sending a student to special education, calling for police backup, referring to a psychiatrist) are important generalist skills, competencies of exquisite importance for effective human services, but that receive far less attention and approbation than finely honed skills in very limited areas of professional service.

Education is a domain in which these issues have a long history of debate. As young people progress through school, their education tends to move from the general toward the specific. Never again will students be as generalized as they are in, say, the sixth grade, when it is fair game for the teacher to ask questions about Egyptian history, the division of fractions, the chemical composition of salt, and the Spanish word for table.

As grade school progresses into high school, students begin to specialize by selecting some disciplines and avoiding others. General knowledge takes a back seat to a growing store of special knowledge in the sciences, or the arts, or in automobile mechanics. By the time a student enters the workforce, her realm of competence usually has become quite focused, and knowledge from other fields is considered of marginal importance.

The role of general education at the university level has been debated hard over the years. Should post-secondary education produce graduates with a broad exposure to knowledge and the ability to further educate themselves, or should it train individuals with specific vocational capabilities to assume places in the workforce? Although areas of concentration ("majors") are the norm, virtually all American colleges mandate some quantity of general education—the dreaded language, or science, or humanities requirement. These requirements represent the educational establishment's effort to hold the line for generalism amid the ubiquitous and powerful pressures to specialize.

Similar tensions exist in business, with many executives building careers in one or another aspect of management—finance or human resources or communications—and climbing toward the top with little sense of the corporate whole. The organizational strategist Peter Senge opens his popular book *The Fifth Discipline* with the following: "From a very early age, we are taught to break apart problems, to fragment the world. This apparently makes complex tasks and subjects more manageable, but we pay a hidden, enormous price. We can no longer see the consequences of our actions; we lose our intrinsic sense of connection to a larger whole. When we then try to 'see the big picture,' we try to assemble the fragments in our minds, to list and organize all the pieces. . . . The task is futile—similar to trying to reassemble the fragments of a broken mirror to see a true reflection."[7]

THE HISTORY OF PRIMARY CARE IN AMERICA

Throughout the twentieth century, the practice of medicine in the United States was marked by a struggle between the specialist and the generalist. Specialists have harvested the products of the rapid growth in science and technology over this period and put them to work in clinical practice. Although the practice of generalist physicians has likewise become more sophisticated, generalists have tended to labor in the backwash of the specialty surge, continuing to provide care to much of the population in a relatively uncelebrated fashion. While the first fifty years of the century were characterized by the relatively uncontested retreat of the generalist physician, the next fifty saw generalists identify and redefine themselves in a variety of ways and initiate a fight for their position and role in medicine. By the century's end there was substantial intellectual, political, and commercial support for the generalist concept.

When the twentieth century began, the vast majority of American physicians were general practitioners treating, as well as they could, all of the maladies that patients brought to their doorsteps. They were, perforce, generalists wrestling with the medical, surgical, obstetrical, and psychiatric problems of people young and old, urban and rural, well heeled and not-so-well heeled. By current standards their science was limited, but they were present in significant numbers throughout the country, accepting payments in cash and in kind for their labors.[8] The concept of specialties in medicine did not exist to any great extent in the nineteenth century. Although an occasional urban physician might achieve a reputation for expertise in one or another area of medical practice, formalized training beyond medical school did not really exist, and most doctors went to work as general practitioners on receipt of their diplomas. Rapid developments in medical science in the latter years of the nineteenth century, however, set the stage for dramatic changes in medical practice in the twentieth. Anesthesia, antisepsis, the germ theory of disease, and the development of the diagnostic X ray were among the most significant of these developments.

The formal differentiation of specialty practice began early in the twentieth century with the formation of the American College of Surgeons in 1913. Surgical leaders argued that the skills and techniques involved in surgery required special training and competencies different from those practiced by the general practitioner. Internists followed suit, forming the American College of Physicians in 1915. The course followed by most ensuing specialty groups was to establish a "college" or "academy" whose membership was limited to physicians who had received training in the field and who specialized in the area. In the 1930s board examinations were introduced as measures of special competence and as requirements for membership in specialty organizations.

The norm, nonetheless, remained the GP. In 1932 the Committee on the Costs of Medical Care, sitting as the first national body to study health care in the United States, concluded that "each patient would be primarily under the charge of the family practitioner . . . (and) . . . would look to his physician for guidance and counsel on health matters and ordinarily would receive attention from specialists when referred."[9] Yet the pace of change was to increase dramatically with World War II and its aftermath. The organized use of medical manpower by the armed services during the war favored specialty-trained physicians and, in fact, provided training to many in areas such as surgery and anesthesia. Following the war, the G.I. bill was made available to physicians leaving the military and entering residency programs, providing financial incentives for postgraduate training that had never existed before. The twin postwar forces of the rapid growth of employer-sponsored, private health insurance and continued technological developments moved medical care toward the hospital and away from the community—an evolution that greatly favored specialists.

Between 1942 and 1954, the number of residency positions in the country jumped from 5,796 to 25,486, and the number of specialties grew to nineteen.[10] The majority of students graduating from medical school were choosing residency programs of three or more years that would qualify them to take specialty board exams. Those who entered practice as GPs after a single year of internship became the exception rather than the rule, and the GP was replaced as the principal provider of care for the family by various specialists, many of whom were hospital-based and none of whom treated the whole family. By 1960 specialists outnumbered generalists in practice.

The rebound of the generalist started in the 1950s with the idea that a generalist could be trained as a "specialist" with a broad set of competencies. In 1961, Kerr White published an essay in the *New England Journal of Medicine* titled "The Ecology of Medical Care," in which he used epidemiological analyses of patterns of medical care to show that in a population of 1,000 people, 250 would seek some form of medical care in the period of a month.[11] Of those, nine would be hospitalized, but only one in a university teaching center—and yet that setting was where virtually all of medical education took place. He argued that we needed to pay more heed to training of "primary physicians" who in fact worked where most medical care took place. This conclusion received concurrence from three national committees that were impaneled during the mid-1960s by leadership groups in medicine. The Coggeshall report (1965, the American Association of Colleges of Medicine), the Millis Commission report (1966, the American Medical Association), and the Willard Committee report (1966, the American Academy of General Practice) spoke variously about the need for reviving, defining, and upgrading the training and practice of the generalist physician.

The first substantive moves in the revitalization of the idea of a primary physician came from general practice. As early as the mid-1950s, the AMA undertook an examination of general practice, releasing the Sawyer Committee report in 1955 which called for the expansion of GP training and led to the first GP residency programs in the early 1960s. These programs developed slowly at first, but following the establishment of the American Board of Family Practice in 1969 and the advent of federal funding for family medicine residency training in 1971, they grew rapidly. In 1971 the American Academy of General Practice renamed itself the American Academy of Family Physicians, formally completing the molt of the old GP into the new family physician.[12]

The second phase of the generalist resurgence was the recognition in the 1970s that training programs in internal medicine and pediatrics had largely become way stations on the road to subspecialization. If generalism were to persist in medicine and pediatrics, attention and legitimacy would need to be given to generalist values and capabilities in these well-established disciplines. During the mid-1970s, the federal government, through its health professions funding (Title VII of the Public Health Service Act), and several private foundations—notably the Robert Wood Johnson Foundation—began providing explicit support of training programs in general pediatrics and general internal medicine.

The third phase of the new generalism was the emergence during the same period of two new, nonphysician disciplines in primary care—the nurse practitioner and the physician assistant. Jointly seen as additions to the medical workforce to deal with the widely perceived shortage of physicians, these two disciplines sprang from quite different roots.[13] The nurse practitioner discipline successfully tested the premise that nurses could be trained at an advanced level to take on certain diagnostic and treatment activities once held to be the exclusive domain of "medical practice." The physician assistant idea was triggered by the return from Vietnam of military medical corpsmen who had rendered major medical care on their own but could find no employment or career tracks in civilian life. Federal Health Professions Act support was also important to the growth of these disciplines, which occurred slowly at first, but at an increasing rate in more recent years.

These achievements, however, did not mean that the generalist ideal was once again securely planted at the center of the health care system in the United States. The steady growth in specialty residency programs and the continued decline of the GP meant that generalists, outnumbered by specialists by about 1960, fell to 37 percent of physicians in 1970 and to just under 33 percent for the decade 1990–2000. The actual number of generalist physicians grew during this period because of a doubling in the number of medical school graduates in the United States, with the net effect of a slight increase in the ratio of primary physicians to population ratio. The numbers of nurse practitioners and physician assistants in practice grew steadily, with most of the former and about half of the latter engaged in primary care. Through the 1980s, however, these five groups of consciously generalist practitioners, possessing federal funding, certifying authorities, and professional academies, could do no more than hold the line against the predominance of specialist practice. The nadir in medical education was reached in 1991 when an all-time low of 14.6 percent of graduating students indicated their intentions of becoming primary care physicians.[14]

It was increased public debate about expense and inequity in the medical system that led to the health care reform movement of the early 1990s and provided new impetus for the generalist movement. The continued escalation of medical costs in the United States troubled both patients and the business community. The continued presence of a large uninsured population and, not insignificantly, poorer health indices than those of many other developed nations expanded the debate. Both in general public deliberations and in President Clinton's Health Care Reform Task Force, the importance of primary care as a foundation for cost-effective medical care received broad endorsement. Simultaneously, the growth of managed care in the country accelerated, stimulating the employment market for generalist providers and adding palpability to the pro–primary care policy arguments.

Suddenly, primary care was "in." Medical student interest rose rapidly, hospitals and health systems competed to purchase primary care practices, and the number of nurse practitioner and physician assistant training programs grew quickly, with 58,500 N.P.s[15] and 40,000 P.A.s[16] estimated to be in practice by 2000. Some physician specialties reported difficulty finding positions for their recent trainees. Many specialists and their organizations began asserting that they in fact practiced primary care, in the hopes of favorable treatment in future compensation or training systems. The primary care provided by various specialists in the course of their practices was posited by some as a good strategy to meet care needs. Many specialties began to worry about competing with themselves and considered controlling their own numbers. For a moment, the generalist was in an unaccustomed position of approbation and demand.

The failure of President Clinton's health care reform legislation did not relieve the pressure for change in the system. The business community, payer for much of the cost of employment-based health insurance, wanted reform—by which it principally meant cost containment. If government-led reform was not to be, business was prepared to invoke "the market," a powerful distributional mechanism from which health care had previously been relatively protected. Managed care became the instrument of that "reform," the agent of the market, the institution with which increasing numbers of patients and physicians had to deal. But managed care was not a fixed entity. It began to evolve quickly, offering a staggering variety of "products" covering service delivery, finance, and risk. Some health plans, such as those with a long history of providing HMO-based care, represented serious efforts at restructuring the health care system in a financially responsible way, with a focus on systematizing quality care. Others were unapologetic business schemes designed to wring profits from the inefficiencies found everywhere in the delivery of health care. Both versions saw primary care as key to a rational and efficient system and together, often touting the "gatekeeper" model, they succeeded in moving primary care to the center of the health care stage and gave the generalist a visible if somewhat ambiguous prominence. Primary care providers were at the core of most managed care arrangements—as clinicians, as care coordinators, and sometimes as gatekeepers empowered to make decisions about specialty referrals and procedures. Some arrangements actually provided personal financial incentives to the primary care provider to limit referrals, hospitalizations, and lab work, thus creating a constant conflict of interest. It was this latter role that contributed to primary care's sudden reputation as medicine's designated miser, limiting procedures and pinching pennies. This, in turn, contributed to new patient demands for "choice," meaning the ability to opt out of primary care. "Choice" quickly became one of the planks of "patient rights." In the process, some critics labeled primary care as bureaucratic, unfriendly, or unnecessary— attributes contrary to the ethos of primary care and ones that generalist practitioners vehemently disavowed.

Ironically, then, the move to managed care in the United States made the "primary care provider" a much better known but also a much more controversial idea. The very success of primary care as a central player in the delivery of health care also burdened the concept with the problematic responsibility of cost containment. Medical student interest in primary care peaked in the late 1990s and started to decline.[17] Managed care plans began promoting options that allowed patients to circumvent primary care and go directly to specialists. Despite the two-to-one pre-

dominance of specialists nationally, some began to argue that the United
States had too many primary care providers and training programs should
be cut back.

The managed care environment prompted changes in the way medicine was practiced in virtually all settings. Primary care providers, in particular, reported that they were required to see more patients per hour,
per session, and per year, often for incomes that were falling. As with
other physicians, the advent of prior approvals, specified formularies
(limitations on drugs that could be prescribed), and practice profiling
(computer-generated analyses and criticisms of physicians' prescribing
and test-ordering habits) raised the hackles of many in primary care.

But managed care was not the only force creating uncertainty. The
"hospitalist"—a physician caring only for hospitalized medical patients—
emerged as a new player in the 1990s and was cautiously adopted by a
growing number of institutions.[18] The hospitalist idea firmly divided the
worlds of inpatient and outpatient medicine, aligning primary care with
ambulatory care and inserting the hospitalist as a formalized practitioner
of "secondary care." From one perspective this change clarified and simplified the role of primary care, but it also impinged on continuity of care
for those generalists with hospital as well as ambulatory practices. Hospitalists have made the argument that they are generalists in the hospital setting and that practice as a hospitalist is an opportunity for primary
care practitioners. It is likely that the efficient division of labor inherent
in the hospitalist idea will continue to prove attractive to some hospitals
and that the concept is here to stay. Although it may be difficult to decide whether the hospitalist is "us" or "them" from a purely generalist
point of view, most primary care physicians have adapted to the presence of hospitalists and find them to be an asset in patient care.[19]

One area of internal challenge for primary care is the increased clinical authority asserted within the field of nursing. Throughout the country nurses have been successful at amending state clinical practice acts
to expand the scope of practice and prescriptive authorities, as well as
direct compensation provisions for nurse practitioners (and physician assistants). Although this has led to increasing numbers of bush wars with
state medical societies and the AMA, these legislative changes have en-
abled the increasing numbers of nurse practitioners (and physician assistants) to realize their clinical potential in a way that would never have
been possible under the old statutes. In 1999, Dr. Mary Mundinger and
associates at Columbia University published a study comparing the experiences of a group of patients whose primary care, including hospi-

talizations, was completely managed by nurse practitioners with those of a matched group who were treated by primary care physicians. On balance, the outcomes for the two groups were without substantial difference.[20] While there are questions about the generalizability of the study, its implications raise a new set of issues for primary care—and for medicine and nursing. Can nurse practitioners actually supplant physicians? Should nurse practitioners supplant physicians? The situation raises philosophical questions as well. If nurse practitioners can "practice medicine," are they not doctors? If nurses are being trained to be doctors, what will become of the traditional stand-alone values of nursing? And if doctors and nurses engage shoulder-to-shoulder in the practice of medicine, are there two professions or one?

"Alternative medicine"—treatments from chiropractic to aroma therapy, from multivitamins to massage therapy, on which patients spend billions of dollars annually—emerged in the 1980s and 1990s as an important element of patient self-care that variously perplexed, angered, and chastened physicians. The increased availability of information (good and bad) and ever growing patient expectations for desired outcomes have contributed to the growth of alternative medicine. Dissatisfaction with physicians and the often inscrutable, fragmented system has spurred it on as well. Here lies an important opportunity for primary care as custodian of the doctor-patient relationship. By attending to the frustrations of patients and by being generally versed in the more popular "alternatives," the generalist can provide protection, instruction, and an affirmation of good doctoring.

While all of these recent developments challenge the field of primary care in one way or another, they all relate closely to it and derive credibility and energy from it. Primary care—how we care broadly for people and populations—is, in fact, at the center of many of the most important health and health policy debates of our time. As these controversies demonstrate, primary care enters the twenty-first century as an integral and important part of health care in America. Despite the unimaginable growth in medical science and technology that has taken place over the past hundred years and the inevitable demise of the GP, the offspring of general practice are well established today in medicine and in nursing. Within medical schools, primary care teaching is the basis on which all medical education is built. In policy deliberations, primary care is seen as the key to future strategies to provide service to the underserved and, ultimately, health care coverage to everyone in the country.

The men and women whose lives are chronicled in *Big Doctoring in*

America tell us where primary care has been and what it has done. In their stories, some themes of the future emerge. Most of these people find great satisfaction in their work and receive enormous appreciation and affection from the patients they care for. These basic themes of human effectiveness and gratification are omnipresent. The practitioners speak with pride about their work, a sense of common utility in their practices, a satisfaction with the teaching that they do, and a general sense of having come up the hard way, sometimes having gone against the advice of their mentors in school who counseled against primary care. They report problems as well. Managed care has tipped almost everybody off balance, including many of those who have chosen to work in managed care settings. Primary care incomes are decreasing in some quarters, and the market is tighter everywhere. But all across America there are physicians, nurse practitioners, and physician assistants who are dedicated to the science and art of primary care, who day and night use their minds, their technologies, and their hearts to practice big doctoring. They are busy building the future of primary care.

CHAPTER TWO

The New GPs

The Family Physician Comes of Age

In 1940, three-quarters of America's physicians were still general practitioners. World War II provided a huge boost for specialization, as board-certified physicians received higher rank, more pay, and, in consequence, higher status in the military. Following the war, the G.I. Bill covered medical education, providing an instant subsidy for young doctors pursuing specialty training. The rapid development of employment-based health insurance in the postwar period also stimulated specialty practice by providing much of the population with a payment system for care that was increasingly procedure-oriented and hospital-based. By 1970 only 20 percent of America's physicians counted themselves as GPs.

Through much of this period the GP was a passive player, an increasingly rare victim of what many believed to be a kind of medical Darwinism—a species of practitioner no longer adapted to the world of medicine. The term GP had become a default definition, largely a role that characterized what a practitioner was not. Although the country doctor who took care of Granny and the baby still held a Norman Rockwell appeal, it was the specialist whose image was now celebrated. Facing dwindling numbers, the absence of residency training programs, and the prospect of the loss of hospital privileges, general practitioners began to organize, in 1947 founding the American Academy of General Practice (AAGP) dedicated to improving the fortunes of their discipline.

The next two decades engendered intense conceptual and political debate over general practice. What exactly was the GP of the future to be?

If general practice was to be saved from extinction and revitalized as a competitive discipline amid the proliferating specialists, it would have to make some tough decisions about itself. Many older GPs opposed the idea of expanded residency training and board certification on the grounds that they themselves would not qualify. Some argued for the importance of surgery and obstetrics in the training of GPs while others favored a new emphasis on psychology, community medicine, and family dynamics to educate what was increasingly being called the family physician.

By the mid-1960s, there was general agreement that the idea of a formally trained family physician was a good one. In rapid succession over the next several years, the AMA approved a specialty board for Family Practice, the AAGP became the American Academy of Family Physicians, and family medicine residencies sprang up all over the country. The family practice curriculum maintained surgical and obstetrical training but emphasized the physician-patient relationship and the sociological elements of medical practice. In the 1970s, substantial federal support was provided to family practice residencies to assist in their start-up and maintenance, resulting in growth from 150 programs early in that decade to more than 450 today. Between 10 and 15 percent of medical students choose to train in family medicine each year, making it among the most popular of residency programs. (For a more complete discussion of the history of general practice, see chapter 1.)

General practice has not so much been saved, as it has been reborn. The idea of family practice carries on the tradition of the GP but has a new identity of its own, a set of quantified capabilities, and a vision of the medical future. The continuity, nonetheless, between the GP of the past and the family physician of today provides a strong, clear, central legacy to primary care in America.

The story of Eugene McGregor, M.D., of Lisbon, New Hampshire, is a bridge back to the roots of family medicine. Having practiced for forty years in the community where he grew up, he is a reminder of the continuity and connectedness of the rural GP and the spiritual grounding for the family physician of today. Fifty miles to McGregor's west, Connie Adler, M.D., carries on his legacy, but from dramatically different conceptual roots. Urban, feminist, and consciously political in her upbringing, she has migrated to a rural family practice that picks up, in many ways, where the GP of the past left off. A residency-trained family physician, she exemplifies the same principles of continuity and availability practiced by McGregor and his colleagues.

Armed with the same values, Neil Calman, M.D., has reentered the city—in his case New York City—which, like so many areas, had seen the virtual demise of general practice. Using a blend of family physicians and nurse practitioners, Calman has constructed a network of family practice delivery sites that are active in training family physicians as well as delivering care in many poor and working-class neighborhoods. Wrestling with managed care, trade unions, and academic health centers, Calman has led a resurgence of urban general practice.

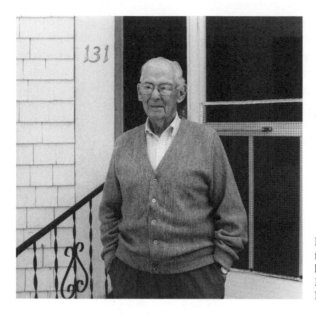

Eugene McGregor in front of his long-time home at 131 South Main Street in Lisbon, New Hampshire.

EUGENE McGREGOR, M.D.

A LEGACY OF GENERAL PRACTICE

Lisbon, New Hampshire
Gene McGregor was born in 1916, six years after Abraham Flexner, the great medical education reformer, published his critical report on the weak condition of medical education in the United States and three years after the founding of the first medical specialty organization, the American College of Surgeons. His life has spanned a period of enormous change in the theory and practice of medicine in the United States, most of which he has observed from the vantage point of Lisbon, New Hampshire—his birthplace and still the site of his medical practice. Spare of words and direct in response, Dr. McGregor displays an alertness and a power of recall that belie his more than eighty years. He sits comfortably on the porch of his green-shuttered white house on Main Street in Lisbon, recalling his days in practice, some fourteen thousand of them. He apologizes for the regular interruptions in his reflections caused by the gearing up of lumber trucks passing noisily out Main Street and by his occasional trips inside the house, necessitated, he explains, by diuretics.

He reminisces about life as a general practitioner in northern New England, about the days well before beepers and cellular phones, when his wife would wait out front to flag him down as he sped by or the local telephone operator would ring all over the county to locate him for an emergency. He thinks medical life for a country GP grew easier as the century progressed, with the arrival of surgeons and obstetricians to share the load, but he has mixed feelings about the advent of medical insurance and is deeply suspicious of Medicare. He doesn't see how managed care will work in rural areas and thinks many in the younger generation are "gypsy doctors," moving from place to place, looking for the best deal.

Dr. McGregor is no gypsy, having left northern New England only for two years of medical school and four years in the army. His lifelong practice in his hometown is atypical by today's patterns but represents a genre of traditional practice that is an important line of heredity to the values of current generalists. Continuity, community, intergenerational care, and home visits were all part of the work of Dr. McGregor. He never used a horse and buggy, but he is a bridge to those generations past, their fledgling science and their powerful art.

⟜

IN 1948 I CAME BACK to Lisbon, New Hampshire, the town where I was born, to start medical practice. I was getting older, and my children were getting older. A woman in Lisbon offered to lend me a sum of money to buy a house and to start a practice. I decided I'd better do it. I was going to be thirty-two that year, which I felt was too old. Lisbon had three doctors in the 1930s, but only Dr. Pickwick was left and he was getting older. This woman didn't like Dr. Pickwick very much. He was a very crusty character, and I'm sure they quarreled.

Coming home to start practice was nice and it was bad. It was nice because I knew the backgrounds of a great many of the people I saw, and I didn't have to spend a lot of time trying to figure them out. But I'd been away from Lisbon for fifteen years, and there was quite a turnover of people. I realized that I didn't really know as much about these people as I thought I did. Many of the names were familiar, but much of the social activities had changed during those fifteen years.

My parents were still living in Lisbon, and I think they were glad to have me home. My father had been a banker and my mother started as a schoolteacher, but later she stayed home to take care of the family. Both of their families came from this area. I had two great-uncles who were physicians, but the idea of becoming a doctor didn't really occur to me until the 1930s, when I was in high school. I think one of the reasons, probably, I went into medicine was the Depression and watching my father struggle. Banking in the early thirties was a difficult, sad business, and he had a very hard time. I think the idea of being a physician and being one's own boss was extremely important to me. It may also have been the fact that physicians didn't have to bear arms if we went to war, and certainly there was some suggestion of war in the thirties. I liked chemistry and the sciences and did reasonably well at them.

When I graduated from high school in 1933, a lot of my classmates couldn't go to college because they couldn't afford to. I found that with the scholarship that Dartmouth offered, I could go there cheaper than I could go to the University of New Hampshire. Dartmouth also had a program that required only three years in college before starting medical school, so I entered Dartmouth in the fall of 1933. I worked all the time I was in college, and summers too. I "hopped" bells every summer at the Mountain View House, which was a big resort up in Whitefield. For those of us who worked, there wasn't much of a social life. The premedical curriculum was very much prescribed. We had only a few elective courses so I took history, which I enjoyed very much.

That was a tough time. I think the main worry was the question of war. There was a war in China at that time, a war in Ethiopia, and a war in Spain. A lot of people had to worry just about their existence. When you have 24 percent unemployment in this country, you're in trouble. For instance, my father's salary had been cut in half during the very first part of the Depression. He had some stock holdings, and they had become worthless. Even at that time, though, there was a great deal of wealth around Dartmouth, although I had very little contact with people who had much wealth until I reached medical school.

I applied and was accepted into the medical school at Dartmouth, probably because they wanted to encourage medicine among the residents of New Hampshire. I did have the idea then that I would be a general practitioner, but I didn't really know where. I do remember that I didn't want to be subservient to anyone if I could help it, except my patients maybe.

Medical school was very, very enjoyable. We had a class of twenty, and there were only two classes since it was just a two-year school. Dartmouth did a deluxe job of teaching. We had some of the best teachers I ever had. In anatomy, there was a corpse for every two students. Spent all year working on it. It was a great time. I believe I am the only general practitioner from that class.

We all had to go on to another school for our clinical training after the two years at Dartmouth. I went to Rush Medical College in Chicago. At that time it was a part of the University of Chicago. It was quite an experience to go from Hanover to the west side of Chicago. I was in a class of 105 at Rush. There were eight or ten women in our class. I'm sure that out of our class of 105, probably 25 percent or 30 percent became general practitioners.

We were in the most impoverished part of Chicago. I'd never seen poverty such as that, not in New England, even at the worst of the Depression. I lived in the YMCA right across the park from Cook County Hospital. I used to walk in town every now and then, and I'd see fifteen or twenty drunks lying on the sidewalk near the entrance of run-down buildings. There were gangsters too. The Mafia was taking over restaurants, bombing and so forth. We were told when we were in obstetrics making home visits that we should never have more than a dollar in our pockets, and a dollar watch, because we might be robbed.

At that time, obstetrics for the poor in Chicago was practiced by the method of Dr. DeLee, I think it was, who established clinics for charitable delivery of obstetric services. The women came to the dispensary for their prenatal care, but when they delivered, they were delivered at home by teams of medical students. We went to tenements and apartment houses and followed the routine of trying to establish a somewhat sterile field with rolled-up newspapers, some hot water, and a pair of gloves. That was about it. The first time you went out, you went out with a student who had been out before, and he taught you what he knew. You could call an assistant resident from Presbyterian Hospital, who would come out and try to help you, but sometimes there were disasters. I had one, actually. A girl was pregnant with her first baby, which was in a posterior occiput position, and she couldn't deliver. Finally we got the assistant resident out, and he tried to put on forceps and rotate the head. I was giving her ether, which I had never done before, and I was scared to death. We were using the dining room table. Friends of the patient came in to hold her legs. One guy crawled under the table and vomited. I was running around the table trying to give ether, or holding up a leg. It was an awful mess. We got the baby out, but I'm not sure how well.

Most of the poor we dealt with were from all over Europe. At that time Chicago had the largest Czech population outside Czechoslovakia, the largest Polish population outside Poland, and so forth. And that was one of the reasons I didn't stay in Chicago, because I had to deal with people with a foreign language. We had to use an interpreter to get a history or a physical from them.

In general, Rush was excellent. We had some very good teachers, but the classes were big. The dispensary was excellent. Rush treated largely low-income patients for free. We worked on the wards at Cook County Hospital, where we really learned. We saw patients at Presbyterian Hospital too, but they were mostly private and we did less with them. I think the tuition was $400 a year. The school helped me a little and my parents chipped in. I borrowed some money, about $2,000 I think, while I was going to Rush.

When it came time to apply for internship, I wanted to come back to the Northeast. I went to Maine General Hospital in Portland partly because I wanted to get away from the foreign languages in Chicago. It was an eighteen-month rotating internship with no pay. Interns got room, board, and laundry, and that was all.

There were ten of us interns, and we were all as poor as church mice. We were on call every other night, every other weekend. I was only at Maine General for a year because the war came along. I had joined the Reserves and got called up in June 1941. I was married in May of that year, so it was kind of a busy time. I spent time in Panama toward the end of the war at Gorgas Hospital, a 1,000-bed hospital run by the Panama Railroad and staffed by the army. I was assigned to the contagious disease section, where I saw people with leprosy and typhoid fever. I did rotations on several other services and came home in December 1945.

When I was discharged from the service, I decided I needed more training, particularly in obstetrics, if I was going to be a general practitioner. So I returned to Maine General Hospital and started a surgical residency. I stayed for two years before deciding it was time to start my practice and to take the offer from the lady in Lisbon.

Getting the practice going in Lisbon turned out pretty well. I guess the fact that I probably had more training than almost any of the local doctors helped. Then, some people apparently didn't much like Dr. Pickwick, and they came to me right away. There was a woman doctor up the road who was getting along in age. I didn't know it at the time, but she was also becoming an alcoholic. As a result, I acquired practically all of her patients. I hired Miss Isabella Smith to do my bookwork, my laboratory work, and so forth. She was a graduate of Lisbon High School two years ahead of me and trained as a bacteriologist at Simmons College.

My wife, Phyllis, was a tremendous help to me in the practice right from the start. She was a nurse, and I would say that any general practice physician who doesn't have a nurse for a wife is crazy as hell. When we first began, she was the housekeeper—took care of the office, the floors, everything—and helped with the patients. She'd listen to my gripes and answer the phone for me at night when I was away or otherwise busy.

I used the Littleton and Woodsville hospitals, both a bit of a distance and in different directions. It could be nerve-wracking, keeping everything covered. My wife used to have to come out and flag down my car at times to try to stop me, or she would leave messages. I used to call up the operator and tell her, "I'm going to Lyman today, and I'm going to stop and see so-and-so." If she needed me she would call me. She'd track me down. It was great—far better than most answering services these days.

I made house calls all my life. I think that's the way medicine should be practiced. A doctor should be able to see people in their homes, to see what their hygiene is like, to look in the refrigerator. I probably made three or four house calls every day.

I used to try to get to the hospital by about nine o'clock so I didn't interfere with breakfast and the cleaning up of patients. Then I'd go to the other hospital, maybe make a house call or two. Then office hours in the afternoon. At first I had open office hours from about one until four, and then in the evening usually from seven until eight. In certain seasons, flu season, for example, the waiting room was packed, and other times I had nothing to do. Eventually I went from open office hours to scheduled appointments, sometime in the 1960s.

Lisbon has always been a pretty poor town. We had a woodworking mill and later a shoe factory, and during the last twenty years we have been making wire, at Lisbon Wire Works up the road. The mill did not offer any coverage, so people had to pay as best they could. Blue Cross came along in the 1950s, and I think probably 15 percent or 20 percent of my patients had it. By 1985, when I retired, maybe 75 percent of my patients had insurance, including Medicare and Medicaid. A lot were still not covered, though. Health insurance made a great improvement in many ways, but the whole thing became so complex, it drove me nuts. First of all, go back to the fifties. I can remember when I first began practice, I realized after a while that some of these patients owed me a fair amount of money, which they didn't bother to pay. I looked at their homes, and they would have TV at a time when I couldn't afford TV. So I remember I got pretty angry at one time, and I told Miss Smith to send the bills to a collector.

It didn't work worth a damn. I told her in 1960, "I'll be damned if I'm going to bother with that kind of stuff anymore," and I didn't. She used to admonish me, "You must do something about these bills!" I'd reply, "The hell with it." That's the way we worked, and it worked well enough. She stayed with me until she retired in 1982.

As time went on, I was seeing a crosscut of patients from Lisbon and the surrounding towns too. Around 1956 a very well-trained surgeon named Harry McDade came to Littleton, and I realized immediately that it really was foolish of me to do surgery since he was here. I kept on with obstetrics, delivering babies until the middle seventies. At that time fetal monitoring came in and caused quite a commotion. It irked the hell out of me, and quite frankly I despised it. I gave up obstetrics about 1976.

When I retired on July 31, 1985, I tried to get someone to take over my practice. I even advertised. But no one was interested, so I simply closed it up. Eventually Littleton Hospital took over my old office and arranged for two Littleton physicians to use it on a part-time basis. Someone must be there about every day of the week. The office is being renovated and will be a satellite of Littleton Hospital. But I tell you, I don't like it. I think it's producing a nation of gypsy physicians. They go where the best money is, and they stay a short time. Then they're off and away.

I have seen general practice become family practice, and that's been for the good. When the American Academy of General Practice [now the American Academy of Family Physicians] was founded in 1947, I joined immediately and kept up. I thought it was an excellent thing. When I started practice, there wasn't this whole array of specialists. So as a result, you were forced to take everything on and try to do the best you could with it. The old-timers, if they had had a year's internship they were lucky. They had to learn on the job for the most part. I'm sure I did. These physicians had to learn a lot of things very quickly. Most of us were aimed at small towns and rural areas and were going to take care of everything. When I began I was probably taking care of 95 percent of everything that came along. A general practitioner today ought to be able to manage 85 percent of everyone he or she sees; the other 15 percent he probably ought not to be managing. The real question is to know who are the 15 percent you should refer.

As a general practitioner, you could experience some real problems, even when you were careful. A girl had a baby. After the baby was born, she came back to see me several times with minor complaints. I didn't think too much of it. Then she showed me some personal journals—just stream of consciousness stuff. I tried to encourage her; her husband was a minister. The next thing I knew she had taken the car and disappeared with the baby. Everyone was looking for her. She was eventually found and brought home, but in a rambling, florid state. At that point, I sent her down to Hitchcock [the Mary Hitchcock Clinic at Dartmouth Medical School]. She continued into a psychotic state and eventually died. It was a sad case. Oh, you get some awful messes at times.

Over the years, of course, I dealt with a lot of family problems and the like. Drugs were practically a nonproblem when I first began practice. I don't think there were so many sexual problems either. I remember one patient telling me a problem she had of a sexual nature and how shocked I had been that she came out with it! At that time, I'm darn sure I didn't offer her any advice whatsoever. I occasionally saw women who had been beaten up by their husbands, and I would try to get them to prosecute, but they never would, even those who said they might.

There were a lot of other things in a small town that militated against this sort of thing. The Masons, for instance, the Boy Scouts, youth groups, religious groups, and so on, exerted quite a bit of power in getting kids not to do things that they ought not to be doing. In addition, the police were not inhibited by some of the things that have gone on in the courts. They had no compunction about beating somebody up if they felt he or she was doing wrong. They did. I think people knew it. If someone was to beat a child, for instance, the father or whoever did it could get one hell of a beating from the police.

Alcohol certainly was a problem. Even when drugs for the treatment of alcoholism came along, they didn't help much. As a matter of fact, years ago, in the fifties, one of my patients—a very wealthy woman— was a terrible alcoholic. She had married a guy who was a drunk himself. One night I was called to her house and found her standing in the middle of the room, not moving. "He's down there," she said. "Who's down there?" "Louis is down there." Turned out that her husband hid his liquor in the cellar. He had gone down to get some and she put the trapdoor down and was standing on it and wouldn't let him up. Well, now she wanted a drink. She tried to get me to get her riding boots, which were in a corner of the room; one boot had a bottle in it. Well, I was pretty irked, and I wouldn't do it. I think I just said, "You've got to let him out of there!" She eventually let him come up, and they were calm and peaceful and then had more drinks together, and I just left. I took care of her for many years after that. She caused a lot of commotion and kept on drinking.

I enjoyed my years in practice, but I wasn't sorry to get out when I did. The number one reason was the litigiousness of patients, physicians, everyone. It had gotten much worse over the years. The second reason

goes back to the late sixties, when Medicare came along. Medicare—
and by association Medicaid—got us into a bookkeeping system that I
think is probably the most monstrous thing I've ever seen in my life. These
people make you continually sign documents that say everything is true,
and if it turns out not to be true, I'm likely to be sent to jail for ten years
or fined $2,000 or whatever. Signing that used to irk the hell out of me
every time.

I'm glad I don't have to practice today because of the choices involved,
the idea of joining an HMO or a PPO, particularly for a physician in a
small town. Some of them want you to sign exclusive contracts. That
would really pose a problem in a small town. How can a physician possibly function that way? I can see how an HMO can save money, but the
only way to save money is if the physicians who are the gatekeepers are
the most honest characters that have ever been created, and I don't believe they are.

I've been asked from time to time, "Isn't general practice boring, seeing the same thing all the time?" Actually I think it's the reverse. When
I was a resident, I thought about going into urology. But the problem
with urology was that I just couldn't believe that I would spend the rest
of my life looking at penises and bladders and kidneys. In general practice, you're looking at a tremendous range of medical conditions. It's true
that you can't have every bit of knowledge at the end of your fingertips,
but you can find it relatively quickly. No, I thought that general practice
gave far greater diversity and much more enjoyment. I saw eyes, I saw
hearts, I did rectal examinations, I did feet. I pared corns and I delivered
babies. Everything. The whole works.

Work as a general practitioner is not necessarily easy for your own
family. Phyllis was a great help to me, and we had three wonderful children: Eugene, Jr., born in 1942, who is now a professor of political science at Indiana University; James G., born in 1947, who is a nuclear technician for a radiologist in St. Johnsbury, Vermont; and Kathryn, born in
1950, who is a Methodist minister in Colebrook, New Hampshire. I think
my wife felt at times that it was all too much, because we were up all
hours of the day and night, with deliveries particularly, and it was a very
hectic schedule.

I probably didn't see my children as much as I might have. But I think
my family would agree it's been a good life. I think about it a lot. I remember it well. But I am glad I retired.

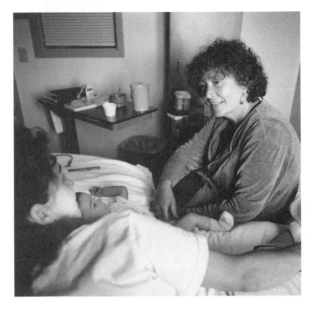

Connie Adler with a
new mother and child.

CONNIE ADLER, M.D.

LIVING RURAL MEDICINE

Farmington, Maine

Connie Adler quotes Marian Wright Edelman: "Service is the rent we pay for living." And she means it. For twenty-five years she has been dedicated to the care of women—women and those important to them, children and families. Working in a free clinic and as a lay midwife in Seattle, Washington, in the early 1970s, she was caught up in the burgeoning women's movement and has never really left it. Her commitment carried her on to medical school, training as a family physician, five years of service in the National Health Service Corps in a migrant health clinic in eastern Washington, and now a family practice specializing in women's health in western Maine.

The daughter of a Jewish immigrant psychoanalyst and an Irish American mother, Dr. Adler grew up in an environment that valued intellectual achievement but discouraged women from entering medicine. It took a degree in history and ten years of vocational wandering before she found medicine and gravitated rapidly to family practice. Primary care was not valued at her research-intensive medical school in the mid-1980s, but with a few colleagues, including her soon-to-be husband, she made it through school with her generalist values intact, graduating close to the top of her class.

She is upbeat and loquacious in discussing her life and her work, chuckling easily and telling stories about herself. She understands what she has accomplished, and she describes it with clarity and a sense of continuing mission. Dressed in brown clogs and burgundy scrubs with her wedding ring and watch neatly pinned to her collar, she is at home in the obstetric suite of the Franklin Memorial Hospital in Farmington, ready to deliver one of the scores of infants she brings into the world each year. She pauses for forty-five minutes in her chat about her career, delivers a seven-pound infant to a sixteen-year-old girl, reflects on the challenges awaiting them both, and returns to her own story. She is never far from giving service to someone.

⟜

IN MY MID-TWENTIES IN the early 1970s, I was "called." That was when I knew exactly what I wanted to be doing—working with women in labor and delivering babies. That was one of the clearest moments in my life, and since then I have known that's really where I belong.

I had moved to Seattle after college and was active in community organizing. I helped to start the Country Doctor Clinic, a collective that was one of the first community clinics in Seattle. A group of ten or so people got the clinic built and going. Then another woman, Margie Joy, and I started the prenatal clinic there. She was doing home deliveries, and I was helping and became sort of an apprentice. She was a lay midwife and had a physician for backup. I started doing deliveries, always with somebody else. The only ones I ever did by myself in those days were by accident when nobody else came out or got there on time. Within a year, though, I felt that I didn't want to be a part of doing what seemed like inadequate medicine to me, that if I was going to say I had some skills, I really needed to have them. And it wasn't enough to know one body system. Women would come in who were pregnant but who also had a sore throat or some other problem, and it just wasn't enough to know only the reproductive system. That's when I started thinking again about going back to school.

The other major and more important thing that happened during those years was that I had a baby. My daughter was born in 1973, and so of course I was involved with raising her. I was in a variety of different collectives at various times, but I did not have a partner. So I was single parenting. At that point came the beginning of a crackdown on lay midwives. I was definitely worried about supporting my daughter and more concerned about consequences like jail once I became a parent.

My father was a physician, but I don't think that had a lot to do with my decision about medicine. He escaped from Germany in 1937, a German Jew. The rest of his family was killed in the camps. My father was a product of European Jewish intellectual culture between the two world wars, and he brought this incredible Renaissance-man character to everything he did. He died recently, so I think about him a little bit more right now. He was a psychoanalyst trained in Austria, France, and Germany. He taught neuroanatomy in Turkey for a while. He actually practiced both neurology and psychiatry for a time, and then stopped doing neurology as he got older. During World War II he was in the U.S. Army, practicing largely as a neurologist.

My mother came from an Irish-English family that had been in New York for a century. An interesting combination. The two families would probably not have spoken to each other had my father's family survived, but it never was an issue. My parents shared their love of the arts and took us to the ballet or the opera or museums almost every weekend. Just as an interesting snapshot of my parents, when my father had three months off between when he was demobilized after the war and when he started practice again, he and my mother visited every church and museum in New York City. That's what they did with that time. That's who they were.

I grew up in Queens; later we moved to Upper Brookville on Long Island. My parents were Democrats, but not terribly political. From the time I was very young, justice was an overwhelmingly important concept for me. There certainly were things that promoted that feeling, including learning other languages. My father spoke eight languages, and we all started by age seven taking French lessons, and then, when I was thirteen, I went on my own to France for the summer. When I was fifteen, I went to Guatemala and learned Spanish, and later I went to Germany. Both learning languages and traveling to other countries were politicizing experiences. When I was in Guatemala, I witnessed incredible poverty next to incredible wealth. Guatemala has 95 percent illiteracy, and 5 percent of the people own 90 percent of the land: a tremendous eye-opener for a fifteen-year-old.

We grew up in a racially mixed neighborhood in Queens, which felt completely normal to me as a kid. Later I discovered that people didn't think that was normal. By the time I was in ninth grade, on Long Island, I was getting kicked out of class for being a Communist. During my high school years, of course, people were starting to organize in the South, voter registration and so on. That's when a lot of my intellectual and political activities started.

I loved my science courses—except physics. We had aptitude tests. Each time I took one, people said I ought to become a doctor, and every time that happened, they also said, "But that's silly. You're a girl." And so I went to college as a history major because it was "silly" for me to think about being a doctor, because I was a girl. That was 1965.

I went to Cornell and liked it a lot. I actually loved my history courses, American cultural and intellectual history. It was an exciting time with the antiwar movement and the black student takeover of the Student Union. Dan Berrigan was there; we had Seder with him. But then I went to Yale to do graduate work in history and just hated it. It was the beginning of the women's movement in New Haven, which I became involved in. Actually what I wanted to do was oral histories of women, especially women in the labor movement. The history department was very much Old Guard and thus a real conflict. I left after a semester, eventually moving to Seattle and getting involved in midwifery.

After Seattle, I came back east to start on my uncertain but determined journey to medical school. Women's health was my focus, my goal. The sixties and early seventies, of course, were a time when the women's movement was just taking off. I was a middle-class kid and hadn't suffered any horrible economic discrimination. But I knew from my own experiences the unequal position of women and the violence against us. I had already been involved in some antiviolence issues, violence against women, as well as the abortion issue. I ended up in Boston working different jobs, raising my daughter, taking premed courses. I remember sitting on the beach with my three-year-old so she could play in the water while I studied organic chemistry.

It was 1979—ten years after I graduated from Cornell—when I started Tufts Medical School. I was ten years older than almost everybody. The very first day I sat in class next to this kid who looked like a kid. I said something about my daughter, and he said, "Oh? What does your husband do?" And I said, "I'm not married." And he said, "But I thought you said you had a daughter." I felt like I had to explain to him that those two were not necessarily related. I met Mike Rowland, who is now my husband, in the first few weeks of medical school, and that actually helped quite a lot. We had each other to get through school. He was also an older student. He had taught high school in Maine and Vermont, and he was the one who first started talking to me about family practice. We got married in the spring of our third year in medical school. Mike and I had a second daughter our last year in school, which was also a challenge.

When I started in medicine, I assumed I was going to do obstetrics and gynecology. While learning the science of medicine, though, I became much more interested in how the art of medicine happens and felt that primary care was the way to go. Being there for the family as a unit was the way I could be there for people, and also help steer people in positive directions. But no one was teaching that at Tufts. In fact, both Mike and I got a lot of flak about wanting to do primary care. It was a very specialist-oriented kind of place. People kept saying things like, "Why do you want to be a family doctor? You're a smart person. You could do something really interesting." But it became just clearer and clearer to me that the unifying of care made a lot of sense.

When I did OB, I felt that way even more. I love OB. It is still the thing I love most in medicine. There's something about that interaction of several hours of labor and coaching and birthing that's special and wonderful, but it's a lot more wonderful when it's somebody you've seen before and you will see later, seeing the child grow up, interacting with the mother throughout her life cycle, or throughout the child-raising years. I wanted to take care of that unit. The further I got into medical school, the clearer it became that I wanted to be able to take care of the whole life cycle. There were about five of our class of 150 who became family doctors.

Mike and I both received National Health Service Corps scholarships to get us through school. Mike needed the help and had planned on doing rural practice anyway, so it was up the right alley. For me, similarly, I was on my own with a child and had to find some way to support her. I really did not want to pile up big debts to influence how I practiced afterward, because I wanted to do shortage-area medicine. I felt that no matter where I went with the National Health Service Corps, I'd be doing shortage-area medicine. I never wanted to do suburban practice.

We had to do residencies before we started our payback practice. We chose the Maine-Dartmouth residency in Augusta because it was a good place—a great place—and we got them to agree to let us do it in four years instead of three because we had the new baby, as well as my eighth-grader. So we split our internship year. We alternated months: one month at home, one month at work. So we both did the internship year over two years. I loved it. We also chose the Maine-Dartmouth program because of the great people there and their attitudes. It was the only place we found where people could be openly gay in the residency, and where women were valued for who they were. The program's commitment to training physicians for rural areas was very clear. I learned a lot about family counseling. My practice has always been a lot of women. Women want to come to a woman physician. I did more deliveries during my residency than anyone had ever done in residency there before. The obstetricians really came to trust me, so I got to do a lot—C-sections and other procedures. Obstetrics was always a focus, but I loved every part of it. I did a lot of work with family counseling with kids, family counseling with the families of children who were diabetic, and teaching and learning how to cope with chronic illness. It was a wonderful time for me.

When we finished residency in 1987, Mike and I owed the National Health Corps four years. We liked the idea of working on the Zuni Indian reservation, but we ended up going to Moses Lake, which was a migrant farm worker site in eastern Washington. The practice was about 70 percent migrant farm workers, 30 percent indigent people from the area. Moses Lake is a town of about 15,000 to 25,000; depending on how big an area you count. We were the only two docs in the clinic when we got there, and there was one physician assistant. There had been two NHSC doctors there before who waved good-bye as we rode into town.

There we were. It was very busy, but the clinic was wonderful. The people who staffed the clinic are still very close friends, fabulous people, very committed. We worked in Spanish half or more of every day, which we enjoyed. It was a very busy obstetrics practice and a lot of pediatrics. The first year was like a fellowship in perinatology. We had a lot of high-risk OB, a lot of very sick babies, a lot of kids with congenital heart defects and congestive heart failure. There was a fifty-bed hospital in town where we did deliveries and hospitalizations. The hospital had a medical staff of about twenty-five; the others were all in private practice. So we took care of everybody who didn't have any money, and they took care of people who did. Some of the specialists supported us but we did almost everything for everybody. I had eight hemophiliacs in my practice, and in fact ended up being sort of the hemophilia expert in eastern Washington. There were several families where I was taking care of four generations of people.

We stayed in Moses Lake for five years. The first two years we were alternating call every other night—with each other! It was ghastly. We never saw each other. Basically the way to change that was to build the practice so we could hire somebody else, and we eventually did. We were seeing lots of patients, we were busy, we took all comers and built up the clinic. By late in the second year we went to every third night on call, which was glorious. The clinic's reputation in the community grew steadily so that the other docs were more accepting. By the time we left, there were four physicians and two physician assistants working at the clinic. We had a new building.

Moses Lake was a very, very conservative town. I was the only woman I knew who had kept my maiden name, and people gave me a lot of grief about it. It was an atmosphere that was stuck in the 1950s. People mostly identified by their church, and that's how they socialized, by church group. So we were almost never asked out because we didn't belong to any of the local churches. The Hispanic community was very open, and we went to lots of "balls" and parties with our patients and staff. But the Anglo community was not all that open to us, with the exception of the clinic staff and one very supportive obstetrician.

The high school was a trial for our older daughter. She didn't fit in very well in town either, but she ended up doing a lot of independent study. During her first week of school she came home in tears saying, "They have mandatory pep rallies here." So there was some culture shock, but she got over it. She did well and went on to Columbia University.

At the end of five years, we decided to go back to Maine. We still had a lot of friends there and wanted to do rural shortage-area medicine. We chose Farmington because it has an excellent school system for our youngest daughter, with a lot of emphasis on music, which is her interest. I found two obstetricians here who were willing to let me do family practice and as much obstetrics as I wanted. We certainly saw a lot of communities where there were turf battles: the obstetricians didn't like family docs. I do primary care, but the three of us share call. I do my own C-sections, tubals, and D&Cs, and I share call with the obstetricians. I enjoy surgery and do a lot of it. I also share call with the pediatricians and do all of the pediatrics I want. People talk about a women's health care specialist, and I guess that's what I am, except I do a lot of pediatrics too. I was chief of staff last year at the hospital in Farmington. I get along with most of the specialists. People have idiosyncrasies, God knows, but there is not a lot of turf fighting here.

Farmington is an interesting community because it's very rural, but we do have a college, the University of Maine at Farmington, so there's some element of college professors and students. We have a lot of farmers and people who work in the woods. Maine is a poor rural state, with many folks who have nothing. There's a big ski area nearby, and there are yuppies who work there. It's an interesting cultural mix. Almost everybody is white, but I think that every Mexican American in Maine knows I'm here, and they come to see me because I speak Spanish.

I hate private practice, except for being able to make decisions about my schedule. But I think it's a dumb way to do medicine. I hate doing the business part of private practice. I'm good at it, I'm doing fine. In OB, a lot of people become eligible for Medicaid, so the OB part tends to pay for itself. The folks we see in the office who can't pay, we write off. It all works out. We have some people who will pay over time, or pay with their services. I'm making a perfectly good living, got my kid through college. That's all I care about. I hate having to think about insurance companies and reimbursement problems. I would much rather be working in a community clinic.

I have been active in shelters and domestic violence work for almost twenty years. It has been very exciting in the past few years to see violence against women become more recognized as the tremendous medical problem that it is. Farmington has united in extraordinary and dynamic ways to combat violence against women, and I have found it challenging and affirming to be a part of that process. We now have universal screening in our emergency department and obstetrical department; more physician offices are screening for violence at office visits; and we have signs when you enter town on any road that say that Domestic Violence is a crime and will not be tolerated here.

As far as managed care goes, Maine is way behind the curve. We're probably ten years behind California. So a lot of it here is just speculation. I have a group of managed care patients in my practice. I have learned how to use that system and play the gatekeeper role. I think we are going to have to learn how to talk to each other better and manage patients on a community basis a whole lot better than we have in the past. There are a few specialists who do inappropriate things, and as a medical community we have to learn how to control that.

Right now I think we're going from point A to point B in the system as a whole, point A being this nonsystem of independent practice, B being managed care in some form. It's hard to get very excited about point B, but I think there's a point C. Point C will be a lot more involved in patient concerns—which have gotten lost in managed care—and involved in public health but incorporate a lot of the savings and organization of managed care. I think I won't be able to be involved in getting to point C if I'm not involved in getting to point B. I don't exactly see what the ultimate product is going to look like yet. I had assumed it would be a single-payer system. I was very excited about the Clinton health plan and working toward some kind of rational health care system. Managed care can't be the end. There are still all of the uninsured and the problems of "rationing" and the appropriate care of the elderly. But you can't be a part of that dialogue unless you're a part of this one.

I do feel that I'm doing what I set out to do when I decided on medicine. I'm the only woman physician doing women's health in this rural area. The obstetricians are all men and so are most of the family docs. I have patients who are incest survivors, cult survivors, domestic violence survivors, and women with multiple personalities from childhood abuse. These are patients who really want to see a woman physician—and not just a doctor, but a doctor/mom. These are people of all ages. This is the need that I fill in this community. It's important to me to be of service.

I have lot of energy and a lot to give. I get enormous amounts back from my patients—some days. Other days it feels like all out-go, no input. But there are some very special moments with people, with their babies, with people who are dying, with teenagers taking on new tasks and figuring them out, that are rejuvenating, that give me as much energy back as I put into them. So it's very renewing. Not every day. There are days when I drag myself around because I've been up all night and can't figure out which end is up. But overall, it's tremendously rewarding. There's nothing I would rather be doing.

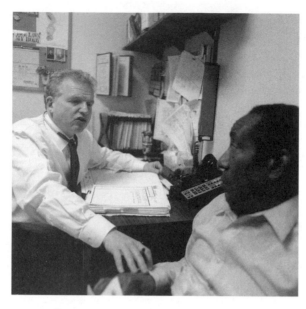

Neil Calman
stresses a point.

NEIL CALMAN, M.D.

URBAN WARRIOR

New York, New York

Neil Calman stands in front of a battered Bronx tenement building, one foot up on its broken first step. There is graffiti on the wall behind him. His hands are in the pockets of his lab coat, and a stethoscope dangles from his neck. This picture, appearing in an article titled "The Urban Frontier," tells a lot about Calman, his values, his strategies, and his chosen battleground. He calls himself "a flag-waving family physician" and "a warrior for urban health." A third-generation New Yorker, he created the Institute for Urban Family Health almost twenty years ago and has run it as a command post for training and placing family physicians and nurse practitioners in community practices all over New York. Clippings from the *New York Times,* the *Daily News,* the American Academy of Family Physicians' *Reporter,* and the Robert Wood Johnson Foundation's *Advances* attest to the tenacity of his technique and the success of his public education campaign.

Calman's grandfather was something of an inspiration to him. An oral surgeon, an attorney, and a socialist alderman for the city of New York, he lived by his ideals and got arrested for them a number of times. Calman practices his ideals running a large and effective enterprise from his office over the Sidney Hillman Health Center, just outside the city's garment district. Recent years have been tough, he concedes, given the changing finances of health care.

⌒⟶

I RUN THE INSTITUTE FOR Urban Family Health, a $20 million business with more than three hundred employees. But I haven't always been so comfortable with institutions. I was thrown out of the University of Chicago as an undergraduate, almost got bounced from medical school, and was suspended for two weeks from my residency program. Politics seemed to get me crosswise of administrations wherever I went. In 1983 I solved my rebel problem by building my own organization, which now enables me to practice many of the principles that got me in trouble when I was younger.

Growing up in New York, I couldn't help being exposed to a lot of politics and a fair amount of protest, too. I was born in New York City in 1949, the oldest of three and then later of five kids—my parents had two more children after I was already in college. When I was about four years old we moved across the George Washington Bridge from Washington Heights to Glen Rock, New Jersey. My father was drafted into the army about a year later, and we lived on a base in Virginia for two years before we returned to New Jersey for the rest of my childhood and adolescence.

Medicine runs in my family. My dad, who retired from practice in 1995, is an oral surgeon, as was his father. They both practiced in Washington Heights through the whole transition of that neighborhood from a mostly Jewish immigrant one to a mostly minority immigrant community today, and they worked out of the same office all those years. My dad now teaches at New York University Dental School.

My grandfather's plaque still hangs in my office. He was my inspiration and a very big influence in my life, passing on to me a passion for political causes. His name was Maurice Samuel Calman, and he was a socialist alderman in the city of New York as well as a dentist and an attorney. An alderman is equivalent to being a member of New York's City Council today. He also had a degree in agriculture, and he was a three-letter athlete in college. He had a philosophy about everything, and he lived by his ideals. As an alderman he was arrested a number of times. One of his arrests was for exposing a fake coal crisis. In the winter of 1918, companies were hoarding huge stockpiles of coal in outlying parts of New York City to drive up prices. As a result, people in tenements were going through a brutal winter because they couldn't get coal. He went around and photographed all of these stockpiles and led a huge protest in New York, eventually buying coal himself to distribute to the poor. That's just the kind of guy he was.

My mother's father was a cantor from the same sort of socialist Jewish tradition. His were more cultural than religious values. He knew everybody that was half Jewish, a quarter, or an eighth Jewish—every entertainer, everybody.

My dad was associated with a small hospital, now torn down, called Jewish Memorial Hospital in Washington Heights. In my dad's day there was an oncologist-hematologist there named Harry Wallerstein who ran a small research laboratory with funds donated by the family of a leukemia victim he had cared for. Dr. Wallerstein allowed the children of hospital staff members to work in the lab during the summer. He literally closed the lab for those months to run his student program, and set up a group of experiments that we would study for weeks. I started working at the lab when I was fourteen, washing beakers and glassware for the first summer and progressing to handling mice the next summer. I learned a bit of biochemistry and became an expert in amino acid metabolism at age fifteen, because Dr. Wallerstein would insist that we learn the basic science behind the research we were doing. By the time I was eighteen, my senior year, I was the second-in-command of the lab's student programs. I don't think this program produced any work of major research significance, but it was responsible for many people going into medicine and assuming leadership positions.

In college I became involved in many political causes, a legacy from my father's father. In fact, when he died during my second year of college, it was a very difficult time for me. My interest in politics led me to the University of Chicago in 1967. An article in *Life* magazine in 1965 about the students forcing the school to deal with issues in the community really caught my attention. That was my first memory of having any kind of real political thought or interest. We could take courses there in any division of the school and we weren't even allowed to have a major until halfway through our third year. I took literature, poetry, music, and archaeology. It was a great educational environment.

At that time I became very interested in the social issues being discussed on campus, how the school was responding, and what role the students had. The university was like a white island on the mostly black south side of Chicago. The school wasn't integrated at all into the life of the community. I think a lot of people felt that the school needed a different vision. But teachers who wanted to design more socially responsible courses were being persecuted by the school and denied tenure, as they were in many other universities at the time. Then the Vietnam War brought other protests to the campus.

During my second year I was involved in a sit-in at the administration building to protest the firing of an outspoken female professor. The school held hearings to determine how to punish us. At my hearing, I basically discussed the need to be true to your values and to act on them. Because I showed up for the hearing and went through the process, which a lot of people refused to do, I ended up only being suspended for the spring and summer quarters. About thirty students who didn't show up at all for their hearings were expelled from school. A number of them joined the Weather Underground. It was a hot time in Chicago.

I spent those two quarters living at home. I didn't want to get totally off track, so I went back to the research lab and talked to Harry Wallerstein. After he gave me a lecture about how stupid I'd been, he gave me a job. I went home and designed an experiment based on the research I had done there years before. Since the experiment was related to work the lab was doing and because Wallerstein believed in it, he spent about $10,000 on special equipment and supplies that I needed. I became totally engrossed in this project, putting in sixty, seventy hours a week at the research lab.

The experiment occupied the period of time that I was suspended from school, and we published four papers from it. I believe the papers were the only reason that I got into medical school. I applied to sixteen schools, but my transcript noted my suspension and I only got two interviews. In a complete quirk, one of the people who interviewed me had actually read one of the research papers I published, on how cancer cells changed their immunologic identity as they became resistant to chemotherapeutic agents over time, as he was doing research in an area very similar to mine.

So, I think I got into Rutgers Medical School for three reasons. First, there were two professors at Rutgers who were really furious about the homogeneity of the student body and the fact that the school was systematically eliminating people interested in political issues related to health care. The admissions committee allowed them to make recommendations for a few slots, and they chose me. Second, the doctor who interviewed me was interested in my research area. And third, the same interviewer was fascinated by my college course work in archaeology, particularly a class I had taken on the Dead Sea Scrolls. His father was actually on the team that discovered and translated the Dead Sea Scrolls and had written one of the books that I read in the course. We talked about that for half the interview and about my research for the other half. So I was lucky.

I really went to medical school to become a researcher. I believed that people with scientific minds had a responsibility to try to solve the big medical problems that people faced. This thought helped me to connect my sense of social responsibility with the fact that I was spending all my time in a lab.

When I landed in medical school, however, I quickly connected with about half a dozen people who were much more socially and politically aware than I had been. This group of medical students used to meet every week or two to discuss political issues in medicine. As I recall, they were very critical of my research interests because the research isolated me from patient care.

At the time my politics weren't well connected to my medicine, but that changed as clinical practice allowed me to integrate these two parts of my life. A pediatric faculty member who ran a free community clinic brought medical students to the clinic in the evenings to learn how to take blood pressures and gain real clinical experience. I went there with the other people in the discussion group and liked it tremendously. The first time, however, I was incredibly frustrated because I spent a whole night being totally unable to take a blood pressure. At the end of the night, one of my colleagues figured out that I was listening with the wrong side of my stethoscope bell.

During my first year of medical school, after I had worked in this neighborhood clinic for a while, I started to get interested in what health care was really about and joined a study group on health care issues. I did the readings and showed up at meetings, but I wasn't a leader. It was all I could do to hang on to the academics of medical school during my first two years because I was never particularly good at memorization. I always looked for logical associations between things, so memorizing the names of bones and veins and nerves was torture for me.

While I loved the clinical experience, I was bored in Piscataway, New Jersey, after the excitement of Chicago. At that time, Rutgers was just beginning to establish itself as a four-year medical school, so most of my class was encouraged to look for another place to finish our program. Leo Hennikoff, a pediatric cardiologist who was then a recruiter for Rush Medical College in Chicago and became Rush's president and chief executive, came to Rutgers to interview students. I'll never forget his interview. He took two or three clinical problems that were clearly beyond what a second-year medical student should know and led me to reason them through for a couple of hours to see how I would approach them. He went through the problems in an incredibly logical way that totally clicked into the way my mind works. I was enamored of that way of thinking and decided I wanted to go to that school. And Rush turned out to be exactly like that. It was a phenomenal two-year clinical experience unlike anything I've experienced since, with brilliant, thoughtful educators and clinicians.

Even so, I almost got thrown out of Rush, too; it is one of my claims to fame. My roommate and I joined a group called Concerned Medical Students at Rush, which started in 1972, a year before we came. The group members were more widely read than I was in political issues related to medicine, but I was very much in tune with them philosophically. In 1973 I became involved in opposing a plan put forth by the president of the hospital, James Campbell, to divide up the city of Chicago into health care districts. My recollection is that the plan showed great disfavor to poor inner-city communities by sending anyone who couldn't afford to pay to Cook County Hospital rather than to Rush. It was great for Rush, but not, many people thought, for Chicago.

This was a major turning point for me at Rush. I was on my ob-gyn rotation and worked on two floors, one largely for paying, insured patients and another for the poor from the community. They were staffed differently and had different nursing models. One doctor was doing experiments on black women having caesarian sections without obtaining their consent. After giving an unnecessary general anesthetic, the staff would start taking blood samples before the baby was delivered. Besides the ethics of doing research without permission, the anesthesia increased the risk that the baby would be delivered sedated. I became concerned because we had been taught to deliver a baby as quickly as possible, so I asked the chairman of OB what was going on. In talking with one of the patients I also discovered that nobody had gotten her consent or advised her that she would be participating in these experiments.

The OB department refused to do anything about it. Another student and I copied a whole bunch of medical records of women involved in this study to show that there were no consent forms and that the delivery times after induction of anesthesia were between eight and twelve minutes when they should have been two or three minutes. When we took this information to the OB director and he refused to change the procedures, we took the story to the newspapers. This was probably not the smartest thing for a third-year medical student to do. A black newspaper in Chicago picked up the story and put it on the front page. The other Chicago newspapers then ran articles about Rush University's illegal experiments on black women.

Since the hospital had been caught in the wrong, they were not in a position to dismiss me, but I was in deep trouble for quite a while. Eventually, they set up their first human experimentation committee at the school in response to this issue and asked us to be on the committee. But inside the school it was clear we had crossed the line. The only thing that saved us was that we had documented every meeting we had with the hospital staff prior to going to the papers. Despite all this controversy, academically I did very well in my third year. Sometime around the end of my third year, when I had to start thinking about residencies, I found out about family practice. Rush didn't open this door to me, however, as there wasn't a single family physician at Rush at the time.

I got my first direct experience in family practice through an advertisement in the back of the *New England Journal of Medicine,* placed by the United Farm Workers [UFW] Health Clinics. A family doctor there, who'd been working in Delano, California, for years without a break, was interested in finding another doctor to come do a locum tenens. I called to find out more and he said, "Well, you have to go and meet with Cesar Chávez from the UFW and be indoctrinated into the union first. Then you can work in the center. Even though you are only a medical student, I have no help out here and we'd love to have you."

After getting permission from the dean, I took two months off, got in my car, and drove to California. It was spring of 1974. I went first to a place called La Paz, headquarters for the UFW union, and got my indoctrination. Then I went out to Delano and lived in the emergency room of the UFW clinic there, sleeping on an emergency room cot for two months.

That, I think, was the single most important experience of my medical career because I learned how poorly the health care system met the needs of this community. We were taking care of people who had no health insurance and no access to the general health care system. They went to the health clinic and got whatever was available, or they got nothing. If they were brought by ambulance to Bakersfield hospital, thirty-five miles away, they could be seen as emergency patients, but they were unlikely to be admitted. If there were questions about their immigration status, forget it. Everybody knew that going to the public hospital in Bakersfield was a direct route to possible deportation.

I took with me several lessons from that place. First, I developed the belief that people in medicine could do much more than just what is done in subspecialty areas. The medical world has this view which, I think, we've all become victim to over time, that you can't do anything unless you're a specialist. But the doctor and I did everything. We did our own lab work and X rays. He had a large number of books that we used to treat conditions usually covered by specialists. We also did complex suturing on some brutal farm wounds, as well as setting fractures and casting. We delivered probably twenty babies during the time I was there.

The doctor had a whole group of liberal-minded, caring specialists who made themselves available free of charge by telephone. So we did a lot of telephone consultations with people all over the state and, in some cases, outside the state, who were sympathetic to the farm workers' cause.

The second lesson I learned, which I recorded in my journal at that time, was that you can't separate the way people feel about their work and their family from their health care. The clinic was right there in the community where the people lived. The people who ran the clinic were enormously political. The clinic closed for half a day every week while we all went out marching through some town or grape fields. Only one of the nurses would stay to staff the emergency room. I've got pictures of myself carrying UFW flags and banners from the clinic through nearby farm towns, where people would cheer the clinic staff on. It was very clear that the health care we were rendering existed within this political context.

I headed back to Chicago for my final year knowing that I wanted to be a family doctor. On my way back east I visited some family practice residencies in Sacramento and San Francisco. Then I visited Montefiore Hospital in New York City, and found a couple of faculty people who were really tuned into the same connection I felt between politics and primary care. In the end I ended up entering Montefiore's third class of family practice residents.

It was at Montefiore that I discovered I had a knack for administration. I was one of three chief residents, and I loved setting agendas for meetings, taking minutes, and writing policies and procedures. A woman pediatrician there, Jo Ivey Boufford, became my model for administrative leadership. As director of the social medicine program, Jo ran a staff of very radical and independent physicians, all of whom were moving in

lots of different directions at the same time. Somehow she maintained a
high degree of flexibility with an established set of values and limits that
gave the program its special richness. I frequently refer back to her model
of retaining control while allowing for distributive decision making.

But I also remained active in politics, and I got thrown out of the residency program for about two weeks during my first year, in July 1976.
The hospital workers' union 1199 went out on strike, and a group of
residents and faculty people within the residency program in social medicine organized to support them. The 1199 strike was a bitter ten-day
strike, one of the longest struggles that 1199 had. Those of us who didn't
have to go into the hospital went out on the picket line and refused to
go to our elective rotations. This was my first experience with a labor
movement struggle, and my grandfather's support of the labor movement
was heavy on my mind. (My father reminds me that when my grandfather died, the gravediggers' union was on strike. Acting against the teachings of the Jewish religion, our family decided to put Grandpa Maurice's
body in storage rather than hire scab gravediggers to bury him!) So I
didn't cross the 1199 picket line then and have not done so since. The
hospital president and some of the faculty members said, "If you don't
show up, you're out." That event dominated my life for about a year
afterwards because we were all fired. Then the National Labor Relations Board came in, supported the faculty people that were fired, and
forced the hospital to reinstate us. Thirty or forty other residents held
a sympathy strike in the hospital to support our being rehired. We even
received back pay and a public acknowledgement from the hospital that
it had been wrong. It turned out that there were laws protecting people
who supported others on strike, which the hospital had conveniently
ignored.

Montefiore Hospital attracted a special cohort of independent and socially committed people and gave them opportunities to pursue some of
their interests. So when they finished their three years of residency, instead of a traditional system where one comes out like processed cheese,
some people actually had an opportunity to put their ideas into practice.

When I graduated from the residency, I knew I wanted a combined administrative and clinical job, so I worked with New York Medical College
for two and half years running the Center for Comprehensive Health Practice, on the border of Yorkville and East Harlem. It was interesting—we
had people who were poor and uninsured and people who had million-
dollar-plus incomes, all coming to the same place for care. Administratively it was a disaster, though. Each of the providers saw six or seven

patients a day and spent about an hour with each of them. The head of the place was a behavioral scientist who believed that the more time you spent with people, the better they would get. The medical school was supporting the center, so finances were not a major issue. After a few months the medical director left and I replaced him. Just three months out of residency, and I was the medical director! I used what I had learned about teams at the Social Medicine Residency Program and I ran back to speak to Jo Boufford every couple of months. During that time I was the only family physician to get admitting privileges at Metropolitan Hospital.

Because I was the only family doctor in the whole center, I was feeling a little isolated from what family medicine was about. I heard that they needed preceptors for a new family practice residency program affiliated with New York Medical College at Kingston Hospital, a hundred miles up the Hudson River from New York City. So every Friday for two years I drove two hours up to Kingston. The most important part of that activity for me was working closely with the head of the Mid-Hudson Consortium for the Development of Family Practice, Dr. David Mesches. He was a very entrepreneurial family doctor who had merged his private practice with those of a few other family docs and set up a family practice network, a department, and a residency program in the mid-Hudson area. He was bringing medical students up from New York Medical College to do rotations there. I was totally enthralled by the idea that he had set up a separate corporation and, in doing so, had gone from being an employee of a hospital to having an independent consortium of family practice people. He even went back and negotiated relationships with the hospitals as an independent entity. Hospitals were dying to attach themselves to him, even though the hospitals themselves would never want to do anything in family practice. I thought, "Wow, this is perfect for New York City."

In 1981 I left the Center for Comprehensive Health Practice and became the founding medical director of Soundview Health Center in the southeast Bronx, a federally funded community health center in a Spanish and black community. The director, Pedro Espada, was a social worker in that community and later became a state senator in New York. He was a brilliant guy, also very entrepreneurial, who had a vision of what services he wanted to provide for the community.

It was my first foray into acting like a CEO. I managed the medical and administrative systems, put together the finance department, wrote computer programs for billing and other things, set up the clinical models, and created the charting systems. When I came, I was the only family physician. I felt we had a good model—a family doctor at the helm with the broadest vision, supported by people in different primary care specialties. Over time, though, we concentrated on bringing in more family practitioners. There weren't many places in New York at the time where family docs could get full admitting privileges, including privileges to do OB. By the time I left there were eight family physicians and two family nurse practitioners.

We developed a relationship with Bronx Lebanon Hospital Center, which wanted to develop stronger connections with community-based health care centers in order to increase loyalty, admissions, and specialty referrals. In my role as the medical director of Soundview, I went up to Bronx Lebanon and started a Department of Family Practice.

At Soundview I also wanted to establish a training program for students and residents, to help sustain the long-term interest of the doctors coming into the practice. Inpatient training was going to be at Bronx Lebanon and outpatient training at the Soundview Health Center, which would serve as the family practice center. But the community board and the executive director of Soundview, Pedro Espada, did not agree with our plan to turn the Soundview community health center into a training center. So we found ourselves recruiting residents without a family practice center in which to train them. That was how Bronx Lebanon became the recipient of a completely grant-funded new department and residency program. Fortunately they were thrilled, and agreed to clear out of an 8,000–square-foot ambulatory care center for us. We ran the residency program there for four years and then moved it to a beautiful new facility. Over time, almost the entire staff of family doctors from Soundview became the core staff of the new residency training program at Bronx Lebanon.

But none of us actually worked directly for Bronx Lebanon. About the time we made the transition to Bronx Lebanon, four of us decided to found the Institute for Urban Family Health, and basically modeled it after the Mid-Hudson Consortium concept of an independent corporation. We proposed to Bronx Lebanon that we would run the residency program under contract to the hospital. The hospital liked the fact that we proposed to run the program on the previous year's budget for the ambulatory care center. Bronx Lebanon gave us a contract, and we received $872,000 in twelve installments. We created the first model for continuity of care between outpatient and inpatient services by hospitalizing and caring for our own patients. Fifteen years ago, these were all new concepts.

The Institute for Urban Family Health represented for me the marriage of a personal issue and a professional philosophy. At that point I saw two choices in my life. One was to continue to be frustrated working for people who didn't move as fast as I did, and the other was to start my own company and gain independence. I'm a developer; that's what I love to do. The four institute founders became the board of directors of a nonprofit, tax-exempt institute with a charitable purpose.

My professional philosophy destined the institute to be a not-for-profit. I describe it as a hybrid between a community health center and a private group practice. It extracts the best of both systems—we take care of uninsured and underserved people but retain our doctors by giving them a real decision-making role. I was sure that the way community health centers employed physicians in the 1970s and 1980s was wrong; they were treated just like clerks. My vision was to create a professional organization that could build on the entrepreneurial spirit of smart people with initiative to achieve our goal of taking care of people who hadn't gotten care before. We had no qualms about not being a community-based or community-controlled organization. We set our salaries according to what people were making in similar positions in the community.

Two months into the program, we heard that the Sidney Hillman Health Center, located off lower Fifth Avenue in Manhattan's Garment District, which served the members of the Amalgamated Clothing and Textile Workers Union, was going bankrupt. This center was supported by a trust fund that was losing a million dollars a year. There was $3.5 million left out of an original $15 million established just six years before. It was clear why they were losing all this money—they had thirty specialty physicians and not one primary care doctor. The specialists would come in and refer the union members to their private offices for surgeries that were covered by their catastrophic coverage. Practically every person that walked in the door ended up in a surgical room or getting an unnecessary procedure. The specialists charged the trust fund $100 an hour to come to the center and do this stuff.

It was the most atrocious health care system anybody could imagine. We called in an independent auditor and found that 78 percent of all of the services done the prior year were medically unnecessary. We proposed that they get rid of the thirty specialists and close their specialty centers—the same type of proposal we'd given Bronx Lebanon Hospital six months before. We offered to make the center financially solvent using just the amount of money lost over the past year and not another nickel.

We met all of our financial projections. I think we lost only $600,000 the first year and then broke even in the second year, two months earlier than expected. We closed down four of the six floors of the building, fired all the specialists, set up a panel of outside specialists we could trust, and brought in four family doctors to run the center. We took about two hundred patients off weekly allergy shots, some of whom had been getting them for twenty years. We opened up to the community, started working with Medicaid, and developed HMO contracts. The building filled up in five years, serving all sectors of the community. Now we have fifteen different programs run out of the building: for HIV patients, the homeless, and many other patients.

When we opened, the union had more than 15,000 members and a hundred shops, and now I think there are only two shops left. The union has shrunk to almost nothing because most clothing is imported now. We still care for the remaining union members, as well as the retirees and laid-off union members. But we guaranteed the union that, after the first year, they'd never have to touch the trust fund again, and they never did. We told them that no matter what the volume of services, we would never charge them more than the amount of interest on the trust fund. Since interest rates were high then, we received $300,000 or more a year from the trust fund interest. By the time interest rates fell and only $100,000 was coming in from the trust fund, the union membership had dropped too.

So, with the Sidney Hillman Center and Bronx Lebanon, the institute inherited two huge projects almost instantly. Then we created a third, a faculty development program. None of our core faculty of community-oriented family doctors had any experience in teaching, so we brought in outside consultants. On the advice of the Health Resources and Services Administration Bureau of Health Professions, the federal agency that provided the funding, we also included spaces for doctors from other family practice residency programs. About 140 people have come through this yearlong training program since it started. We've now started to do advanced faculty development that includes organizational development concepts, budgeting, and some managed care topics, as well as some continuing education for people who've been through the training before. And we have a training program for nurse practitioners, based on a collaborative practice model of how physicians and nurse practitioners should work together—a model very different from that popular in the 1980s.

About a year after we started these programs, we made a pitch to set up another community-based residency program at Beth Israel Hospital, but the hospital leadership didn't bite. In 1991, when the Medicaid managed-care revolution started, we went back to Beth Israel, and the next thing we knew, they wanted to be the first family practice residency in Manhattan—and they were. With the money and resources they were feeding us, we made a swift transformation. By that time we were administering two large hospital contracts, the Hillman Center, and our faculty development program. By 1998 we had thirty residents from Bronx Lebanon and twenty-four from Beth Israel in our programs.

The Institute for Urban Family Health is really a business now. I don't think you can have a $20 million-a-year operation with three hundred–plus employees and not be a business. The institute now includes seven family practice centers, and nine part-time sites that cater solely to the needs of the homeless population. These last are run out of soup kitchens, churches, and shelters. While many homeless people are on Medicaid, and federal reimbursements are available for the rest, they don't have anywhere to go except emergency rooms. We provide them with a care system that doesn't depend just on insurance.

It's important to stay true to your commitment to the people you are out there to care for. We have had a number of opportunities to operate networks and primary care sites that cater totally to a commercially insured population, but we turned them down because they aren't consistent with our mission. As much as I've become entrepreneurial in trying to do new things, my colleagues don't let me stray very far from why they came here. In the end, we don't define our mission around insurance, we define it around people who have difficulty negotiating or gaining access to the current health care system in New York City. I think our mission is defined by our being "Ghostbusters" of a sort. If you need primary care and you have a population that's tough to serve, that's the kind of folks that we try to develop health care delivery models for.

We have totally integrated delivery systems for the care of HIV, for instance, because there are very few places where you can go for these services in New York that don't have AIDS or HIV written on the door. We have hundreds and hundreds of people with HIV at our sites, but they're sitting with everybody else, being taken care of by the same providers. We have two or three people who are real AIDS experts who help us provide quality care.

Through our relationship with the Visiting Nurse Service we deliver primary care to a group of about forty homebound people who cannot get in and out of where they live even with assistance. It's a small population, located in both the Bronx and Manhattan, but that's the kind of special work that we do.

We also have a program in the Bronx for people coming out of prison, many of whom have been diagnosed as HIV-positive. They have all kinds of other medical problems, and nobody wants to open their doors to them. So we transfer their medical records over after their release and begin caring for them.

I have been accused of being a flag-waving family physician, which I accept. We have one of the largest primary care organizations in the country that delivers care exclusively on a family practice model. It is based upon a singular philosophy that if somebody were to wipe out the current health care system in the United States and start over from scratch, they would create a front line that looks a lot like family practice and a back line comprised of subspecialists. The role of the primary care internist or pediatrician would not exist.

Nurse practitioners, physician assistants [P.A.s], and midwives are going to have an enormous new role in a managed care–dominant health system. People are concerned that the physician glut has eliminated the need for these "physician extenders." But in the transition to managed care, I think we will all be depending a lot more on P.A.s and nurse practitioners, who will focus on doing the preventive and educational interventions that most physicians don't like to do. Nurse practitioners are much better at sitting down with people for forty-five minutes and teaching them how to use metered dose inhalers and nebulizers to treat asthma. Doctors usually just don't do this, although it makes a critical difference in whether or not somebody ends up in an emergency room or in the hospital.

Managed care, in my mind, is like nuclear energy. It can be a constructive or a destructive force, and it will always remain a little bit dangerous. On the constructive side, it's the first time we've had a financing mechanism that truly supports prevention, that recognizes that keeping people healthy is in an organization's financial interest as well as its philosophical interest. The entire financing system before was designed around illness and sickness to make money. I think that redesigning the system with the opposite incentives has more potential payoffs than problems.

The real danger is that we're designing a system that the American public doesn't yet understand. We're all familiar with being sold something we don't need, and that's the way the old health care system often worked. But the new system is like having prepaid insurance for your car; there's a danger that the garage mechanic will tell you not to worry about the noise your car is making instead of telling you that you need a new fan belt or muffler. There's really no incentive for him to do anything, because the price of the fan belt or muffler comes out of his pocket. Most Americans don't realize that the health care "garage" they now go to also has a financial incentive not to provide care. So even though I'm a big supporter, I'm glad the media keep running stories about managed care abuses. After the transition is complete, we'll have a protective mechanism for the public and a much better financing system. Both managed care companies and family doctors want to keep people healthy, and thus can be said to have similar goals. They want to keep people out of the hospital; limit hospital stays to the shortest time necessary for good health; and use tried and true, less expensive, medications wherever possible instead of new designer drugs. The danger is that the entire country is trying to reduce what it spends on health care, and that *cannot* be done. The population is aging, technology is expanding, and treatments cost more every day. If we try to save money while we convert to managed care, the system will surely collapse.

At the institute we're working to improve our medical records systems to keep pace with patient and practice needs for immediate information related to drug recalls and interactions. In the future, we will use the Medicaid managed-care company we started to help figure out how all these special-needs populations fit into managed care—HIV-positive patients, homeless people, and others, who will be the most vulnerable during the transition. I would like us to have a network of sites in each of the boroughs and in the neediest communities.

I would know my life was successful if a large number of people from very poor communities in New York City received care at our centers on a par with or better than that dispensed on Fifth Avenue. If we do this right, at least in certain model places, we're going to end up with a truly first-class system of care, serving the people who need it most. My job continues to be to fight the system, but now on behalf of an organization that is trying to serve those who are truly left by the wayside in our health care system. But now I also have to worry about meeting our payroll obligations, raising money for our work, and planning for a future in a health care environment being starved for resources.

I have always believed that one's professional life mirrors one's personal life, and my family life has been both a challenge and a blessing. My father provided stability to my family of origin, teaching by example the rewards of hard work and perseverance. He went to work six days a week and later recruited my mother to work in his office. My mother was a Holocaust survivor and struggled, as many do, with the memories and terrors she faced as a nine-year-old fleeing the oncoming Nazi army. She survived but with a legacy of nightmares and memories that would come back to haunt her whenever life's stresses became too great. Perhaps because of her childhood experiences, she developed a knack early on for emotional sensitivity and could never pass anyone less fortunate without offering a helping hand. Our family home frequently had boarders—orphans from the local institution where she volunteered or children of family friends in need.

My relationship with my wife, Renée, started in the midst of the 1199 strike in 1976. Her parents were also Holocaust survivors, and we shared many interests. Though she was nonpolitical, a fact that disturbed some of my more radical friends, she always supported me in my struggles with the system and, I think, was more afraid for me than she let on. We were to face many challenges together—first infertility, then the adoption of two boys, and, many years later, divorce. I often wonder if some of the same issues that caused me to challenge authority in my life and work didn't cause me problems as a parent and husband. I recognize that every human trait, like every new drug, has potential ill effects as well as benefits. What keeps me going is a belief that my shortcomings at home and at work are the results of the same traits that have driven me professionally to prove wrong all those who said that the centers we built and the doctors and nurses we trained and the models we created for inner-city health were impossible to do. The remaining challenge is to be able to teach that perspective to my children.

Roots Rediscovered

The Internist and the Pediatrician as Generalists

The philosophical difference between "medicine" and "surgery" is a time-honored one. Surgeons have long been distinguished by their use of knives for manually removing disease from the body. In contrast, practitioners of medicine have relied on their powers of observation and analysis to make decisions about therapeutic interventions. Early in the twentieth century, as medical science progressed and the tendency toward specialty training and practice gained momentum, several important developments occurred. The first was the formalization of the distinct professional identities, organizations, and, eventually, certifications for medicine and surgery with the founding of the American College of Surgeons in 1913 and the American College of Physicians in 1915. Next was the emergence of pediatrics as a distinct discipline and its formal separation from the field of adult medicine (increasingly known as "internal medicine") with the founding of the American Academy of Pediatrics in 1930. During this period increasing numbers of physicians were choosing to do nonsurgical postgraduate training as "internists" or pediatricians but with the principal intent of entering practice in the general care of adults or children.

Continued developments in medical science, however, created more and more clinical possibilities and stimulated the birth of a spate of subspecialty fields rooted in the traditions of "medicine" but focused on specific organ systems and patients with diseases of those organs. By the 1970s, two-thirds of internists and one-third of pediatricians were training and practicing as subspecialists, leaving general or comprehensive medical care as something of a subsidiary enterprise undertaken only by those not ambitious or well-positioned enough to get specialty training.

Internal medicine and pediatrics were becoming holding companies of subspecialists who had divided up the body, organ by organ—all of whom were highly competent in their respective organ systems, but none of whom took responsibility for the human being as a whole. Questioning voices began to be heard, lamenting the balkanization of internal medicine and pediatrics and calling for the recapitalization of the idea of the "general" internist and the "general" pediatrician. As early as 1952, a group of pediatricians convened at the annual meeting of the pediatric academic organizations to discuss the state of teaching and practice in outpatient departments, the indisputable center of primary care pediatrics in training programs. In 1960 they formalized their group as the Association for Ambulatory Pediatric Services, stating that their goal was "to improve the teaching of general pediatrics, to improve services in general pediatrics and to affect public and government opinion regarding issues vital to teaching, research, and patient care in general pediatrics." The organization, which was subsequently renamed the Ambulatory Pediatric Association (APA), has grown over the years and has continued to be a force for generalism in pediatric education, research, and practice. In addition to sponsoring an annual meeting, a journal, and a variety of regional programs, the group collaborates regularly with kindred organizations in internal medicine and family medicine.[1]

The challenge of supporting generalism in internal medicine was in some ways harder than in pediatrics—and in some ways easier. Because specialization was far more prevalent in medicine than in pediatrics, the challenge of organizing was more difficult. Without a real revitalization of the idea of adult primary care, it was altogether possible that internal medicine would become exclusively a land of specialties, with the residual generalists absorbed by family practice. The 1960s saw an increase in interest in the teaching of generalist principles in academically affiliated programs such as clinic-based teaching practices, neighborhood health centers, and area health education centers.

Increasing numbers of academic internists who embraced generalist values found that fields such as clinical epidemiology and health service research provided areas of scholarly pursuit that dovetailed with their generalist practices. In 1972 and again in 1976, Congress passed versions of the Health Professions Educational Assistance Act, which provided support for training programs in general internal medicine and general pediatrics. The new Robert Wood Johnson Foundation, under the leadership of Dr. David Rogers, an internist and former medical school dean, gave priority to funding primary care initiatives in internal medicine and pediatrics. In 1978, one of those grants was awarded to the American College of Physicians to start a new organization called the Society for Research and Education in Primary Care Internal Medicine. This organization had been in the planning stages for more than three years, led by a group of academic internists including Drs. Frank Davidoff, John Noble, Thomas Delbanco, and Robert Lawrence.[2]

The Society, which simplified its name to the Society for General Internal Medicine (SGIM) in 1987, has been a strong and articulate force for generalist values and careers in internal medicine. SGIM has supported federal generalist activities, including the founding and development of the Agency for Health Care Policy and Research (now the Agency for Healthcare Research and Quality) and has worked extensively with other groups such as the Primary Care Organizations Consortium and the Public Health Service Primary Care Policy Fellowship. Patient-centered medical care, evidence-based medicine, ethnic diversity, and cultural competence are among the values promoted by SGIM and the movement of general internists.

The line of demarcation between generalists and specialists in internal medicine and pediatrics is crossed frequently and argued about a great deal. All specialty internists and pediatricians have completed basic residencies in those fields. Many who have gone on to training in specialties continue to treat patients for ailments that fall outside their chosen domain and many, doubtless, do a reasonable job of it. Some specialists, of course, choose not to work outside their areas, and others are sufficiently out of date or out of practice that their competency is not what it should be. Debates continue about the division of labor between generalists and specialists and about the training requirements for both. These issues will not be decided easily or by fiat, but it is worth reflecting that the central issue is not one of simple skills but one of perspective. Generalism requires an attitude, an interest, a degree of patience, an element of human curiosity—a perspective—in addition to a set of special skills that cut across all of the specialties and enable a practitioner to reach out to the whole person. It is a vocation, not a subsidiary or passing occupation. It is an attitude of practice that goes back to the roots of the profession and to the roots of the individual practitioner.

Beach Conger, M.D., is a general internist in the heroic mode—a solo practitioner in a rural area, practicing a care-taking and individualized

form of medicine. He earns respect for both his principles and his idiosyncrasies. His independent practice probably tells more about the general internist of the past than the one of the future, who will undoubtedly rely a great deal more on systems of care. Linda Headrick, M.D.,
spends much of her time thinking about systems, clinical systems. An academic general internist at Case Western Reserve, she is hard at work on
the language and ideas of the future—words and concepts that will bring
physicians and patients together in more effective practice groups. Selma
Deitch, M.D., M.P.H., has devoted almost five decades in practice to the
care of children. Her work extends well beyond the examination room
to the family, the school, and the community, demonstrating the population medicine potential of primary care. Her concern with the forest
as well as the trees is a hallmark of the true generalist.

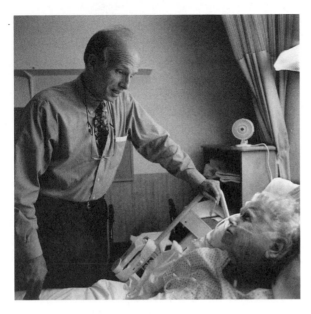

Beach Conger engaging
in spirited dialogue.

BEACH CONGER, M.D.

CARETAKER AND CONTRARIAN

Windsor, Vermont

Beach Conger started into medicine with an eye on public health. He worked in Mississippi as a medical civil rights worker, led a job action at the Boston City Hospital to improve patient care conditions, and spent two years as an epidemic intelligence officer for the Centers for Disease Control. Thirty years later, though, he is the quintessential personal physician, practicing in a small town in Vermont, watching illnesses come and go, families grow up, and the elderly pass on. When he finally began practicing medicine, it turned out that he loved it.

His vocation is internal medicine, but his avocation is professional contrarian. He enjoys gently telling people the truth about their health (some day they're going to die), the doctor (he doesn't know everything), and their part of the world (it has some strange medical habits). His hands-on engagement with life and his eye for the humorous started him writing, first a column for the local newspaper and then two books of autobiographical musings. The cover of the first book, titled *Bag Balm and Duct Tape*, advertises itself as "How a doctor taught a town to be proper patients and how the patients taught the man to be a doctor." The second is called simply *It's Not My Fault,* a tongue-in-cheek comment on Conger's chosen role as the medical custodian of thousands of lives.

Conger counts himself an activist generalist who happily handled all manner of medical challenges that face a small-town physician. After adjusting to life in the country, he came to take pride in his ability to cope with most of the medical problems that came his way, calling on specialists only occasionally. But the environment is changing, and a determined generalist such as Conger is finding mounting pressures to join networks, to refer, and to rely on technology for diagnosis and treatment. "Today I feel more like an endangered species than a role model," he observes. "Kind of like the gray wolf or the cougar. It seems my feeding grounds are gradually being replaced by multispecialty clinics and CAT scanners. Still," he concludes, "I can't think of anything else I'd rather do."

⌒

I HAVE ALWAYS BEEN INTERESTED in public health. I used to think that I would wind up being the Surgeon General. Who wouldn't want to battle the scourges of history—tuberculosis, infant mortality, malnutrition? Medical school reinforced my interest. We studied salmonella outbreaks, cholera, and clean water strategies in the second-year epidemiology course, and I loved it. This was the era when we thought we had beaten infectious disease, before AIDS, before Legionnaire's disease and hantavirus and drug-resistant TB. Smoking wasn't much of an issue then, and diet and exercise were still the concern of health food types. We had no idea how important public health would become to medicine and to all of us.

But it turns out that medicine involves a lot of acting, and I'm a bit of a ham. You can't crack jokes when you're trying to solve the problem of infant mortality, but I can with my patients. I have spent time working in public health. I enjoy the problem solving and dealing with public issues like access to health care, abortion, and prevention. I've been active in local politics and, for a while, served as chairman of my local school board. But it turns out that for me it isn't as much fun as the one-to-one with patients. As things have developed, I'm a country doctor, not the Surgeon General—and I love it.

I started in the city. I was born in 1941 in New York City but was raised in suburban New York, first in Hastings-on-Hudson, and then in Pleasantville, a suburb about thirty miles outside New York City that is known as the home of the *Reader's Digest.* My parents were both writers. My father worked for the *New York Herald Tribune*. It was the only job he ever had, until the *Tribune* died, and then he died about six months later. My mother wrote children's books and then worked for *Reader's Digest*. They had lived in New York City before I was born, then moved out to the suburbs. That was their upward mobility. My mother edited condensed books. When she first started she felt it was presumptuous to edit other writers, but after a while she began to realize that even the best writers could be improved upon.

Pleasantville was your basic town, all that its name implies. In the 1940s it had about 5,000 people and was just far enough out that most people who lived there did not commute to New York City. We had one African American in town. His name was Sidney Poitier. I went to a small high school, where about 40 percent of the kids went on to college. They tended to be the ones from educated families who worked in New York City.

My decision to become a doctor was basically the result of my doing well in school; that was one of the things that kids who did well in school then were supposed to do. I went to Amherst College, where I majored in Russian and traveled to Russia in 1962. I thought it would be more interesting to become a Russian scholar than a doctor, but I couldn't see far enough on the horizon in that field, whereas medical school was pretty clear.

I went to medical school at Harvard. I found the first two years tedious, and I didn't apply myself much. I'm not good at compulsive learning, so if it wasn't interesting I tended not to study it, with the result that I didn't do very well. One day after I got a D in physiology, I was called into the dean's office. Since you've been accepted to Harvard they assume you're smart, so if you're not doing well they think you're having some problem at home. Just before entering medical school I had married. The dean asked me if my home life was happy. I replied, "Yes, I think that's fine." After that I realized it was in my interest to have been a little bit unhappy, otherwise they thought there was something wrong with me. The second two years were better. I enjoyed the practical stuff.

During my junior year I did my medicine rotation at Boston City Hospital, which I loved. A city hospital setting is much more egalitarian than places like the Massachusetts General and the Brigham Hospitals [now the Brigham and Women's Hospital]. It's much more forgiving, both in terms of what the patients expect from you and the way people treat each other. I did my medicine and surgery rotations there, as well as my internship and residency.

Between my second and third years of medical school, in the summer of 1965, I went to Mississippi. Jack Geiger, one of the leading spokesmen for the Medical Committee for Human Rights, gave a talk in Boston. As a newspaperman turned doctor, he envisioned health care as an instrument to raise people out of poverty. This appealed to my public health instincts. Geiger was very charismatic. He'd gotten a grant from the Office of Economic Opportunity to set up a clinic in Holmes County, Mississippi, and he was looking for summer volunteers to go south. I signed on.

After a week of training at the University of Pittsburgh School of Public Health, they sent me to Holmes County. My wife, who was similarly politically inclined, was teaching math that summer at Tougaloo University in Jackson, Mississippi. I wound up living in the house of a sharecropping family that was about five miles outside the county seat, Lexington, Mississippi. I was full of grandiose concepts about what I was going to do as a medical civil rights worker but I wound up working on voter registration and school integration—not the stuff of medicine but historic movements of the time. It was a remarkable experience.

The one medical experience I had was being called to the home of a child who was lying on a bed seizing. At that point, I probably knew something about the idea that children may have febrile seizures, but that's about it. "We'll have to take him to the hospital. This is terrible," I said. The mother put him on the floor so he wouldn't hurt himself. "It's just a seizure," she said. "And besides, they won't see us at the hospital." I was horrified. I assumed that something drastic was going to happen to the child if they didn't get him to the hospital, and the family accepted it. They thought I might have a pill I could give the child. They never asked me anything again.

For my wife and me—as for many others who went south to work in the Civil Rights Movement—the experience was a politicizing one. Once back in Boston, we decided that we wanted to be active in local politics, so we moved into the Cabot Street Housing Project in Roxbury. We were the only white couple living there. The rent was $44 a month, which was a nice benefit, and my wife served on the board of the local Community Action Agency. I worked on the Boston arm of Dr. Geiger's project, which was opening a clinic in the impoverished Columbia Point section of the city.

Living in the ghetto at that time was very different than it would be today. People used drugs and alcohol and fell asleep on the sidewalks, but violence and fear, regardless of your ethnic group, were much less a factor than they are now. It was just a very poor place. I lived very close to where Louis Farrakhan lived when he was growing up. I was there when Martin Luther King was killed, and I remember sitting on the stoop of our housing project watching the local convenience store burn, but nobody felt at personal risk. These were old, dilapidated buildings burning down.

When I was a fourth-year medical student I still didn't know much, but I came and went in a white coat. My neighbor was a taxicab driver. One day, his wife came over to see me and said, "You've got to see my husband. He needs to go to the hospital and he won't go." So I went over. He was sitting watching television with a Band-Aid on his forehead. "What's the matter?" I asked.

He said, "I've got a headache."

Being a dutiful medical student, I began asking him a recently learned list of questions about a headache. "When did it start? Did it come on suddenly or gradually? Does it radiate, or do you feel sick to your stomach?" We didn't know each other very well, but I think he figured this was something he had to go through. Then I asked, "What's the Band-Aid for?" I thought it was some kind of funny thing he did to make him feel better. So he took it off and said, "That's the bullet hole."

"What do you mean?"

"Well, I was driving my taxi and I went to let my fare out, and the guy put a gun to my head and said, 'Give me your money or I'm going to shoot you.' And I said no, so he shot me."

"He shot you in the head?"

"Yeah."

"With a bullet?"

"Yeah."

I said, "You've got to go to the hospital! You've been shot in the head!"

And his wife said to him, "See, I told you he'd say that. Listen to the doctor."

He says, "No, if I go down there, I'll sit around for five hours, they'll take an X ray, they'll say there's nothing they can do, and they'll send me home again."

I said, "No, no, no. You've been shot in the head. I'll call an ambulance."

He said, "I'm not going to take an ambulance."

He went to Boston City. Five, six, seven hours later, he comes back. "What happened?" I asked.

"They took an X ray, they said there's nothing they could do, and they sent me home."

So now, whenever anyone comes in for a headache, the first thing I ask them is if anybody shot them.

We lived in the project for the last two years of medical school and into my internship. My son was born while we lived there. We moved out of the housing project because we were no longer economically eligible after I began to make a salary. Because of my background, living in Roxbury provided me with a perspective I hadn't had. It gave me an understanding that, even in this country, there is a way of life that has nothing to do with what goes on in places like Pleasantville, where I grew up, or Vermont, where I have lived since 1977.

Going to Mississippi and practicing at Boston City Hospital were conscious decisions I made to work with people who were poor. Working with the poor was more rewarding for me. I was not comfortable as a student at Boston's upscale hospitals. I didn't feel smart compared to the doctors there, but also those hospitals seemed a little too classy, too detached. The Shah of Iran was a patient at the Mass General when I was there. That wasn't why I was in medicine. In contrast, I felt at home at Boston City Hospital, which was falling apart.

In 1967, while I was a fourth-year student at Boston City Hospital, we held a "heal-in" to protest conditions at the hospital. The heal-in was an alternative to a strike where we continued to admit patients but didn't discharge anyone. Interns were paid only $100 a month and wanted a raise. We also wanted better laboratory services, more nursing, and improved patient care all around. The city said, in essence, "Listen, we'll give you pay increases and some lab technicians, but we're not going to address nursing and patient care. We don't have control over that. If you fight this, you may not get the money you want." The house officers were getting tired of the heal-in, so we settled for our money and the promise that they were going to work on our other demands.

In 1968 I became president of the house officers' association, and we became the first labor organization of house officers in the country, although I didn't find that out until I attended our thirtieth anniversary this past year in Boston. We hired a lawyer and, full of righteous zeal, we sat down to finish the business of improving patient care. At the time I felt I had really accomplished something. Now, years later, I am ashamed. The real tragedy of Boston was not how they treated the house officers, who would soon go on to rich and prosperous careers, but how they treated the poor people of the city of Boston and the health care workers who took care of them day after day. Like the heal-in, when we were done what we mostly got was a little more money. I can't remember anything substantive we achieved in improving patient care.

I was at Boston City Hospital for two years, then I joined the Public Health Service and was assigned to the Centers for Disease Control in Atlanta in a special program called the Epidemic Intelligence Service. Practicing public health appealed to me, especially given the choice of going to Vietnam or an assignment in the Public Health Service. My intent was to stay in the Public Health Service permanently, and the time I spent at the CDC substantially raised my estimation of the federal government. The dedication of some medical staff at the CDC was improved by the sense that if they weren't at the CDC somebody would be glad to take their places, and they could always be sent to Vietnam as medical officers.

This was pure public health work in a public health agency, and I liked it a lot. When I began, the entire focus of the CDC was infectious disease, but they were at the point of applying epidemiological principles to other aspects of health. I went to work with a gynecologist who was beginning a program of contraceptive evaluation using data from family planning clinics. I staffed rural health clinics in southern Georgia, where the local doctors, who were all white, wouldn't go, because public health clinics were believed to be a Communist plot. I traveled to these clinics, where a very pleasant, condescending white nurse would usher in her black clients, whose faces I would never see. When I would come into the room they were already in the stirrups, covered with a sheet, draped around so that it was physically difficult for me to talk to them, which was intentional. I would be either checking an IUD, or putting an IUD in. That was what these clinics were doing.

In 1970 New York state passed a law legalizing abortions, and I was sent there in 1971 by the CDC to conduct surveillance of outpatient abortions in New York City, tracking down complications and deaths. People came to New York from all over the country to get abortions, so it was really a national issue. For the first time the CDC recognized that the morbidity from abortions needed to be treated on a par with tracking down salmonella outbreaks and eradicating smallpox. Abortions had finally become part of the mainstream political debate in this country. This was 1969 and 1970, long before AIDS arrived on the scene.

We were still based in Atlanta, and we had had our fill of the South. My wife was involved in a class action suit against AT&T because she was one of many women who were being paid less than their male counterparts. I had been arrested for operating a dive because my neighbors couldn't stand the fact that we had a black friend from Mississippi staying with us while he went to a summer program in Atlanta. A night in jail and a civil rights countersuit later, it was all dropped, but it left us less than satisfied with our time in Atlanta. At that point my wife wanted to go to San Francisco and start law school, so I left the CDC and resumed residency at the University of California–San Francisco. During that last year of training I spent time working in a methadone maintenance clinic in a ghetto area, trying to help a group apply for federal support. Subsequently, this same group received a grant to take over a failing community health center and asked me to run it. I accepted and started working there while finishing my residency, in 1972.

The clinic, called the South of Market Health Center, was just off Mission Street, smack in an area of dilapidated housing, soup kitchens, and run-down hotels. We saw people on a first-come, first-served basis and, often when I arrived in the morning, I would see my patients sleeping on the sidewalk, waiting to get in. Medical care at the clinic had been terrible before we started—Vitamin B-12 shots and antibiotics for everything. We came in with new money, new employees, and outreach programs. We treated patients with respect, practiced preventive medicine, and went door to door. Besides homeless alcoholics and heroin addicts, there was also a large immigrant Filipino population living in the same area who, in contrast, were very stable and upwardly mobile. Many had come from the upper classes in the Philippines, including some doctors who were working as housekeepers. Tension existed between these two populations over the clinic. The Filipinos wanted it to be their clinic, and after a while many of them joined the clinic staff. The alcoholics then tended not to show up as much.

I worked there for six years and discovered, somewhat to my surprise, that I liked practicing medicine. Although public health planning had been a lot of fun, I really enjoyed patients. At that time, of course, I had the illusion that you could do both population medicine and clinical medicine. I was no longer planning to become Surgeon General. But if someone said, "Would you want to become director of the city's health clinics, at some point?" I might have said yes. This was an activist time in San Francisco with many free clinics and a lot of federal money available to set up neighborhood health centers. The budget for our clinic doubled about every two years.

By 1977 I'd gotten an amicable divorce and married Trine Boh, who was first year law student at Golden Gate University. My focus changed after I met her. I was no longer thinking, "What am I accomplishing with medicine?" but was thinking about my life and my kids—two from my first marriage and then one from my second. And Trine, Norwegian by birth, wanted to be closer to snow, which was an important part of her cultural life. That, together with a horrendous drought in 1976, drove us east to Vermont. Trine needed to finish law school. She discovered the Vermont Law School in South Royalton, a tiny town about twenty miles south of Burlington. At the same time, I found an ad from a community hospital looking to replace a retiring internist in Windsor, Vermont, which turns out to be twenty-five miles from South Royalton. I was dubious but decided to take a look. All of my real experience had been at huge city hospitals and, by comparison, the hospital in Windsor seemed like a doll hospital. It had twenty beds, and everybody knew everybody. But I liked what I saw and, it turned out, they were excited to see me. I took the job.

The doctor who was leaving told me, "Oh, you don't want to come here. There are no patients to see." I thought, "Why not? They're going to guarantee my salary, and I can do this for two years. In the meantime, we'll figure out what we're really going to do." That was nineteen years ago.

For the first six months I was petrified, because I was used to places where there was always somebody around to help you deal with a problem. If somebody got sick, I sent them to the hospital. I might visit them, but I didn't start the IVs, insert tracheal tubes, put casts on people. I prescribed drugs, and I talked. Suddenly I was dealing with everything— train wrecks and broken wrists, things I'd seen a hundred times and things I'd never seen before. I was the doctor. There were no diagnostic radiologists, no backup orthopedic surgeons, no backup anything. It was anxiety-provoking.

And then I got used to it, and realized that you do what you can do. For instance, I was treating a man with chest pain. I don't remember what went wrong, but he died suddenly. I told the family I felt just awful, and they could see it. "Doc, don't feel bad," they said. "You did the best you could. He would have died anyway." They were understanding of the idea that doctors don't always succeed. People in Windsor back then accepted the idea that doctors could fail or even screw up.

An example of the kind of thing I had to learn on the spot was caring for a patient with a fracture. In all my years of medical training, I was never taught how to place a cast. Internists didn't do that in city hospitals. When I worked in the emergency room at Boston City Hospital, for instance, I never even saw the broken bone. The patient was sent somewhere else long before they saw me. One day early in my practice in Windsor, a man arrived with a clearly fractured wrist. "You've got a broken wrist," I told him. "You need to see Dr. Shoemaker, the orthopedic surgeon over in Claremont." Claremont's about half an hour away. He retorted, "I'm not going over to Claremont. Can't you set it?" I said, "No, I've never set a broken wrist before." "Well," he said, "I've never had a broken wrist before, either." I put on a cast that must have weighed 150 pounds. The nurse warned me, "You're going to have to take that off." When he came back a month later I realized what she was talking about. It must have taken me half an hour to cut through that cast.

There were a lot of things I just gradually started doing. I practiced more intense medicine than many internists do today, largely because people expected me to. I referred very few patients out unless they needed a surgical consultation.

We now have six internists in Windsor, two pediatricians, a general surgeon, a full-time orthopedic surgeon, and a variety of visiting specialists. The specialists visit from the Dartmouth-Hitchcock Medical Center twenty miles to the north, or they've set up a private practice in which they circuit-ride to a series of community hospitals, of which we remain the smallest. So specialists are all around me again. Patients are now more likely to consider a specialty referral option, so I do a lot more referrals than I did when I first arrived here and a lot more than I would otherwise want to do. Several of our physicians have become employees of a huge physician organization whose brochure states, in essence, that "Primary care is the doctor you go to, to help you figure out which specialist to see."

Fifty percent of my patients are on Medicare. Of the other 50 percent, everybody has managed care of some type. The only difference it makes to me is that I have to fill out more forms. Part of the reason it's not a problem is that there is no competition here in primary care. The patients who live in this town are going to have to come to see someone in this group, by and large, unless they hate us all, in which case, they could travel some distance. Managed care will never have the same impact here as it does in a place like California, where you have plans competing with each other, and there are real issues about patient jumping. I have patients who have gone through three plans in the last five years. I'm always the doctor. If they're in California, they would be changing doctors. But here there's nobody else for them to see.

What has changed is that if somebody came in with a headache nineteen years ago, I would have talked to them and, unless I had been really worried, I would not have ordered any more tests. Now, the chances are better than fifty-fifty that the same patient with a headache knows about CAT scans and expects one—regardless of the fact that I don't think one is indicated in the vast majority of cases. When I first came here, patients were not as educated about health issues as they are today. "What are you here for?" I'd ask them. "That's what I came to find out," they'd respond. "You're the doctor, you figure it out." This sort of attitude gave me latitude in where to go with things, but also showed that the patient remained marginally involved in what was going on.

Poverty in this area is not concentrated, the way it is in what's called Vermont's northeast kingdom in the northern part of the state, where people have no money and live in shacks with no electricity. Isolated poverty is quite common here, but most of my patients get by okay. Windsor is distinctive in that we had a maximum-security prison and several factories. Once the factories left town, a large apartment complex, initially designed for factory workers, became home for the wives and children of the prisoners, and that brought in an underclass. The apartment complex looks like something that was airlifted out of the Bronx. It's a huge brick structure. There's nothing anywhere like it in Vermont. So we have this small underclass population. I handled a case of lead poisoning when I first got here, a kid who lived on a back porch and ate lead, just like in an urban setting. Outside of the prison-related population, some immigrant Vietnamese, and a few adopted black children, it's still a white culture.

I have more access to specialists than I would like to have. It's kind of like having too many restaurants to choose from. You're also more likely to eat out when you have a lot of restaurants, and I'd really rather eat at home. For every disease there's someone who is smarter than I am. I could send every patient to somebody else for every complaint, but that's not what I choose to do. My practice is made up of patients I've known for a long time, and they tend to look primarily to me for guidance. An irritated cardiac surgeon to whom I had sent one of my patients called me once, saying, "We think your patient needs to have his mediastinum opened up because he's gotten a postoperative infection, and he wants me to check with you." That's patient loyalty.

There's a group practice of younger physicians in a nearby town who don't even come into the hospital when they're on call. When somebody gets sick they send him to Hanover to the medical center. If somebody has chest pain, they send him to the cardiologist. These doctors are quite content with that kind of relationship. Many primary care internists today do substantially less with patients than older GPs and old-style internists. My partner is fond of saying that we older internists are dinosaurs: we once ruled the earth, but our habitat is shrinking and we're becoming extinct. Today's younger internists will never set a broken bone or take care of a patient in an ICU—they'll transfer the patient to the orthopedist or the pulmonologist.

When I was in medical school, cholesterol wasn't much of an issue. If you identified a patient with high cholesterol, it was really high—like 500 and they'd have huge globs of fat hanging from their eyeballs. You'd call people. Big hoopty-do. Now, everybody is potentially a patient because we've lowered the cholesterol standard so that nobody will pass. This means that there are people trooping in and out of the office all the time who aren't sick. People have gotten used to going to the doctor on the premise of not being sick—which is okay. But when they get sick, they think, "I've got to see a different doctor. This is not my doctor for sick. This is my doctor for cholesterol, and blood pressure, and maybe Pap smears. Now that I'm actually sick, I need a specialist." Many younger internists and family practitioners collaborate in this by focusing on health maintenance and avoiding more intensive forms of patient care. And since everybody does get sick sooner or later, this kind of thinking has led to a doubling in the number of specialists in the country. A cynic might say that we were training too many doctors in this country and we didn't have enough sick people to go around. Since lots of the new doctors were becoming specialists, we had to find something more for them to do, so we invented diseases in well people.

One way to stem the tide of expense and futility in medicine would be to admit students into medical school who aren't quite so smart. Why don't we just conclude that we have enough medicine right now? We won't make any more improvements, and we'll live with what we've got for a while. Maybe thirty years from now we'll start working on it again. If our doctors were not particularly smart, sort of nineteenth-century doctors, we wouldn't invent new procedures. We'd just muddle along, and things would stabilize. The rest of the economy would grow for a while, and we'd stop spending larger and larger chunks of it on medical care.

When a patient arrives in my office I put this cuff around his arm and pump it up. "You've got hypertension," I say. The patient says, "That's the silent killer," and we start down the long, long road of antihypertensive treatment. Now the fact that everybody's going to die, and that there may be a point in the patient's life when having hypertension is the best option available because it's better to die of a heart attack than get Alzheimer's disease, is not an option that's discussed. I had an eighty-nine-year-old woman come into my office and ask to have her cholesterol checked, and I refused. She said, "What do you mean? You can't refuse." I said, "No, but can I talk you out of it?" She said, "Well, I don't want to have a heart attack." I said, "Why not?" "I don't want to die." "What are your options at this point? You're eighty-nine years old." "Well, I'd like to die in my sleep." "How do you die in your sleep?" "I don't know." I explained, "Your heart stops. You need to have a heart attack, and high cholesterol is the best thing you can have. This is what you want!" I'm joking, but in another sense, I'm not.

I think that the evolution now is toward primary care as very distinct from secondary care. Primary care, as I see it, is really wellness care, secondary care is general sickness care, and then tertiary care is caring for people with special sicknesses. Wellness care means dealing with the "pre-sick" who have yet-to-be-determined diseases. I see my general internist role as doing secondary care as well as my own brand of primary care. That's what I was trained to do. What I like best about my practice is the interaction with people but, I have to admit, there still is a part of me that likes disease. I get energized when somebody comes in with an abnormality. But I've known most of these people for a long time, and it's always upsetting when I pass along a bad diagnosis. I had a medical student with me one day when a patient's CAT scan came back with an ominous spot in the right lung. The student was excited. "This person's going to have lung cancer." I responded, "If your sister had this CAT scan you would not be very excited."

I've lived in the community and know everybody here. A woman on chemotherapy just came in with a sore ear, terrified. I looked in her ear and it was okay; she felt great and so did I. I like that. I have to have a certain number of sick people to fuss with or I feel that I'm betraying my training. But I don't need a lot of it; I don't even need it every day. People in Windsor give doctors so much benefit of the doubt—more so than anyone else including the local clergymen. I can make a fool of myself, and people don't mind; I march in parades wearing wild outfits, I write crazy stories in the newspaper and, because I'm a doctor, people like me.

I'm an ex–Epidemic Intelligence Service officer, and I keep up with infectious diseases. In 1983 I made the diagnosis of Legionnaire's disease in a hospital patient. After another case was diagnosed and we found the source in the hospital's water heater, we were credited with what has been humorously called the world's record for terminating a *legionella* outbreak—two weeks. A big press conference was held locally, and the hospital administrator asked, "Would you talk about the outbreak?" Legionnaire's disease in Windsor was a big deal.

At the press conference I joked, "This is nature's revenge. You put people in buildings and nature says, 'This is not what you're supposed to be doing,' so it's got germs to try and combat you with this." A guy there from the local newspaper said, "You've got a strange way of looking at things. Will you write an article about this?" So I did. They then asked if I'd write some more, and I did. The paper is called the *Valley News* and has a circulation of around forty or fifty thousand. I wrote a piece on herpes, and something on why doctors lie. A couple were sort of whimsical. Eventually, I wrote a column every other week under the heading "The Second Opinion." It was never serious, though I always told the truth. I enjoyed the writing, and after three or four years my editor suggested I collect the pieces into a book. I sent them to a publisher, who responded, "I don't know how we're going to use this. There's no market for it. But maybe you want to write it into something that fits together." I turned the articles into a sort of diary that, in 1988, came out as my first book, *Bag Balm and Duct Tape*. After that, I was off and running. My second book, *It's Not My Fault,* was published in 1995.

I really enjoy writing. It imposes a kind of discipline on me that medicine doesn't. My first and second drafts are usually gibberish. I have to rewrite probably six or seven times to get what I want. In medicine you don't usually have that chance. I'm working on a book that is much more difficult than my other two, which were just stories I wrote from my everyday experience. This one is about a doctor who practiced in my town one hundred and seventy years ago. She was a woman, but because women weren't allowed in medicine she had to practice as a man. It has been a real challenge to set myself in a time where doctors knew almost nothing and the only two medicines of any definite benefit were morphine and quinine. I'm not sure I am good enough to write it, but I'm working at it.

Trine and I have three children. Our youngest, Nadya, teaches Spanish in the Boston area and the oldest, Matt, teaches science in Woodstock, Vermont. He lives about one mile from us. Our middle daughter, Dylan, lives in Brooklyn, New York, with her husband. She is a research analyst for the Vera Institute, which does analytic work on social service programs. None of my children ever showed the slightest interest in medicine, which is okay.

Trine is a recovering attorney. After she got her degree here she went into private practice, which is not what she really wanted to do. One of the problems in the country is that you feel left out of the real problems of the world. She went into family law and had an extremely busy and successful practice for twelve years. In 1990, she became a family court magistrate. Then she quit it all in 1994 and went to Baltimore as an Annie E. Casey Foundation Fellow. She worked as a consultant for the Rhode Island Department of Children's Services and now for the state of Vermont trying to bring some sense into the way the courts and the social services deal with abused and neglected children. Unless Trine takes a job elsewhere (which is a possibility), I plan to practice here until I retire, because at this point there's nothing else I can do. I have an excellent practice, and I'm the senior physician in town. Everybody looks up to me, except the people who can't stand me. It's a very small pond, but I'm the biggest frog in it. In ten years, if I'm still in good health, I'll cut back my practice and start writing more.

I'm fond of telling patients something that is very clear to me. "You know, if I treat you long enough only two things can happen. Either you die or I die." So I keep treating sick people, and I recognize the futility of it because they're going to die. But I keep at it because it's what I do.

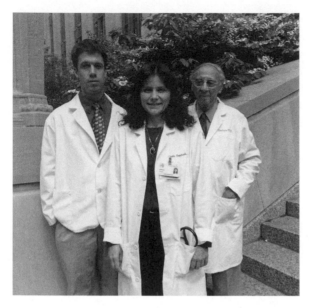

Linda Headrick with her colleagues in quality improvement, medical student Kenan Sauder and faculty member Jack Medalie, M.D.

LINDA HEADRICK, M.D.

SEEKING A COMMON LANGUAGE IN PRIMARY CARE

Cleveland, Ohio

Linda Headrick is an academician—a teacher, a clinician, and a trafficker in new ideas. She is a member of the "academy" by dint of being on the faculty of Case Western Reserve University Medical School in Cleveland, Ohio. But she is not a classical academician by traditional standards. Her patients tend to be those with common problems rather than those with esoteric ones. Her teaching addresses the problems of the system and the population in addition to the biological problems of the individual. Her research subjects are neither patients nor laboratory animals but rather the system that makes the medical center and health care delivery function—or malfunction.

She is a quiet but constant warrior against complacency in medicine. Her passion is "quality" or "quality improvement," but these well-worn terms do not do justice to her mission. "What is the aim of our work?" she asks. "How do we know when it works and how well it works?" Satisfying the doctor or the institution or meeting some long-outdated goal does not mean that "our work" is "working." Her research and her teaching bear on measuring the success of the clinical enterprise by patient satisfaction, clinical outcomes, and community change. These are not indices that medical researchers are seasoned at measuring or, in fact, inclined to examine. Yet they are at the heart of what payers, policymakers, and the public are asking of our medical system.

Dr. Headrick's base of operation is one of the nation's most prestigious medical schools—one that is increasingly open to her mission but still uncertain what to make of it. There is growing respect for her ability to interpret the powerful industrial forces that are buffeting academic health centers across the country, but for many the enthusiasm for applying this wisdom at home is tempered by a reluctance to abandon age-old institutional behaviors.

The daughter of a career agricultural extension agent, articulate and enthusiastic, Dr. Headrick speaks with gusto about her work. She is applied and practical in her vision, and she has a growing cadre of allies around the country in education, practice, and business. She believes that the generalist physician and nurse are well positioned to lead a quiet revolution in how we do our medical business in this country, how we improve it, and how we keep on improving it over time.

⌒

RIGHT FROM THE START I wanted to be a primary care doctor. I was going to take care of folks over time. I was going to be there for them, the first contact person, whatever they needed. I liked the science, but it was the relationship part of medicine that I found most appealing and where I thought I had the greatest skill.

I think my dad's work influenced me, although I didn't realize it until I was talking with a medical student a couple of years ago. He asked me about what my folks did. I told him about my dad. My father worked for the University of Missouri Extension Service, helping community businesses and community development in general. He started as a county agent after World War II and spent his career in the extension service. I tried to explain to the student what that was. "Well, basically he was part of the community and used the resources of the university to try to make things better." The student responded, "Oh, that's interesting. That's sort of like what you try to do." This huge light bulb went on, and I realized that the extension ethic was a big influence on me.

The Protestant ethic—literally, the Protestant ethic—was a factor for me too. My mother's influence was very important there. Her father was a Baptist minister, although our own family was Methodist. Responsibility for the collective good and responsibility to the other guy were core values. And that's how I saw my role as a physician.

I'm from Missouri. I grew up in Chillicothe, a little town of about ten thousand people, a hundred miles northeast of Kansas City. When we moved to Chillicothe, my dad was promoted to director of a nine-county area for the Agricultural Extension Service. It was in seventh grade I decided I wanted to be a physician. There were no doctors in my family, but I came from a family where it was, "Sure, whatever you want to do. Education is important, and if you want to go for that, that sounds good." Except my grandmother, interestingly enough, who got this downcast look on her face and said, "Linda, I always thought you'd be such a wonderful nurse."

I went to the University of Missouri–Columbia and majored in chemistry for, what I'm embarrassed to say now, were pretty typical premed reasons. This was 1973, and at that time the competition for medical school was tough. I went to a meeting—one meeting, that's all I could tolerate—of the Pre-Med Society and they had us, all the freshmen, stand up and look at the people on either side, and they said, "Only one of the three of you will actually get into medical school." That was the competitive atmosphere.

Everything wasn't premed at the university. I met my husband there. He was a year ahead of me, a molecular biologist. When I started looking for medical schools, I was trying to follow where he'd gone to graduate school, which was Stanford. I started there in the fall of 1977. But Stanford was different, filled with people with very different backgrounds from mine—prep schools, Ivy League, and cultural experiences I hadn't had. I found the first two years difficult, but I felt that I blossomed in the clinical years because I could draw upon all of my skills, not just my ability to read a book and memorize what was there. Stanford has a reputation of not being supportive of primary care. I didn't feel that so much because it was not difficult to find people who shared my interests. There was a growing group of general internal medicine people, and they had a small but valiant group of family medicine physicians. I didn't feel particularly discouraged in my interest in primary care, except that I clearly didn't match the specialty and research focus of many of the faculty.

My husband got his degree in molecular biology and accepted a postdoctoral position at the Carnegie Institution in Baltimore. That meant I needed to find a residency in the Baltimore-Washington area. I had to decide between family medicine and general internal medicine. The fact that there weren't many family medicine programs in that part of the country contributed to my decision to go to the University of Maryland in internal medicine. I really liked Maryland because it was a house staff–oriented program where we had many opportunities to make decisions and do things on our own. I found wonderful faculty mentors there and became a chief resident in medicine. It was my chief resident year that made me realize how much I loved to teach and that I wanted an academic job.

My husband was also looking for faculty jobs at that time. He was offered a position in Cleveland. On his second visit, he was invited to bring "the wife" along, and they tried to find "the wife" a job. Interesting position to be in. It worked out quite well, in fact. I wound up joining the Division of General Internal Medicine at Metro [Metro Health Medical Center, formerly Cleveland Metropolitan General Hospital]. All of the physicians there were full-time faculty of Case Western Reserve University [CWRU]. My job was as a half-time practitioner and a half-time educator, helping to run the residency program and a fourth-year primary care medical student clerkship. This was 1985.

I started out in practice, loved it, and got so busy that, after about two years, I couldn't take any more new patients. Everybody wanted us—the general internists—for everything. The specialists wanted to refer their patients to us because once they controlled a specific problem, they recognized that the patient needed long-term primary care. They were delighted to send patients to us. The surgeons grew to value our contributions in doing perioperative consultation. The house staff said they thought that the generalists were the best teachers in the wards.

When I became involved in the larger educational programs, though, I began to encounter some of the more negative attitudes about primary care, particularly from people in other fields. I'm afraid I was surprised that other faculty didn't care about the same things I did. Why isn't it a good idea to teach physical diagnosis in the first year so people can be learning with patients at the same time they're learning in the classroom? That's not a primary care–oriented issue on the surface, but it has a very primary care–oriented flavor to it. Why shouldn't we have students learn from generalists as well as specialists? Don't we learn scientifically even if we can't isolate one variable and have sixteen controls? What I'm interested in is harder to control, harder to experiment with, but so important, so critical to the problems before us.

I also continued my role as an innovator, in that I couldn't leave things alone. There were lots of opportunities to do things differently, and I was in an environment that supported that. This was in large part due to the chief of the Department of Medicine at that time, James Carter, an endocrinologist but also one of the best generalist physicians I know. During his tenure, he strengthened the general internal medicine presence in research, clinical care, and teaching. With his support, I created the first ambulatory block rotation for our house staff in general internal medicine. I did quite a lot of work with others to improve the residency program, and was pretty satisfied doing that for a while. Then I realized that even though I thought I was making things better, I didn't really know. Five years down the line, somebody could very well come along and make cogent arguments about how some of the things we did were not so good anymore and reverse everything. No evidence would exist to support one approach or the other. I realized that everything I thought was important was vulnerable to being blown away in the wind over time. That's when I changed my mind about research and realized I wanted to find ways to evaluate what I was doing, and do a better job of saying whether the changes were better.

I decided to evaluate and write about some specific education projects that we had done that others seemed to think were interesting and unique. I was frustrated by my inability to do that very well, and particularly by my lack of preparation with respect to quantitative and research methods. Early on, I started going to national meetings. In particular, the Society for General Internal Medicine helped me see that people were defining careers for themselves in academic general internal medicine that were education-focused. With those role models, I began to think of myself as an educator, a primary care physician and an educator. Eventually, I also arranged to work part time to get a master's degree in health services research.

It was great luck that Duncan Neuhauser was here at CWRU in the Department of Epidemiology and Biostatistics. He has a Ph.D. in business administration and was interested in teaching students about the costs of medical care in the context of primary care. We designed a project in which students wrote case studies of patients with asthma and shared what they learned about how to think about measuring quality and cost of care in asthma. Initially, we focused on cost. We asked the students to simply go out and find out how much it cost for what they prescribed for a particular patient with asthma. That was astonishing. Students had no idea it cost $40 for a steroid inhaler, for instance. Duncan kept saying, "You know, Linda, it's a very interesting thing about cost. We can't think about it alone. We can't talk to our class about cost without teaching them about quality." So I began to learn how one thinks about quality in health care. I became interested in the methods and principles in continuous quality improvement. Suddenly, I found a way to get at some of the systems problems that kept us from doing things well, both in health care and in education.

With tremendous help from the chief of general internal medicine, Randall Cebul, I did a randomized controlled clinical trial, an education trial about cholesterol screening and management with the residents at Metro. None of it worked. Resident behavior didn't change. I thought, I wonder what happened? The residents picked up a chart, and there would be a bright yellow piece of paper on the front that stated, "Patient's last cholesterol was 270. According to the guidelines, the next thing to do is . . . "and all they had to do was fill out a form to do it. So I surveyed the house staff. I said, "Was the yellow form there?" "Yes." "Do you agree that this is an appropriate thing to do with your patients?" "Yes." "Do you agree with the recommendations?" "Yes." "How often do you do it?" They thought 75 percent of the time. The real answer was only half the time, which was no different from the residents who received no coaching and prompting. "Why didn't you do it?" It was all systems issues. "There wasn't enough time." "I didn't have enough help." "I couldn't find the form." There also was no difference in performance of residents who scored well on the test of cholesterol management knowledge and those who did poorly.

I was stuck. Until I learned about quality improvement, I had no way of getting at the systems problems that kept us from being able to do what we knew how to do, and we'd like to do, but just couldn't do consistently, patient to patient. Then I met Edward McEachern, who had been a medical student at CWRU, and was working as a consultant for hospitals that were trying to improve quality. He taught me a lot and helped me identify what to read. Duncan helped me connect with Donald Berwick and the Institute for Healthcare Improvement [IHI],which has sponsored our work using and teaching quality improvement in medical education. I've been learning like crazy ever since. Paul Batalden, who leads IHI's work in health professions education, has become my most important mentor in this area. Now working out of Dartmouth, he is one of the country's best thinkers about the improvement of health care. I'm constantly finding other people who have also been influenced by his work.

What I want is to have medical students finish medical school, or residents finish residency, ready to actively improve the care that they're delivering—not only to deliver excellent health care, but to be able to improve the care as they go along, and have that as part of what they see as their job. That includes being able to work as part of a team, in a meaningful way, with people from other disciplines—nursing, health administration, and so on—because that team is needed to make improvement. The language for all of this is difficult because the field hasn't matured enough in medicine to have a common language. More and more I'm using the words "continuous improvement" or "continual improvement," but not everyone's satisfied with that. And the receptivity to these ideas has changed considerably over the years. When we first started talking about this in 1988, some students had a fit about attempts to measure and improve quality. One example was their reaction to guidelines, "cookbook guidelines." "Don't tell me what to do. Every patient's different. You can't give me guidelines about how to take care of patients." That's largely disappeared because people became comfortable with the idea that a guideline is only a place to start.

Physicians now seem to be fairly accepting of the fact that cost is something they're going to have to deal with. Improvement methods allow them to deal with the cost issue by focusing on quality, and that is very attractive. But many physicians, and particularly academic physicians, are still negative about thinking of the people we serve as customers. They don't like the idea of transporting business ideas into medicine, they don't think they belong. Generally, though, I'm finding now that a lot of academic leaders are asking me about quality improvement. People seem more friendly to the idea of thinking in systems—including managed care systems. I've been asked to travel all over the country to consult for medical schools and hospitals on teaching quality principles in medicine. Many physicians recognize in their everyday lives now that they have to work as part of systems. Otherwise the system will roll right over them.

I think that the natural leaders of systems in health care are generalists, because they have the broad perspective needed to have a systems view. The same personality types and the same sort of worldview fit both places. But even if you're not a leader, if you're a practitioner working with your office nurse, your receptionist, and the pharmacy, you're going to be better off if you can be thinking about that as a system and figuring how to deliver better care in that system. And you have to, because people are going to be asking you what your outcomes are.

One of the critical tensions that is going to be important in my lifetime as a health care professional is the tension between reductionist thinking that breaks things into small parts and broad systems thinking

in medicine. We in medicine have been at the altar of reductionist thinking for a long time, and we have mined enormous benefits from it. But
we've also lost many opportunities because of what we have ignored.
We devalue the importance of working with systems, and we don't know
how to do it.

For a while I was trying to learn how to play the banjo. I was very serious about it. My teacher was trying to get me to learn how to play by
ear, but I had picked out a couple of songs on a record that I liked a lot.
In my typical reductionist way, I tried to listen very carefully to write the
song down so I could understand the chord structure, exactly what the
notes were. I was going to try to tape it, and write it down, and break it
down into pieces, learn the pieces, and put them back together again. I
completely blew my teacher away. He thought that was the dumbest approach to learning how to play a piece of music he ever heard in his life.
He was trying to get me to try to think of the music as a system, to really hear the music and have it come out in my fingers. And he had no
better way of describing it to me, and I had no idea how to do it.

I would argue now that a good generalist needs to be able to do both—
reductionist thinking and systems thinking. In fact, I think that from the
perspective of a system of care, one has to ask, why are internal medicine and family medicine separate? What are the roles here? The goal is
to deliver the best primary care. It doesn't make sense to divide it up between medicine, family medicine, and pediatrics. We have to sort of
scramble, depending on the environment we're in, to define how we're
different from one another. I also think that it's nonsensical and, frankly,
foolish not to take advantage of what our colleagues in nursing and other
disciplines know about doing primary care. I'm a general internist. There
are things that family practitioners know, that physician assistants know,
that I'd be a much better primary care physician if I knew. There are things
that nurses do that the ideal primary care physician of the future would
be better off knowing how to do—such as listening, counseling, thinking about families, and thinking about the caring part of care. So why
are we not teaching them together, and why are we not combining our
strengths rather than splitting them up? What I would like to see in the
future is a new kind of primary care provider who is the product of the
best in all those fields.

As I look to the future, I know I want to be in a place where I continue to have the freedom to explore and learn, and have a laboratory
in which to do that. I think that I'll stay in academic medicine because
of my devotion to education. Some days I think I'm better off staying

as a fairly independent faculty member. There are other times when I think that pursuing leadership roles, more central and mainstream to the organization, might be a way to go. And there are other days when I think, well, maybe it would be useful to spend some time outside these institutions. My department chair thinks I should become a department chair, and my former dean thinks I should become a dean. It's a great compliment that they want me to do what they do, but I worry about those standard organizational leadership positions because of the fact that it's so easy to be distracted from what I think are the most important agendas.

At home I'm still married to the same biologist who enticed me west to Stanford years ago. My work is way out there at a systems level. He spends his days on a molecular level, working on the precise factors that control RNA transcription. He's a good bellwether for me because he is a very thoughtful guy who cares about the world and shares my values of what would be good for the community and the country. The kind of thinking I do is so different from what he does. He respects me and my work and is willing to explore my professional interests—ideas that otherwise might make him very suspicious. He's a key reminder to me about important parts of my audience in the academic medical community.

Recently I heard a senior physician, a family physician, describe his career to a group of medical students. He talked about all the different paths he has taken, and he did so with considerable excitement about every step of the way. I was listening to him and thinking, you know, I can do that. I think when I'm seventy, I will still get excited about these things, because so far I've been challenged and excited by new questions and new solutions that I think are important—and will remain important. That's the one thing that I absolutely can be sure about, that I'm going to be an avid learner, and have fun doing it. I will continue to work hard to move us closer to a world in which all physicians finish their educations ready to assess and improve the work they do every day, with a clear focus on the individuals, families, and communities they serve.

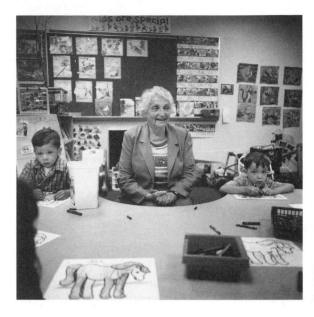

Selma Deitch
brings pediatrics
to the classroom.

SELMA DEITCH, M.D., M.P.H.

CHILDREN FIRST

Manchester, New Hampshire
One hundred fifty years ago, when the first American children's doctors began calling themselves pediatricians, some 200 of every 1,000 infants born died before the age of twelve months. Today that rate is 7 in 1,000, a monumental accomplishment of pediatrics and of public health and a marker of dramatically improved child health in the United States.

Selma Deitch is a practitioner of both of these disciplines, and for much of the latter half of this century she has devoted her training, her energies, and her personality to the cause of improving the health of children. At seventy-three, she remains in full stride as the founder, executive director, and chief booster of Child Health Services, a nineteen-year-old, innovative pediatric clinic for low-income families in downtown Manchester, New Hampshire. Part clinician and part public health zealot, she sees patients, raises precious support funds, and consults nationally on maternal and child health issues. "I work two weeks a week," she states simply.

Born in Manchester to immigrant parents, she grew up wanting to be a veterinarian but gravitated toward medicine under the influence of her

physician father. Her training in Boston in pediatrics and public health
provided a formula for returning to New Hampshire as the state maternal and child health director in 1966 and the start of a thirty-year campaign waged in both the public and the private sector to improve the
condition of disadvantaged children. The diseases prevalent when she
trained—polio, pneumonia, and lead encephalopathy—have been replaced by what she sees as the new scourges of inner-city children: drugs,
alcohol, and children having children. "These 'morbidities,'" she says,
"result in dysfunctional human beings in far greater numbers than the
children who have physically disabling conditions."

Child Health Services occupies a large storefront on Manchester's Elm
Street in the city's old business district, which surely has seen no elm trees
in many decades. The offices are newly refurbished thanks to a $1 mil-
lion community fundraising campaign. Energetic and grandmotherly, carrying a stethoscope and a notepad, Deitch points with pride to the
mini–jungle gym in the waiting room, the engaging animal prints on the
walls, and the new, multipurpose teen room. Her enthusiasm for her creation is palpable.

Deitch is not without her adversaries—individuals or institutions
whom she considers rigid or not clear about the needs of children. "Child
Health Services," she observes, "has given me the privilege of being a bit
of a free thinker, of having the luxury of being my own person and being able to push the system. That really is a privilege."

⟿

I HAVE SEEN A LOT of children over the years, including many sick ones.
Some of the things that make me happiest about my work, though, don't
have to do with medicine in the traditional sense. Recently I was able to
arrange for a photography shop to donate a camera to a thirteen-year-
old patient and to get him enrolled in a photography camp. He's having
a wonderful summer. But I know that he was born to a thirteen-year-old
girl and that he bounced from day care center to day care center while
his mother tried to stay in school. His mother finally quit school because
she just couldn't get coverage for her baby. At age five he was molested
by a boyfriend of his mother. Now his mother has settled down, is married to a stable man, and is working full-time. But along the way, terrible things happened to the little boy.

With a little help now from the staff of Child Health Services, he was
enrolled in a summer program for gifted students for the previous two
years and is showing real promise as a photographer. He brought me his

portfolio the last time he came for a checkup. It was beautiful. Then we talked about acne, tobacco, drugs, and sexuality.

This is a critical part of pediatric care in the 1990s in Manchester, the city where I was born, the adopted city of my parents. My father came from the Ukraine near Kiev, and my mother was from Lithuania. She was eight years old when she arrived with an older sister to stay with relatives in the Boston area. My father came to Boston when he was eighteen or nineteen. He had been a premedical student in Odessa, Ukraine. When he arrived, he enrolled in high school and then went on to medical school at Tufts, graduating in 1918. My mother became a nurse. In those days that was a pretty special thing for an immigrant woman. Her relatives expected that as soon as she could speak English, she would work in a button factory. She was head of an operating room where my father was the intern during the influenza epidemic of 1919. The day they married in 1919 was the end of her nursing career.

They moved to Manchester in 1921, where my father went into practice as a GP with a special interest in surgery. After that, my mother was responsible for answering the telephone when the office was closed. I used to imitate the way she answered. "Hello," she used to say angrily. She was not really an angry person, but the role tied her down. I think that was characteristic of the time. Women were not getting out to do their own thing. When I was thinking about what I wanted to do with my life, she shook her hand at me and said, "Don't ever be a nurse."

I was born in 1924, the second of three girls. I was going to be a veterinarian because I loved dogs. I think my father gave me subtle encouragement to pursue medicine, support that made it easier for me to keep going to school. I went to Jackson College, which was the women's part of Tufts, and took mostly premed requirements, all those courses that have labs. I was even advised to take scientific German. Scientific German! I snuck in a few liberal arts courses, but the rest was science. It was wartime, and we were encouraged to go to school summers and get through quickly. I was nineteen when I graduated in 1944 and too young, they told me, to go to medical school, so I was accepted for the following year. I moved into the Elizabeth Peabody House, a settlement house in Boston, where I taught neighborhood kids to build airplane models as my contribution as a tenant.

I started at Tufts Medical School in the fall of 1945. There weren't many women in our class but more than in earlier years. There was some sense that the war provided an extra opportunity for women, since it wasn't clear how many men would be available. Although I'm very gender-aware now, I wasn't then. I was sort of one of the boys. Medical school got better as it went along. I liked radiology, surgery, and general medicine. Pediatrics really didn't occur to me. The rotation that I found the most exciting was home medicine. It wasn't just ambulatory care. We were assigned to a district—East Boston, in my case. We did follow-up care in the homes of patients from the clinics at the Boston Dispensary. We'd start from our preceptor's car with addresses and medical records and make house calls. The neighborhood was poor, but it wasn't obvious. Homes were well-kept, and people were home when we went to visit. Safety didn't seem to be an issue either. Nobody troubled us. I loved the work. I think home medicine had a big influence on me and what I have ended up doing.

I wanted a rotating internship. I couldn't go to Boston City Hospital because they had no place for women to stay. Mount Auburn was the other hospital that I wanted to go to, but they wouldn't take women in rotating internships. I finally accepted a position at Springfield Hospital in Springfield, Massachusetts, mostly because the man I was going to marry was taking a surgical residency in Boston, and Springfield was the closest rotating internship I could get.

One of my first rotations was in ENT; I had to give anesthesia for tonsillectomies. Kids. I felt sorry for them. I remember dropping ether on the gauze over their noses while they were lying on stretchers and rolling them into the OR. In Springfield I was inspired by a very bright pediatrician, Hy Schumann. He taught me an awful lot about hospital pediatrics, and I enjoyed the way he practiced. This exposure got me thinking about pediatrics.

I came back to Boston after the year of internship and did what was called a fellowship at the Boston Dispensary—the outpatient department for Tufts teaching hospitals. I worked as a preceptor for the same home medicine program that I had taken as a student, this time in the Irish neighborhoods of South Boston. I still loved the work. I began to see pediatric patients on my own under the supervision of the pediatric staff from the Boston Floating Hospital. I had decided that pediatrics was what I wanted to do with my life and, in the summer of 1951, I began two years of pediatrics residency followed by a year as chief resident at the Boston Floating Hospital. It was an intensive exposure to the hospital treatment of sick children. Penicillin was a new and exciting drug then, and we had chloramphenicol with its benefits and complications. We saw a lot of things that you don't see often today; replacement transfusions were common for Rh incompatibility, acute epiglottitis, meningitis, poorly treated seizure disorders, acute rheumatic fever, and carditis. Polio was seasonally endemic.

I saw my first and most tragic case of lead poisoning in my first week as a resident. The child came in with acute encephalopathy, the only child of older parents. The anesthetist put four burr holes in his head to relieve the pressure, but the boy died. He'd been eating his crib paint, and his parents kept repainting it. We knew about pica, but people didn't know that most paint contained lead at that time.

I was amused to read recently about a professional athlete who had raised money to make a floor at the New England Medical Center into a residential facility for families of patients with cancer. The article said something like, "Farnsworth Five, a dilapidated part of New England Medical Center that has tile falling down, and floors that need repairing, and rugs that are torn." When I was there, female residents didn't have a place to stay the nights we were on call, so we all shared one room on Farnsworth Five. Sometimes there were more of us than there were beds. It could be crowded, but we thought Farnsworth Five was a pretty spiffy place in those days.

When I finished my residency, I moved to Needham and went to work covering the practice of a pediatrician who was called up during the Korean War. I continued doing this kind of part-time coverage until he returned, but I kept up my affiliation with the dispensary. In 1958, I became the director of the pediatric outpatient department of the Boston Dispensary, which was the Boston Floating Hospital outpatient department. It was a general pediatric outpatient department for low-income patients from South End, South Boston, East Boston, and Charlestown. The pediatric residents rotated through. The attendings were physicians who had privileges at the Floating, who gave their time for a month or two a year to precept the residents and the medical students.

I did a lot of teaching, and I learned a lot. One thing I never forgot is not to assume that a person who's in training knows how, for instance, to look at an ear. I always had to look for myself. I also learned about the role of social work from a woman named Liz Wheeler. She taught me a great deal about families and how they function. We also had the benefit of a nutrition service in the outpatient department. Right there in our outpatient department was an ongoing nutrition program where they served food to the kids and taught people how to budget and purchase, to do all those basic but important things.

The chairman of pediatrics at Tufts at that time was a wonderful generalist named James Marvin Baty. Those of us who worked with him still chuckle about him. He made wonderful rounds. You saw the whole child. He was instrumental in starting a child psychiatric unit at Tufts as well as an attractive playroom in the hospital so that hospitalized children didn't have to stay in their beds all the time. Most children got to go to the playroom, pulled in something like grocery carts or wagons if necessary. The playroom was staffed by an early-childhood education specialist who was one of the most wonderful people in the world, Kris Angoff. I learned a great deal about pediatrics, clinical environments, public health, and developmental pediatrics from her and also from Dr. Baty's orientation to that sort of thing. They taught me about the importance of behavioral and psychosocial pediatrics.

These experiences had a lot to do with shaping me as a pediatrician and determining what I would do in the future. But a lot also went on in my own family life during these years. I married my classmate in 1950 and had my first child when I was finishing my residency in 1953. We were divorced in 1957. Through my extended family, I met a wonderful man, a chemical engineer back in Manchester, and we were married in 1960. He had three children, and we had one more together. I actually commuted to Boston until 1965, when I finally settled down in my old hometown after being away for nineteen years.

During this whole period, I believe I was beginning to use a different language about health care. From what I had learned in the outpatient department, I was much more aware of things that had to be brought together based on the role of communities in health care. I became more of an advocate for kids in school and families who didn't get care at all. I didn't know what public health was then, but in retrospect I had become a public health–oriented pediatrician. When I left my work in Boston, I enrolled at the Harvard School of Public Health, commuting daily for a full year and graduating in 1966. It was a wonderful time at the school with fabulous faculty and students from all over the world. I wrote my master's thesis on day care in Manchester, a system previously unknown to me, resulting in my growing interest in child care policy.

My first real job in public health was as a part-time, volunteer medical director of the Head Start program in Manchester. We had Head Start only in the summertime then, and it gave me the chance to get to know people in Manchester whom I hadn't really known before, an entirely white, poor population who were largely French Canadian. We started programs in three different public schools. I got to know school principals in a nice way that held me in good stead as life went on. In 1966, the director of the New Hampshire Department of Health hired me as director of the state's Maternal and Child Health [MCH] Program, a program with an expanding national mandate as part of the Great Society strategy of the Johnson administration. The concept was that children's health care should be comprehensive and include social support services and nutrition as components of general health care. Family planning and prenatal care were to be included, and all those delicious things were going to be funded for populations that hadn't had access to care. It was a terribly exciting job. When I started, there was only one well-child clinic in the state of New Hampshire. It had been organized by a very competent pediatrician who couldn't handle poor people coming into his office, so he started a free clinic that met once a month in a fire station, in an adjoining town. My challenge was to establish programs where parents could bring their children for complete care, including promotion of growth and development.

It had always been difficult to use federal funding to build programs in New Hampshire. The basic philosophy was against accepting any federal money because the federal money would eventually "go away" and the state would be stuck with the program, so the attitude was "Let's not do anything the government pays for." Nonetheless, we did get some new MCH money and were able to start many programs, including well-child clinics, all over the state and the real jewels, four comprehensive Children and Youth [C and Y] clinics in North Conway, Exeter, Charlestown, and Suncook. We established family planning sites in many places and, despite much opposition, they survived. People associated birth control with abortion, and still do. If you don't talk about one, you don't talk about the other. Many decision makers were against family planning—period. My strategy always was to start programs first by going to where people were receptive. There was need, goodness knows, everywhere. In the Dover and Rochester areas, we started prenatal and family-planning programs *together* because there was good community support and good local leadership. The federal Community Action Program came in at that time and collaborated well with us.

While I was MCH director, I worked as a pediatrician in one of our clinics at Suncook. I also saw patients in the Crippled Children's Clinic, a multispecialty service for children with problems like cleft palate, seizure disorders, and cystic fibrosis. It kept my clinical hand in, and I got to know physicians and public health nurses around the state. I learned a lot from those public health nurses.

I left state government in 1974 because I wanted to spend more time laying on hands. I'd become much more aware of underserved populations because of my experience in day care and through the state clinics. We were seeing kids with special needs all right, but many poor children weren't getting any primary care. And I wanted to do something here at home in Manchester. May Gruber, an industrialist in Manchester, had known me for some time, and I knew she liked my work. I told her I was interested in starting a program that focused on low-income children and families with an emphasis on developmental issues. So she agreed to underwrite my associate Ruth Butler and me, and we started the Institute for Child Health and Development. We provided consultation and staff training to day care centers, preschools, and programs for children with special needs, focusing on the identification of parent strengths.

The Institute did well enough for three or four years, but I really wanted to be able to provide primary health care services to low-income families with children in need here in Manchester. Mrs. Gruber pushed me to look for more backers because she was restless about being our only resource. A number of foundations had turned me down, but suddenly two grants came through simultaneously—the federal Bureau of Maternal and Child Health and the local United Way. At about the same time I called the Children's Defense Fund in Washington, D.C., and they were able to provide me with articles that showed that comprehensive programs (like Head Start) were far more effective in the long term than piecemeal programs. The Manchester superintendent of schools at the time was my classmate from high school. I asked him to go up before the mayor and board of aldermen with me, using the data I had collected, to argue that even if 10 percent of the children we saw in our clinic were more healthy and ready for school, we could reduce the cost of education because they were not going to need special help later on. It would save the city money. Amazingly they voted to fund us and have continued to supply about 8 percent of our budget ever since.

In November of 1979 we opened Child Health Services on Elm Street in Manchester as a nonprofit agency with one pediatrician—me. We also had a program administrator/community organizer, a social worker, a family-support worker, a part-time nutritionist, a secretary, and a board of community doers. Our aim was to provide full-service health care to children from low-income families. From the very beginning we limited our enrollment to families that had at least one child younger than two or a child younger than seven with a special medical need. We did this because we planned to promote parenting functions, to support family strengths, and to be in a position to intervene when necessary.

Almost twenty years later, we are following the same model, more or less, with a staff of five part-time pediatricians, two social workers, ten family-support workers, and three nutritionists. The family-support workers are a unique and key part of what we do. They make "follow-up" happen. Two workers do mostly transportation, one runs our bicycle safety clinic and seatbelt and helmet education programs. During the summer, they place kids in camps and in art classes, get them tutors, museum passes, and music lessons. Our nutritionists cover all the clinics, working with children and families who have conditions like diabetes, galactosemia, feeding disorders, and tube feedings. They also arrange for food in school for kids who are not being fed at home and send snacks over to the boys' and girls' clubs for children who are not growing well. Optima Health Care, an alliance of the local hospitals, is our largest sponsor, but county and state government, foundations, service clubs, the United Way, and fund-raising activities of our board help a lot. Only 20 percent of our funds come from insurance.

We get a high percentage of referrals from other agencies, hospital emergency departments, intensive care units, and nurseries, plus private doctors, neighbors, and relatives of current clients. We have a waiting list, but if we get a call saying, "This mother's going to be discharged, and we doubt the family's ability to provide consistent parenting," we arrange to take that family right away. We have one social worker who meets the family at the hospital. Her job is to project to what extent that family will need our involvement as an agency. Meanwhile, we collect all of the medical information so that we can go over it prior to the first visit. We do the same with a child born with spina bifida, for example, or an infant with an enlarged liver. We try to make all the needed connections: education, transportation, and treatment. Local pediatricians provide our hospital backup.

Over a third of our clients are now teenagers, just by virtue of the fact that they've stayed with us since infancy. So we do a lot of adolescent health, both through a Planned Parenthood/Teen Options program that meets in our office space in the late afternoon or evening and through our regular clinic program. But our adolescent strategy isn't working well. Our way is still too traditional for adolescents. We knew we needed more staff to be able to have drop-in discussion groups, "hang-around" sessions for teens, peer counseling–type activities. We needed to shake up our system for teens and, for that matter, for their parents. We needed a much more casual, flexible approach with much peer influence. Our space became too small for the "hang-around" approach. A grant from the American Academy of Pediatrics got us started on a new teen program, and with support from our board and many others in the local community, the program opened in July 1998 at the YWCA.

I think Dr. Robert Haggerty had it right a few years back when he began talking about the "new morbidities"—what we now call psychosocial health care. I mean young people using drugs and alcohol, and risky sexual behavior resulting in part from more and more dysfunctional families. Young people not finishing school, not being able to provide for themselves, and not being able to take care of their own families. These are the problems that are tearing our families and communities apart. These "morbidities" result in dysfunctional human beings in far greater numbers than the children who have physically disabling conditions—especially among the poor.

This is the part of pediatrics that I see as the major forte of the generalist pediatrician. It takes the skilled generalist together with support staff and a caring community to deal with these problems. I want every general pediatrician to be a good diagnostician and well trained so as to be able to treat illnesses properly. But the generalist also needs to be able to recognize simultaneously other aspects of that child's environment and development that are key to that child's health. How old are the parents, are they well, do they know how to use resources, what is their level of education, what are the community resources, and how does one access them? From the beginning, it has been the intent of our staff and board to promote this model of practice—the Child Health Services model—so it could be adapted in more traditional settings.

I think that over the past twenty years I've learned that I knew less about the health of people who were poor than I thought I did. I used to say that no child in New Hampshire was sexually abused except "up north in the wintertime." That was naive and wrong. We have held parenting classes for young mothers who came to talk about how to raise children. By the second or third session these young parents want to talk about themselves, and often they begin to talk about how they were abused in their own lives: "This is what happened to me. I thought I had the big secret." Spousal abuse is a big problem too. Just recently a teenaged mother with three small children—all my patients—was with her drunk husband and two or three of his friends. He picked a fight with his friends and then got out a knife to go after her because she was telling him to stop. So she called 911, and he went to jail. Two days later he got out again because he said he was sorry. And the children witnessed the whole thing.

There is an increase in family violence. It's not just that we've scratched the surface and found more. More is going on. People have more access to drugs and alcohol. Poverty is more prevalent, and with it comes more stress in the population we see. I have learned an enormous amount about how children are handled in families and how the community itself has not always responded to the needs of children. I simply didn't appreciate how rigid and provincial some people's attitudes can be in the face of the actual pathology that takes place. It's sort of like, "Oh, the plane crashed in Guatemala. Glad it wasn't here." Many people aren't really accepting the fact that the kinds of things we're talking about are happening in our town, and they need fixing.

I have been blessed with a good and supportive blended family. My second marriage was a very good one with love, compatibility, and fun things, but my husband died in 1982. My youngest son is a lawyer here in New Hampshire and active in state government affairs. My older one is a lawyer in Boston. The youngest of my three stepchildren is a social worker in an HMO in Minnesota, the second teaches school in Barbados in the West Indies, and the third is a psychiatrist in Boston. All of their spouses and my grandchildren are a great pleasure to me.

Seeing Child Health Services grow and flourish has been a source of real satisfaction to me. I really try very hard to stick to what I feel is close to the truth, and to say what I feel has to be said. That's a privilege. I know there are some people along the way who think that I have been a troublemaker. Maybe I have been. I do know that for the sake of the program and the people supporting it, I try not to go out on a limb alone and risk the limb being chopped off.

But still, the system can be so rigid. I have a teenaged patient with tattoos who never did anything wrong to anybody. She got a little bit defiant regarding the dress code and piled up a bunch of administrative absences halfway through her junior year in high school and got expelled. She was born to a fifteen-year-old girl who works and who loves her daughter. We have provided her health care since infancy. She is a very bright girl and a talented musician, but she's determined to be herself. She loves hard rock, wants to play the piano professionally, but she needed to be in school badly. I called the principal, and I went down with her mother to see the superintendent but they said, "Look. She just doesn't fit the model." So now she has her GED, works as a stock clerk, and plays the keyboard with a local band as we help her pursue other educational opportunities and keep healthy.

I went to my fifty-fifth high school reunion—the same high school—shortly after this girl's rejection. The high school principal was the featured speaker and was telling my classmates how wonderful the high school is now. They all were listening to him, pleased to hear what he had to say about "our" school. It really angered me because this was the same guy who wouldn't keep our patient in school. These graduates were told just what they wanted to hear, and then they went off to dance.

I think there's a lot of work still to be done.

CHAPTER FOUR

The New Clinicians

Nurse Practitioners and Physician Assistants

Well past the middle of the twentieth century, every state had a medical practice act that granted qualified physicians a license to practice "medicine and surgery," with little in the way of further requirements or definitions. At the same time that these acts ushered physicians onto the terrain of medical practice, they served to keep the rest of the world out. There was, in theory, a clear division between what doctors did and what, say, nurses did, though in practice there was always some amount of overlap, which tended to increase in areas with fewer doctors.

Two phenomena in the 1960s challenged the arbitrariness of the traditional "practice of medicine" statutes and concepts. The first was the development of a broad consensus that the United States was a doctor-poor country and needed to move rapidly to boost the capacity to deliver health services. This conclusion allowed physicians, nurses, educators, and legislators to think more creatively about who might provide medical services. The second development was the emergence of movements for the rights of individuals, particularly the women's rights movement. The intellectual and political environment was conducive to nontraditional thinking and to the birth of ideas and new professions such as the nurse practitioner and the physician assistant. Although these disciplines were technically and educationally new, both, in fact, built on the largely unacknowledged work in advanced care delivery that many nonphysicians had been performing for years.

The first nurse practitioner training program was started quietly in the mid-1960s by the nurse-pediatrician team of Loretta Ford and Henry Silver at the University of Colorado. The focus of this program was pediatric, with a nursing emphasis on health assessment and health promotion, but with training in physical diagnosis and basic interventions for common health problems. The original nurse practitioner role was envisioned as complementary to the physician's and limited to practice in a supervised setting. According to Ford and Silver, the role of the pediatric nurse practitioner was to provide "comprehensive well care to children of all ages, to identify and appraise acute and chronic conditions and to evaluate and temporarily manage emergency situations until needed medical assistance becomes available."[1]

Although some in nursing opposed the nurse practitioner idea as a capitulation to medicine and an abandonment of nursing, the concept caught on quickly, and new programs around the country began to provide training in adult care, family practice, and ob-gyn as well as pediatrics. Congress provided early support—which continues—for nurse practitioner educational programs, starting with the Nurse Training Act of 1971. The Robert Wood Johnson Foundation also funded nurse practitioner training activities throughout the 1970s. In the early years many of the programs awarded certificates rather than formal degrees, but gradually the academic hierarchy of nursing adopted the nurse practitioner idea, and the programs today are almost exclusively at the master's degree level. Nursing programs award degrees to nurse practitioners by area of specialization, such as "F.N.P." for family nurse practitioners. National certifying bodies offer exams to graduates which, when passed, attest to the abilities of the practitioners who may then use the designation "certified," represented as "C" before "F.N.P." Studies have shown repeatedly that nurse practitioners are well accepted by patients and get particularly good marks for communication skills and patient education.[2] The vast majority of the estimated 58,500 working nurse practitioners have remained in primary care.[3]

Nurse practitioners have always had to struggle for independence in their practice. State professional practice acts, with rules that determine the scope of practice and prescriptive authority for nurses, have been the principal battlegrounds for these issues, with nurses pushing for expansion of their authority and some physicians battling to hold the line. Liberalization has proceeded steadily, though irregularly, and some states allow nurse practitioners a greater scope of practice than others.[4] Nurse practitioners have also worked hard to secure direct compensation for their services, negotiating with HMOs and insurance carriers and, where necessary, lobbying for explicit inclusion in any legislation pertinent to provider compensation.

The physician assistant as a new profession emerged at almost the same time as the nurse practitioner. The first documented reference to the physician assistant concept appeared in a 1961 article in *Journal of the American Medical Association* by Charles Hudson, in which he called for "an advanced medical assistant with special training, intermediate between that of the technician and that of the doctor, who could not only handle many technical procedures, but could also take some degree of medical responsibility."[5] In the mid-1960s, Duke University Medical Center in Durham, North Carolina, was experiencing a severe shortage of both physicians and nurses. The chairman of the Department of Medicine, Dr. Eugene Stead, had tried to train and employ clinical nurses for advanced roles on specialty units, but the effort failed because of opposition from the National League for Nursing. In April 1965, Stead proposed a two-year program to train former military corpsmen as "physician's assistants." That fall he enrolled four ex-Navy corpsmen and, with funds borrowed from an NIH grant, he inaugurated the nation's first physician assistant training program.[6]

The idea took root quickly. In September 1966, *Look* magazine ran a spread on the Duke students entitled "More Than a Nurse, Less Than a Doctor" touting the emerging physician assistants as representatives of "a new career that promises better care for the sick." Multiple programs followed the Duke lead, including the Medical Extension (MEDEX) Program run by Dr. Richard Smith at the University of Washington that made heavy use of an apprenticeship model and began placing physician assistants throughout rural areas of the northwestern United States and, later, the Pacific basin. Funding for new physician assistant programs came from the Comprehensive Health Manpower Training Act of 1971 (initiating a stream of federal funding that continues today) as well as a number of private foundations. By the late 1970s, some fifty programs had opened; by the 1990s that number had more than doubled in response to rising demand. All programs are now academically affiliated, and most offer degrees at the bachelor's or master's level. To obtain state licensure, PAs must pass a national certifying exam after which they have the option of using the credential P.A.-C., reflecting their status as certified. Today there are estimated to be almost forty thousand physician assistants in practice.[7]

In name, history, and practice, physician assistants as a discipline are "derived" from physicians and medical practice. Over the years, the profession has been unambiguous in defining its relationship to physicians as dependent. To put it succinctly, physician assistants believe that dependence and performance autonomy are compatible. In this regard, the philosophy of physician assistants is quite different from that of nurse practitioners, for whom conceptual independence has great importance and for whom the notion of subservience to physician authority is objectionable. Nonetheless, the liberalization of the medical practice acts around the country has provided the physician assistant, like the nurse practitioner, with the potential for far more practice autonomy today than in the past. This phenomenon, coupled with their relatively easy working relationships with doctors, has contributed to a drift by physician assistants away from their conceptual roots in primary care. Today physician assistants are found throughout the health care system, with only about 50 percent engaged in primary care.

The future of the physician assistant and the nurse practitioner disciplines is not without uncertainty. Rapidly increasing numbers of schools and graduates over the last ten years have raised questions about practice opportunities in the future. Growing clinical autonomy, due to increased levels of training and reduced legal barriers, has raised the possibility of new categories of independent health care providers—a development welcomed by some and decried by others as further crowding and complicating the world of medical practice. For the past forty years, though, physician assistants and nurse practitioners together have provided enormous new capabilities and flexibility to health care in the United States. This contribution has been particularly important in primary care, where they have frequently been key clinicians in practices and systems. The stories in this chapter testify to that history.

Therese Hidalgo, C.F.N.P., trained and practiced as a nurse before ever hearing of the idea of the nurse practitioner. When she did, however, she caught hold and never looked back. She works in a practice in a large town in rural New Mexico as part of a primary care team. The route she has traveled is representative of many other nurse practitioners and has brought rich new capabilities to the practice of primary care. Carl Toney, P.A., followed a different, but likewise classical path to a similar point. As a veteran Vietnam medic, he returned to the United States to a civilian health care system ill-prepared to make use of his experience and skills. The physician assistant profession was created specifically to put his sort of capabilities to work in health care. Toney enrolled in an early P.A. at Duke and has gone on to be a practitioner, teacher, and pol-icymaker. Holly Gerlaugh, F.N.P./P.A.-C., has borrowed from both tra-ditions. Trained and employed for many years as a nurse practitioner, she eventually took and passed the P.A. certifying exam. She now prac-tices under both banners, suggesting—to the chagrin of some in both professions—that these new and important clinical disciplines share im-portant common ground.

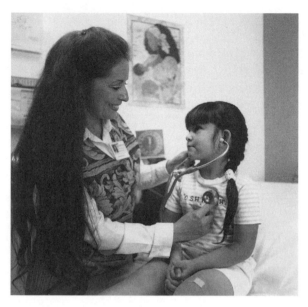

Therese Hidalgo teaching the next generation.

THERESE HIDALGO, C.F.N.P.

PROUD TO BE A NURSE

Belen, New Mexico

Therese Hidalgo will tell you quickly and with pride that she is a New Mexican and a nurse practitioner. Twice a graduate of the University of New Mexico, trained at St. Vincent Hospital in Santa Fe, and now living in the railroad and farming community of Belen, she works at the town's ambulatory care center, which once was its hospital. Hidalgo has been a leader in the successful campaign to expand the scope of practice for nurse practitioners and an enthusiastic proponent of their role in delivering care in rural New Mexico.

Dressed in slacks and a vest, her desk stacked with patient charts, her office walls decorated with children's drawings, Hidalgo is at home in her clinic. When she began practice in Belen in 1991, she was the area's first nurse practitioner and, in her words, she had to "break some ground." Doctors who had known her as a nurse had to adjust to her new role, and patients—many of whom had never heard of a nurse practitioner—had to try her out to form their own opinions. She does believe that doctors and nurses bring different perspectives to patient care, variability she salutes.

⟜⟶

I'M A NURSE PRACTITIONER. I'VE had to break some ground, do some educating, and change some attitudes in both doctors and patients. I trained at New Mexico's premier educational institution—the University of New Mexico—but my practice is in a small town that never had seen a nurse practitioner before. Still and all, I see myself first and foremost as a nurse. I do some of the things that doctors do, but I am and always will be a nurse. I got a letter recently addressed to T. Hidalgo, M.D. The physician I work with saw the letter and said, "Look at that, Therese. Gosh, doesn't that make you feel good?" I said, "Absolutely not." I want people to know that I don't feel I'm bringing something less than a doctor to my profession. I'm happy being a nurse who does some of what physicians do.

A person from Mars could probably tell by dropping in on our practice that doctors and nurses represent two different perspectives and ways to treat a patient. But it's subtle, and it also depends on the individual providing the care. I've seen some physicians who take almost a nursing-type approach to their patients. I remember telling one physician, "Gee, that was just so 'nursey,' the way you intervened with that patient. I'm really impressed." I'd like to shed some of the old stereotypes and visions about our professions.

I began life as a New Mexican, but then detoured to Arizona for my early years before returning to New Mexico. I was born in Las Vegas, New Mexico, in 1955, and grew up in Phoenix. I went to Catholic schools in Arizona through high school, and then moved back to New Mexico to go to college at the University of New Mexico in Albuquerque. I've been here in New Mexico ever since.

My mom worked as a nurse's aide in Phoenix and raised eight children on that income, which was difficult. She was a single parent; my father died when I was in third grade. Later my mother remarried, and we have three half-sisters, so there were eleven children in my family.

My high school in Arizona was mostly white and middle-class. There were very few Hispanics, and I definitely encountered barriers because of my ethnic origin. My original last name was Lopez. When my stepfather adopted me I became Bloyed, but I was clearly Hispanic in appearance. In Arizona, the Hispanic population is treated differently than in New Mexico. I think there's more discrimination in Arizona—and prejudice. Most of the Hispanics had Spanish last names and accents that stereotyped them. I was a good student without an accent, and I didn't even have a Spanish last name—but I was still Hispanic. Some of the barriers were subtle. There was a white nun who knew I wanted to go to college, and she said, "Oh, Therese, I don't know. I think that college wouldn't be right for you. I think you ought to be a secretary." Well, she said that to the wrong person, because that made the hairs on my neck stand up. That was the type of barrier I faced. It didn't stop me, but I know it has affected a lot of other Hispanic women and men.

My mom always wanted to be a nurse, so I thought that by becoming a nurse I could fulfill her dream and mine, too. At first, actually, I thought about going to medical school, but I remember deciding as a sophomore in high school that I wanted to have a family and that combining family and medical school wouldn't work. In those days, in my culture, family came first. So that helped me make the decision about nursing. I had my mom's and my family's support in that decision. I knew when I went to UNM that I wanted to go into nursing, and I graduated with my bachelor's degree in nursing in 1979.

Eventually my mom did start nursing school, but at about sixty-five years of age she switched out of nursing school and went back to college. In 1999 she finally got a bachelor's degree in bilingual education and counseling. There are several other nurses in our family. My brother became a licensed practical nurse and then went on to become a registered nurse. He and I used to have long discussions about L.P.N.s and R.N.s, and I kept urging him to go back for his R.N. When he did, I was very proud of him. I also have a sister who graduated from Arizona State University in nursing and is working on an Indian reservation in Tuba City, Arizona.

I started my nursing career on the floors at St. Vincent Hospital in Santa Fe. Obstetrics was my first love, and gradually I moved toward maternal-child areas, doing several years in labor and delivery followed by a year as the hospital staff educational coordinator. Altogether, I practiced in Santa Fe about seven years.

In 1977 while I was still at UNM, I married Miguel Hidalgo, a fourth-generation New Mexican from Belen. Miguel graduated from the University of New Mexico in architecture and has worked for both the state and in private practice over the years. Currently he is the director of capital projects for the state's Commission on Higher Education. We had the first of our three sons in 1980, while I was working in Santa Fe. Nursing has been very good to me in terms of raising a family because it allows a lot of leeway in choosing shifts. People think working the graveyard and evening shifts can be a real downer on family life but, actually,

I used it to my advantage. When I had a baby, I'd work the night shift three days a week, so I didn't need babysitters. I really felt I was there with my children in their early years. When they got to a certain age, I worked from three in the afternoon to eleven at night. I have primarily worked part-time and been creative with my shifts and the type of jobs I'll do. Although now I am working full-time, I feel very fortunate to have been able to achieve both my personal and career goals.

When I was pregnant with my third son, my husband and I decided to make the move here to Belen, New Mexico, where my husband was born and raised. It's very different from Santa Fe, but it was good for our family goals, including raising the boys in the country. We have a ranch where we all help with breeding Santa Gertrudis cattle. We enter the cattle in state fairs, show them, and travel with them—it's a lot of fun.

In August of 1986, I began to work at the local hospital here in Belen. At first I was fearful about the new job, because I had become very specialized in maternal-child care early on in my career. I had no experience working in a small rural hospital, where an R.N. is responsible for an emergency room. I also had to handle geriatrics and take care of male patients again after primarily caring for women in recent years.

So the transition made me a little bit nervous—but it was probably the best thing that could have happened to me. I was challenged by the diversity of the job and became much broader. Even so, I was quickly driven toward labor and delivery again, and became head of the clinical department for maternal-child areas, including labor and delivery, postpartum, and pediatrics. I became a supervisor as well as a clinician.

Our hospital was one of several satellite rural hospitals owned and operated by Presbyterian Health Services, and it was closely affiliated with the main Presbyterian Hospital in Albuquerque, thirty-five miles to the north. It was a thirty-four-bed hospital with full obstetrical services, including surgery and C-sections. We had a general surgeon here, an ob-gyn, two internists, a pediatrician, and some family practice doctors. We saw some acute care patients, but most emergencies were transported to Albuquerque.

Like many other rural hospitals around the country, however, it was in financial trouble. We served a large Medicaid population at the hospital, and there were reimbursement problems and ongoing financial losses. Finally, Presbyterian decided that, without support from the community, they would be forced to close the hospital. This was tough for the town and tough for me personally.

There was a lot of community discussion and some division, even among those who backed the hospital. To raise funds to support the hospital, an add-on to the sales tax was proposed and put on the ballot. But the community didn't pass the tax; it wasn't even close. After the hospital closed, some physicians attempted to resurrect a coalition to bring another hospital to the area, but the effort was unsuccessful. People were very upset about losing the hospital and the access to twenty-four-hour emergency care. I never heard anyone say they were happy about the hospital being closed. In fact a lot of people were angry with Presbyterian—but not with themselves—about the loss of the hospital. Their attitude was that Presbyterian should have kept the hospital open despite the financial losses. The hospital facility was converted into a clinic after it stopped operating as a hospital in 1990.

The year 1990 was also a year of change for me personally. Since the mid-1980s, as the obstetric nurse director in Belen, I had served on a lot of committees, both in the local hospital and in the larger organization in Albuquerque, which took a lot of time and commitment. By 1989, I wanted to do something for me, so I decided to go back to school for my master's degree in nursing. Even back in the 1970s, when I was getting my R.N. degree, I knew that I eventually wanted to be a nurse practitioner, but the UNM Medical School closed down its nurse practitioner program in 1980. So I had to tuck that dream away for a while, but I never let it die.

When I started looking around in 1989, I learned that the University of New Mexico was thinking of starting up a nurse practitioner program again. Even though they hadn't found grant funding yet, I started telling people I met that I was going to be part of UNM's new nurse practitioner program. I think the school felt sorry for me; in any case I was one of the first seven people chosen for the pilot program. I entered in fall 1989 and finished in 1991.

I had a lot of the same instructors in the UNM graduate program that I'd had as an undergraduate, but there was room for growth, and our group was able to make suggestions that were used to improve the program. There were still no role models in our preceptorships, though. I knew a nurse practitioner in Santa Fe, Barbara Salas Stehling, and asked her to come and talk at some of our educational programs, but I never worked directly with her. She was probably the only role model I had. The physicians I worked with in preceptorships didn't know much about nurse practitioners either, because they hadn't really worked with them.

Despite the lack of a role model or mentor, I did come away from the graduate program with strong ideas about what a nurse practitioner should be. Some of it, a feeling of independence, was just ingrained in our minds, because that was the movement at the time in clinical areas. The work of nurse practitioners was gradually becoming more independent over the years here in New Mexico, with changes in the state Nurse Practice Act. I think all of us evolved in our roles together. The lack of role models is changing now. I try to do a lot of role modeling. I have spoken at Career Day at the high school, participated in a mentoring program here at the clinic, and served as a preceptor for the university.

The role of the nurse practitioner was more limited when I was in school. Prior to changes in the Nurse Practice Act in 1991, nurse practitioners worked only under the supervision of physicians and protocols. But some nurse practitioners were working in very rural areas, with only phone consultation, so physicians weren't really doing direct supervision. And while nurse practitioners have always been able to prescribe, their prescription authority did not include narcotics or scheduled drugs. Revisions to the Nurse Practice Act in 1991 tried to address all the different levels of independence: supervisory, interdependent, and independent. Nurse practitioners still had to maintain a connection with a physician, however, and various affidavits were signed to determine the level of the relationship.

In 1993, the act was amended again and cleaned up to get rid of all the language about differences between independent, interdependent, and doing supervised work. The new language says that we are "independent in primary care, chronic and acute, and will consult as needed." At the same time, we gained the opportunity to apply for a Drug Enforcement Administration [DEA] number to write prescriptions for controlled substances. These changes in the Nurse Practice were supported unanimously by the state legislature in Santa Fe. I tell you, I think the nurses took the state medical society by surprise here in New Mexico. There was a lot of lobbying done on the part of our state Nurse Association. Not all the responses to the changes in the act have been positive, however. The osteopathic society, for example, has some objections on principle and has formally complained that the state legislature didn't give enough opportunity for rebuttal, so the changes slipped past them. I believe the state Medical Society also has made some comments. Pharmacists are also trying to become primary health care providers, and they have raised a lot of flags. The lack of role models is changing now. I have served on the Advanced Practice Committee for the Board of Nursing, and we always worry that although we have made a lot of headway toward independence as a profession, there is always the possibility of legislation aimed to curtail that independence.

As the role of nurse practitioners has evolved, the program at UNM has also been growing. There were seven in our class, the next year about twenty, and this year almost forty. The goal of the program has been to promote rural health care, and much of the funding is linked to that goal. The program accepts people from out of state, and all graduates are encouraged to work in underserved areas. In my class, most of the graduates stayed in New Mexico, or on the border of Colorado and New Mexico, and about half ended up in rural areas such as where I work now in Belen.

After I finished the graduate program, I came back to work in Belen at the clinic in the former hospital, this time as a nurse practitioner. Many of the doctors and some of the nurses were left over from the hospital staff. It was comfortable to know the physicians already, but at the same time I felt a lot of pressure, because they had known me only in my previous role as a nurse. I thought, "Gosh, I'm supposed to know a heck of a lot more now." So I put expectations on myself that I thought they would have for me. Actually, the physicians here have been very nurturing.

I was the first nurse practitioner at the clinic in 1991, and, although we have a number more now, I had to teach the doctors how my role had evolved. It turned out that I was a very welcome addition to the clinic staff, however, because the physicians were trying to handle their scheduled appointments and taking turns doing urgent care. It was very difficult for them, and they weren't happy about it. So I felt needed when I came back. It was hard at first because I was a new graduate, and I did need extra time, but they were willing to make an investment in me for their future benefit. They needed help most with urgent care, so that's where I started, and it really freed them up. I worked Monday through Friday in urgent care for about two years.

Doing just urgent care was challenging and exciting, and I loved coming up with diagnoses and treatments, but I missed having any continuity or follow-up with patients. And although providing urgent care was an ideal setting for learning more, by talking to the doctors and reviewing the charts, I simply didn't have the time for that. I was seeing patients constantly from the minute I arrived until way past the time to leave, and it wasn't fulfilling for me.

I wanted to develop long-term relationships with patients. That's why a lot of us go into health care, for the "Dr. Quinn, Medicine Woman" experience. But working in urgent care was like loving and leaving them. So I proposed to the staff that I move into primary care, and that we could hire the nurse practitioner student who I was precepting to replace me. I had it all planned out, and they agreed. Again, I think it worked because I was trying to teach them what I could do in my role, and I just pushed it, pushed it, pushed it.

It worked, and over time I have developed my own patients, who are pretty much exclusively mine unless they go to urgent care or can't get an appointment. The selection process by which patients and I choose each other is interesting. I've learned to know my own level of skill and experience and to recognize when I'm not the best provider for a certain patient. I can think of some complicated cases, like, the woman with chronic obstructive pulmonary disease, polycythemia, and depression— a lot of health problems. She was fed up with the traditional physician providers that she'd had in the past, and she desperately wanted me to handle her care. Some patients see me as a person they can talk to, who won't talk down to them. But I knew at the time that this case was very, very complicated, so I consulted frequently with a female internist here. When the internist retired and that link disappeared, I felt I needed to direct this patient to another level of care. The process of learning my limitations was just part of the growing process, the learning curve. But it was hard when I first started, because the physicians didn't know quite what a nurse practitioner was, and the public surely didn't. It was different when I did just urgent care, because those patients don't choose who sees them. When patients make an appointment, they're making a selection, so it's clearer.

Then there were the patients who didn't like the idea of having a nurse instead of a doctor, so that was really hard. A lot of older people, especially, felt this way, although they expressed it in many different ways. Some said point blank: "I don't want to see a nurse," while others would say, "Oh, I thought I was seeing my doctor." The first year was probably the roughest, when I still found a lot of people who preferred to be seen by doctors. By the second year the numbers dramatically declined, and after that I hardly ever saw it.

People have a mental picture of a nurse and a physician; they've been socialized into those roles through television and their own past experiences in hospitals, so their whole frame of mind about a nurse is totally different. Once I gave a talk about nursing and the advanced practice role to some high school juniors on Career Day. I did an experiment, going around the room and asking each student to give me a response to the word "nurse." Develop a mental picture, and just tell me the first thing that comes to mind. From their responses, I could see that societal attitudes to nursing hadn't really changed much; they still thought of nurses as handmaidens, assistants. That was disturbing. Nothing I heard indicated that the students saw nurses as independent care providers with their own little bag of tricks.

I've had coworkers say, "Therese, can't we call you something? Isn't there a title we can use instead of your name?" The doctor is called a doctor, and that makes people feel comfortable; people are not used to calling the doctor Rick. We joke around about that, but those comments reflect a real problem in how the public sees advanced practice nurses. I still go by my first name, like most nurse practitioners that I know. A title might make some people feel more secure, but, on the flip side, people feel more comfortable and less distant using first names.

I think physicians often have a different perspective on patients than do members of the nursing profession. When Ford brings out a new model truck, they put it on a revolving table for the cameras. Then they show you pictures from the side, from the front, and from the back, so you can get a feeling for the whole vehicle. Health care providers, in our different domains, also see patients from different perspectives. I can tell you from my early nursing experience, physicians brought more of a disease perspective, while nurses seem to provide the health perspective. Now, because of the changing health care market, we're all trying to work toward disease prevention and health promotion, so those lines are getting more blurred.

I do think primary care physicians are better than specialists and subspecialists at viewing the patient as a complete person, as more than just the disease, the organ, or the organ system. But nurses bring their own skills as educators and communicators to their relationships with patients. The emphasis on education is one of our strongest points. Nurses also definitely bring more of a case-management perspective. I'd like to see everybody really put their money where their mouth was. We all talk about disease prevention and health promotion, but no one is willing to pay for it.

On a personal level, I do a lot of counseling on weight management and diabetes education. This is an arena that's separate and different from the clinical care being provided by physicians. I see patients who, with regular consultations on weight management and nutrition, are able to stop their medicines, with obvious benefit to the patient and to the system as a whole. I think that's a victory. I don't have any hard-core studies to document this, but I can tell you from my practice, I've seen a difference.

The community context is also very important from our perspective. Nurses don't look only at the patient; we want to look at how that patient is affected by or affects the family context, and then at the family within the community. That is part of our perspective.

I'd like to see doctors and nurses take advantage of their different perspectives and look at patients as a team. Some tasks can be done by either, so let's consider cost effectiveness and let the nurse practitioner handle some areas, freeing up physicians for other things. With a health care team, we could improve access. When you sign up for a provider, you should be signing up for a team of providers that shares the responsibility for your care. That's how I'd like to see it evolve, but people need to think in new ways. You don't need a bazooka to shoot a rabbit; a BB gun will work just fine. You don't need that much velocity to get the rabbit, and you don't always need a doctor for primary health care services.

Although many more women doctors are entering the workforce, they are not necessarily more comfortable than men are with the nurse practitioner model. Actually, it has been the male physicians, in my experience, who are more comfortable with the two roles, and it's the male physicians who often show more of the "nursey" qualities at our clinic. I can tell you that many of the female physicians I've worked with have not brought those qualities to their role. In fact, a woman entering medicine and moving through medical education may actually suppress some of the feminine qualities she would normally bring to her role because of the competitiveness of medical school.

Politically, because New Mexico is a rural state, nurse practitioners are very well accepted, although I've been told that not all clinics are as accepting as ours is. One problem in a salaried setting is a certain amount of economic competition. At a meeting in Albuquerque, I heard a family practice physician sounding very resistant to the role of the nurse practitioner in her team, feeling that her income is threatened by the nurse practitioner. It's not the nurse practitioner per se that she's resistant to; it's the fact that physicians are seeing fewer patients because people are seeing the nurse practitioner when they could be seeing her, and her paycheck is based on that.

Nurse practitioners have been in New Mexico a long time, and I don't think they're going to go away, despite competition among different types of health care providers. I think the system will retain a variety of providers: physicians, nurse practitioners, and others. There's even a new physician assistant program at UNM Medical School. There is a lot of controversy over who is more efficient, a P.A. or a nurse practitioner, but I think there is room for all of us.

Here in our practice we provide both primary care and nonappointment urgent care. I see primary care as an ongoing relationship. You begin a relationship by doing a new patient history and physical, and both of you should identify needs to maintain or improve health care of that patient, with ongoing surveillance. Primary care includes health promotion, screening, and episodic care. It's more than just coming in for treatment of a sinus infection or for an annual Pap smear.

Some people here in Belen, including many older people, have a different point of view. Some people show up at a doctor's office and just want medicine. They've been accustomed to thinking that when you've got a cold, you just go in and get a shot. But they don't go in for screenings or for consistent follow-up for a particular problem like hypertension. There's still a large population here that is very episodic, and quick fixes are all they want out of the health care system.

Here at Presbyterian we see an economic cross-section of the community. Honestly speaking, the physicians I work with provide good primary care, meaning more than just episodic care and referrals to specialists. I've actually seen a change in the referral process over the last couple of years, both as a consumer and as a provider. As a consumer, I know when I need to see an ophthalmologist, and I don't want to go to a primary care provider first. I believe a lot of people share that view. But I've also seen physicians roll with the punches. I think at the beginning, when physicians were given the gatekeeper responsibility, they took it very seriously as a way to keep costs down. But in actual practice, the gates are now looser and physician referrals are multiplying because patients have demanded it.

Looking to the future, I don't see primary care being squeezed out by specialists. Consumers don't want to be seen as just a liver, a skeleton, or a heart. They want to be seen as a whole person. And I think that's what primary care and the health care team of physicians and nonphysicians can provide. The hierarchical approach is old stuff. After we have educated consumers about the system, I think they may feel better cared for and not feel this need to reach for the specialist right away.

In the future I'd like to develop educational programs for diabetics and others, in an entrepreneurial sense. I'd like to be able to demonstrate the cost savings and get HMOs to recognize those programs and be willing to pay for them. I also still love doing prenatal care, and there are a number of community-based programs that could be developed in that area as well.

People know what a doctor does, but explaining the distinction between a nurse practitioner and a doctor isn't easy. It's so much easier to say, "I do what a doctor does." But I don't like using a physician as a reference point. My family now basically understands what I do. My husband has been my biggest promoter among his extended family here— about how exciting my job is, and how elevated it is from what they see as a nurse. Some people still see a nurse is a nurse is a nurse. My mother-in-law, God bless her, I think she's just now figuring it out. Attitudes are hard to change. But the family has been very supportive, and they sacrificed a lot when I went to school. So I think they've had just as much commitment to this career as I have.

My boys are really ranch-oriented, and none has shown much interest in medicine or health care. They still have dreams of going into professional sports. My oldest is twenty and a student at UNM. My seventeen-year-old will study architecture or engineering if baseball doesn't work out. My youngest is working his way through high school. I thought that maybe I could get one of the boys to be a veterinarian, but it doesn't look promising. So, it will be interesting to see what they finally decide to do.

Twice recently, I visited Presbyterian Hospital in Albuquerque. The first time was to care for my nephew, who has muscular dystrophy. During my visit, I met hospital's peds intensivist, Dr. Rob Miller, and he told me how pleased he was to meet me finally since he'd been on the receiving end of so many hospital referrals of mine in the past. He really greeted me as a colleague. The other instance was when I traveled to Presbyterian to check on a newborn of one of my special prenatal patients. I walked into the nursery and introduced myself. All of the nurses looked up. "You're Therese Hidalgo?" one of them asked. "All your patients call you Doctor. All this time I thought you *were* a doctor." I reassured them that I tell my patients over and over again that I'm a nurse practitioner. "I'm still a nurse," I explained to them, "and proud of it." One young nurse responded, "Well, you may be a nurse, but being a nurse practitioner is quite an accomplishment!"

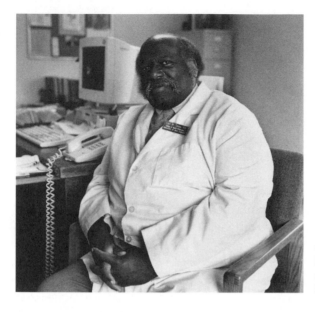

Carl Toney
bringing town
and gown together
in southern Maine.

CARL TONEY, P.A.

BUILDING A NEW PROFESSION

Portland, Maine
When Carl Toney returned from service as an Army medic in Vietnam, where he had patched bodies and saved lives, the only job he could get in health care was as a hospital orderly. The year was 1968. After suffering frustration and a few false starts, Toney discovered a new profession—the physician assistant—whose very reason for being was to put experienced and gifted people like him to work in health care. In 1979, he graduated from the nation's first and most prestigious physician assistant program at Duke University, and he has gone on to be a teacher, practitioner, and leader in the physician assistant movement. In 1993, he moved to Maine to work for the state's Department of Health, and he gained instant—and friendly—notoriety for being the only black in state government. Since 1994, Toney has worked for the University of New England in Biddeford, Maine, providing leadership to the school's Area Health Education program, physician assistant program, and statewide town-gown relations. He is an affable man, with a drooping mustache flecked with gray, and sideburns that conjure an image of earlier years. *The House of God, Disraeli,* and *The National Health Service Corps*

Policy Manual are on his office bookshelf. A plaque stating "It takes a whole village to raise a child" hangs on his wall beside his diploma from Duke and a certificate from the Public Health Service Primary Care Policy Fellowship.

⟵⟶

IN AUGUST 1967 I WENT to Vietnam as a U.S. Army combat medic. There was an urgent need for medics in Vietnam because medics had the third shortest life expectancy in the war, behind officers and radio operators. The enemy's strategy was to identify the officer and kill him to destroy the chain of command. Next, the radio operator was targeted to disrupt communications, and finally the medics were targeted to prevent them from caring for wounded soldiers. The enemy knew that health care was important—a lesson I haven't forgotten.

Two years earlier, just a year after I graduated from high school, my mom had arranged for me to work as an orderly at Columbia Presbyterian Hospital, close to my home in New York City. In 1966, I was drafted by the Army and enrolled in a training program for medics at Fort Riley in Kansas. I thought my training there was superb. The senior noncommissioned officers, who had already served in Korea and Vietnam, really focused on the type of situation in which we would find ourselves. Beyond medical skills, they taught me the importance of pragmatic decision making.

In Vietnam I served with a combat engineering group, a regular infantry unit, as well as a mechanized infantry unit. I served in the field virtually the entire year that I was there, working mostly in the area south of Saigon in the Mekong Delta, which saw a lot of action. I was there during the Tet Offensive, and we did a lot of support work for units in the Mekong Delta and central highlands. While I didn't enjoy the war, I learned a lot of medicine and liked being a medic. I learned how to take control of a chaotic situation. My role at the front line was to provide ongoing primary and preventive care services to allied troops and civilians and in combat situations to stabilize ill or wounded soldiers and arrange for medical evacuation ("Dust-off") via helicopter. I thought that if I had to be there, at least I was doing something life-supporting, rather than life-ending. Those of us who were out in the field saved many lives that otherwise would have been lost, despite high casualties.

About two and a half months into my tour, during an enemy assault at unit base-camp where I was temporarily assigned, I was wounded in the right knee and leg by a rifle grenade. I was pulled from the field for about a week of treatment and convalescence, and then reassigned to my regular unit. The shrapnel wound has left me with some chronic bursitis and osteoarthritis problems. After completing my twelve months in Vietnam, I was reassigned in August of 1968 to Fort Dix, New Jersey, for immediate discharge from active duty. Upon completing my discharge processing, I returned home to New York City.

I was born in 1947 and raised on the Upper West Side of Manhattan in New York City, an area known as Washington Heights. My father, born and raised in Philadelphia, was a high school graduate who had worked for many years as a self-trained and self-employed electronics technician in Philadelphia and Newark, New Jersey. About the time I was born he began work at Columbia Presbyterian Medical Center in New York City and stayed there for twenty-five years as a maintenance supervisor. My mother, also a high school graduate, spent most of her life working as a domestic; my half-sister (twenty-one years older) was a licensed practical nurse; and my half-brother (fifteen years older) was a career criminal. My parents were in their early forties when I was born, and I was raised essentially as an only child.

Our home, on 157th Street between Broadway and Amsterdam, was just a half a mile from Columbia Presbyterian, so the hospital was very much a part of our community. Our local family physician, Dr. Reginald Weir, epitomized what being a physician was all about. He still made house calls in the 1950s, when I was growing up. He was also the kind of physician who included the family in the decision making—in my case my mother, who was basically in charge of our family's health care. So Columbia Presbyterian and Dr. Weir were important factors in my growing up.

I started out in the footsteps of my father, who had been an electronics technician and engineer, by attending Samuel Gompers High School in the Bronx, one of two schools that offered a major in electronics. But the experience in Vietnam changed that course radically. The problem was that when I left the Army in 1968, I wasn't a doctor or a nurse, but I was something more than an orderly. There were no jobs for medics outside the military. I took a few months off and then went back to work at Columbia Presbyterian, essentially in my old job.

With the level of knowledge and experience I brought back from Vietnam, I soon began to feel frustrated as a general medicine orderly at the hospital. So, I left Columbia and went to New York Hospital for a brief stint at the Payne-Whitney Psychiatric Clinic as a psychiatric aide, which is another name for an orderly. I didn't find that job particularly rewarding either, so, in 1969, I went to work as an avionics technician for Pan American Airways at Kennedy Airport. Using the skills I had learned in high school and those I gained in a night school program in which I earned a broadcast engineering license, I did work I loved and work that paid me—by comparison—a small fortune. I was there for a little more than a year before I got caught in a downsizing in December 1970, got laid off, and ended up back in my old job at Columbia Presbyterian. Initially I worked on the general medical service before being asked to join the cardiac intensive care unit [ICU] staff as a technical nursing aide. In that job I got to do more than the usual bedside nursing functions and was able to broaden my technical skills.

While I loved the four years I spent working in the cardiac ICU, I began to realize that this, too, was a professional "dead end." In 1974 I began to rethink my options and considered nursing school, medical school, and something new called a "physician assistant." There were a few P.A. programs around the country at that time, one of which was at Duke University, founded by Eugene Stead, M.D. I had first heard about this program while I was in Vietnam, from an article sent to me by a former head nurse from Columbia Presbyterian. She had been urging me to go to medical school, but sent information to me about this new profession in case I decided not to become a doctor.

In the early seventies, when I was thinking about what to do with my life, after considering and rejecting careers in both nursing and medicine, I remembered the P.A. profession and talked again to my former head nurse. She thought that the P.A. profession had a real future. Through her father, John Loeb, who coauthored the Cecil and Loeb *Textbook of Medicine,* she knew Eugene Stead and the program at Duke. She told me, "You really should become a P.A., and if you want to do it, you need to go to Duke." I decided that the P.A. profession did hold the most promise for me, and I set my sights on Duke.

Having no college credits at the time, I enrolled at City College of New York to obtain the prerequisite courses and credits I would need to be eligible to go to Duke. I was keenly aware I came from a blue-collar background and that I was the first member of my family to go to college. City College was a challenge; I had to work full-time to pay my way, and I studied a lot riding the subway commuting between work and school, but I loved it.

I did two years at City College, as a biology/psychology double major, and then applied for entrance to the Duke P.A. program. When I visited Duke, I remember thinking that it looked like every university I'd ever seen in the movies. It was so beautiful, and I could "feel" it radiating educational energy. I was very impressed by the P.A. program and medical school faculty who interviewed the applicants. Seeing some of the other candidates, I didn't believe I had a chance of getting in, but when I got accepted, I said "yes" without a second thought.

The P.A. program was the hardest two years of my life, without a doubt. I almost didn't make it the first year, which was all didactic. My self-confidence fell so low that I decided to leave when final exams came. Fortunately for me, the faculty did some wonderful crisis intervention and helped me make it to the second year. Because the second year consisted of clinical clerkships, I was back in my element and really blossomed. I went from almost flunking out in the first year to being the outstanding student of the 1979 graduating class. When I graduated I was absolutely convinced that a P.A. was the greatest thing to be, and that a Duke P.A. was the greatest P.A. of all.

There were forty-two students in my class, and more than a third had been emergency medical technicians, paramedics, or military corpsmen—many of the latter with combat experience. These people, along with the pharmacists and nurses in the class, had seen and done a lot. The medical school teaching faculty, from the attendings down to the house staff, had a lot of input in the P.A. program. Duke's philosophy was to teach using an applied model. P.A. students were seen as analogous to second-year medical students because that was when the second-year students did their initial clinical rotations. The program allowed the P.A. students to capitalize on their special skills. An informal collaborative bartering relationship evolved in which the P.A. students offered their technical skills and practical experience in return for in-depth theoretical knowledge from the medical students, along the lines of, "I'll teach you how to start an IV if you'll help me understand acid-base balance a bit better."

Being black, one concern I had about going to Duke was living in the South. Until then, my experience with southern racism had been limited to one brief week in South Carolina. To my surprise, I actually found being in the South a very positive experience. For one thing, people were far more honest in the South than in the North. They let you know their feelings and attitudes, whether they were positive or negative. You didn't have to guess, and, also to my surprise, I found a much greater sense of community, particularly among blacks. Even though I was a stranger with no family, no roots, and no connection to Durham or North Carolina, I felt as if I received a lot of informal support, and that I was a "member of the community"—this was very, very helpful.

In 1979, following my graduation from Duke, I entered a P.A. residency program in emergency medicine at the Maine Medical Center in Portland. This residency program was a pilot project sponsored by the Robert Wood Johnson Foundation. Following a national competition six individuals were chosen for the charter class of residents, including two of us from Duke.

It was now my turn to experience life north of New York, and I loved that too. Maine was absolutely beautiful and the people were extraordinary. It was certainly the quietest place in America I'd ever been. I trained in both urban and rural settings, rotating through six hospitals across the state. Those experiences allowed me to learn a lot about emergency medicine, as well as a lot about the state of Maine, including an interesting social education because there were not very many blacks living in Maine at that time. In fact, it seemed as if I "met" and "treated" most of the blacks during the time I was there. They would hear about this black "doctor," or "P.A.," or "something," who was working in the emergency room, and people would come in for treatment. When I went to a rural area such as Skowhegan, where black people hadn't lived for over a generation, families would come in to introduce their kids to a real black person. Everyone was very welcoming and accommodating wherever I went. Socially it was an extraordinary experience, and educationally it was a superb program.

When the program ended, I planned to stay in Maine and accept a contract I had been offered to staff a small rural emergency room. But at that time my wife, who I had met and married while I was at Duke, decided she wanted to go back to school and become a P.A. She had been a nurse for twelve years and felt she had done everything she could in clinical nursing. She had seen me go through the P.A. program and residency and had decided that being a P.A. would give her the knowledge base and level of patient care responsibility she wanted. She was accepted into the Duke P.A. program, at which time we reluctantly departed Maine and returned to Durham, North Carolina so that she could begin her studies.

Back at Duke, I was invited to join the Department of Community and Family Medicine's faculty at the medical school. I taught in the P.A. program, saw patients, and precepted second-year medical students and first-year family practice residents as a member of the attending staff within the department's Family Medicine Center.

Our chairman, Dr. Harvey Estes, who is a wonderful man and one of my mentors, emphasized education and service, particularly in the area of primary care and family medicine. He assigned the junior faculty members the jobs of teaching, spreading the mission of primary care, and establishing Duke as a deliverer of primary care services. He supported a training philosophy based on the generalist "team model," an idea that was ahead of its time in the early 1980s at tertiary academic health centers such as Duke.

Even those P.A. graduates in the 1970s and 1980s who were increasingly recruited into specialty settings were more aware of primary care issues than typical medical students or residents. Unfortunately the marketplace, including local politics, often made it difficult for P.A.s to find primary care positions in locations of their choice, or at salaries that would allow them to meet their family financial responsibilities. Time and time again I would hear people say that they really wanted to go to a rural area, but either "I can't find a job" or "I've got all this debt, and this cardiology practice is willing to pay me much more; I've got a family to support."

One thing that has been increasingly helpful is support from sources such as the National Health Services Corps. More students are now financing their training and education either through a scholarship program, through federal loan repayment programs, or federal and state partnership repayment programs. These options allow more people to attend and widen their choice of practice. But if the federal government had not stepped in—particularly at the level it did in 1971, when the Nixon administration supported a comprehensive health education bill that covered P.A.s and established family practice and nurse practitioners—I don't think that the P.A. profession would be where it is today. Some programs, such as Duke, were fortunate and quickly developed a significant amount of institutional funding that allowed them to wean themselves from federal support. Other programs, because of a lack of local resources, have had to maintain a close association with the federal government, a relationship that has been essential to the growth of the P.A. profession, but often at the price of financial and operational vulnerability.

My wife graduated from Duke in 1982 and decided she wanted to focus on women's health care. In early 1983 she moved to Atlanta to join the medical staff of Grady Hospital, the only public hospital among the city's forty-six hospitals, as the first P.A. assigned to their gyn emergency clinic. I continued teaching at Duke till the end of the calendar year, at which time I then moved to Atlanta to join her. Shortly after my arrival in Atlanta I joined the faculty of Emory University in the Department of Community and Family Medicine working with their P.A. program on two federal grant projects—one developing a preventive medicine curriculum and text, and the other on minority recruitment.

In June 1986 I decided that I'd had enough of academia after six and a half years and was ready to move back to full-time clinical practice. I was looking for a community-based primary care position. Some of my colleagues at Emory introduced me to Dr. Roy Wiggis, a general internist practicing at Piedmont Hospital, an Atlanta community hospital and a teaching site for Emory. Dr. Wiggins had just turned sixty and had been practicing in Atlanta for about thirty years. He was white; I'm black. He was from the South; I'm from the North. He was a capitalist and a conservative; I'm a socialist-leaning liberal. But our respective past professional experiences at Columbia in New York and Duke in North Carolina brought us together despite our differences. Dr. Wiggins went to medical school at Emory, did his internship and residency at Duke with Dr. Stead, and fellowship at Columbia. He noted during my interview the fact that we both had survived training under Dr. Stead, which said a lot about both of us; and if I was willing to put up with his capitalist, conservative ways, he would try to put up with my "radical socialist agenda."

We had a very, very large practice which combined general internal medicine, occupational health, and geriatrics. Dr. Wiggins had three offices to cover, although he was basically a solo practitioner. When our practice was at its height, we were caring for five hundred geriatric patients spread out in five nursing homes across the breadth of Atlanta. We also had patients in the hospital, admitted through the general practice. So it was challenging and exhausting.

Our arrangement worked pretty well for four years. I enjoyed the patient contact, which is why I took up medicine in the first place. Nonetheless, over time I began to realize that I was feeling unfulfilled. I found that, although I recognized that it was important and relevant, reading medical journals bored me. On the other hand, it was intriguing to read a copy of the *American Journal of Public Health* or similar journals that covered health care and policy issues, because they approached things from a very different perspective. After all these years, I realized that it was the issues related to health care that so enthralled me, more than medicine, per se. So I went back to school on a part-time basis, enrolling at Georgia State University to finish working on my bachelor's degree. I majored in political science with a minor in philosophy to prepare for a career in health policy and planning, and in 1990 I received my A.B. degree.

In early 1991, after leaving Dr. Wiggins's practice, I joined the Georgia Department of Human Resources' Primary Health Care Section, as a "health manpower specialist." In this capacity I was the state's liaison with the federal Bureau of Primary Health Care and the National Health Service Corps—two very important national programs assisting Georgia communities to deliver health care to poor populations. Georgia, a predominantly rural state composed of 159 counties, had a very large community and migrant health center system in place. Shortly after I joined the staff, the idea for the formal establishment of a state Office of Rural Health surfaced amid debate about how to staff it and where to locate it within state government. Fortunately, after a lot of negotiation, the governor decided to transform my office from the Primary Care Section into the state Office of Rural Health. Almost overnight our role expanded dramatically, and I got the opportunity to help take a leadership role in doing community-level primary care systems development statewide.

We made many decisions about the placement and use of primary care clinicians. We also inherited the J-1 Visa Physician Placement Program from the federal government at that time. This program sought to match foreign medical graduates with communities in need of a doctor. The foreign graduates who were completing residencies in this country with a visa obligation to return to their home countries would be given a waiver to remain in the United States in return for practicing medicine in needy communities. Until 1991, the program was administered at the federal level, but federal agencies decided they were being overwhelmed, and it made more sense to hand over the operational level to the states.

At the outset, we had to work hard to convince communities to consider the program, even desperate communities that were having trouble recruiting and retaining physicians. Finding foreign physicians did not prove difficult; in fact, I was inundated with unsolicited phone calls, faxes, and CVs from people around the country trying to find positions. The problem often turned out to be in keeping these doctors in the communities in which they'd agreed to work. The program's structure allowed people to obtain their visa waiver, abandon the program, and remain in the United States with impunity. Unfortunately, the federal agencies did not offer the states any support in pursuing sanctions to prevent this kind of visa abuse. Word that the federal government wouldn't enforce the sanctions traveled quickly through a sophisticated underground network. As a result, communities that had gotten their hopes up and rallied around the program were just devastated. Those of us working at the state level were very angry that participating communities were left medically no better and emotionally worse off than they had been before.

In 1993, I was selected for a U.S. Public Health Service Primary Care Policy Fellowship—a wonderful program that gave me a Washington-based short course in federal health policy and convinced me that I was ready to move on. My plan had always been to return to Maine, so my wife and I decided the time had come to make the move.

In the fall of 1993, following my completion of the fellowship, I returned to Maine and assumed the directorship of the state Bureau of Health's HIV/STD Prevention Program. My principal challenge was to create a greater awareness among policymakers and the general public about a set of diseases, which, though present in the state, were not viewed as significant public health/public policy issues. It was really difficult to convince communities, both people at risk and policymakers, that they desperately needed to deal with these issues. My job was to make that case.

To promote the HIV prevention program I met with infected individuals, AIDS service organizations, other community groups, community leaders, local physicians, and other service delivery folks. I would explain public health and the HIV issue and then listen to them. People were shocked because they very rarely saw anybody from state government, much less someone representing public health. They knew of an 800 number to call for information, but they were literally amazed to have somebody actually come to them and say, "I want to hear what you think about this situation." I adopted that approach out of a sense of survival and because it really fit with my preference for face-to-face communication. Bit by bit people began to understand the nature of the problem and the availability of the program in Maine. With a good staff of ten people that I inherited, the program began to weave together crucial public-private partnerships.

I had a terrific time in that job for two reasons, both of which make me laugh because, while they seem to be liabilities, they actually proved to be assets. The first was the fact that, to the best of my knowledge, I was the only black in the entire state government at that time. There *had* been one before me. Even though I did not have a "high-profile" position, everybody knew who I was. But being black did not prove to be a problem at all. In fact, when I met people, they had more trouble with the fact that I could have lived in Maine before and left than with any racially related issues. The other asset was my belief that you have to go where the issue is located. That had a tremendously positive impact on the success of the program.

My mentor from Duke, Dr. Estes, always told me that when you take a new position, the first thing to do is look around for your replacement and get that person geared up. I identified a person who I felt would probably do a better long-term job than I would. And so I thought, "This is not a bad time. Everybody's excited. Leave while they're still engaged."

In 1994, I left state government and joined the staff at the University of New England's College of Osteopathic Medicine, located in Biddeford, Maine, to become the associate director of Maine's statewide Area Health Education Center [AHEC] program. The AHEC is an exciting program that supports community-based clinical training for practicing clinicians and health profession students. It sends the students into the community where the action is and is very much in line with the work I'd done in Georgia previously. In June 1996, the university initiated a physician assistant program, and from then until January 2000 I served as its first director. We admitted twenty-seven students that first year, two-thirds from Maine and New Hampshire. It received full program accreditation in 1998, and we graduated 100 percent of our first class. In January 2000, I started a new job as coordinator of community projects for the University's College of Health Professions. I'm now based in Portland, Maine. The university is growing, the programs are growing, and I have the ultimate town-gown job, which is just right for me. Additionally, I am pursuing a master's degree in theological studies at the Bangor Theological Seminary.

As a society we continue to face daunting challenges in providing health care to all those who reside within our borders. In poor and rural states such as Maine this problem is particularly evident. Managed care, which seemed to hold such promise for Maine a few years ago, has failed to connect with the rural, elderly, or poor who represent our most vulnerable residents. I believe there needs to be serious consideration given to the future use of nonphysician providers such as physician assistants in meeting these problems. It is fair to say that the "experiment" of creating such a model of health provider has been a success. The lack of a cohesive public policy plan regarding how to integrate these providers into the health care team model, coupled with the dramatic and unbridled growth in the number of training programs (i.e., 1990–99 saw 100 percent increase in the number of P.A. programs nationally), however, creates a scenario of health professionals (physicians versus nonphysicians) competing for practice opportunities rather than collaborating on patient care issues. This is a real problem.

I believe that health policymakers are going to have to develop a rational and integrated approach to the distribution of health care personnel and resources. But, at the same time, health professionals, such as physician assistants, are going to have to challenge themselves to do better at defining our role, documenting our overall professional contributions, and justifying our existence in a competitive marketplace.

As a physician assistant, a health planner, a teacher, and a student I hope to help find the answers or, at the very least, to keep raising the questions.

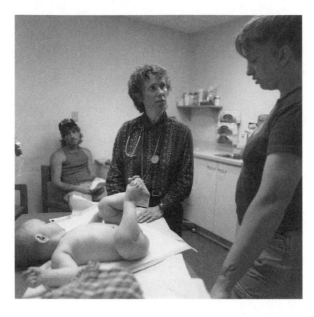

Holly Gerlaugh
working with a family.

HOLLY GERLAUGH, F.N.P., P.A.-C.

A ONE-WOMAN MERGER

Augusta, Maine
Since 1981, Holly Gerlaugh has taken care of patients and taught residents and medical students at the Maine-Dartmouth Family Practice Program in Augusta, Maine. She is a slim woman with bright blue eyes, a comforting smile, and a stethoscope perpetually draped around her neck. The Unitarian church, the Quaker meeting house, Albert Schweitzer, and motherhood have all been important influences on her. Her years as a practitioner and a teacher have been interspersed with work in Nicaragua and Jamaica and recent involvement in a statewide organization providing mediation services to families and groups.

Gerlaugh's professional credentials are unique. She is both a nurse practitioner and a physician assistant. Trained originally as a nurse practitioner, she worked for four years in Rochester, New York, at a community health center before moving to Maine to join the Maine-Dartmouth program. In 1985, worries about the future of independent practice for nonphysician clinicians as well as concern about infighting in the leadership of nursing led her to take and pass a challenge exam for certification as a physician assistant. Since that time she has been able to practice under both flags, giving her an unusual angle on primary care practice and politics. "I guess I'm something of a one-woman merger between professions," she observes.

I READ ABOUT ALBERT SCHWEITZER when I was in elementary school. He became my hero. I wanted to go to a third-world country and be a doctor. But I was a long way from the third world. I spent the first eight years of my life in Ohio, outside Cincinnati. Then we moved to Florida, where my father was an engineer with the Apollo project.

There was a real sense of humanism in my family. Both my parents were very active in the Unitarian church. It was the church that encouraged me to see the importance of being the best possible human being I could and caring about people in my community. That message got transmitted through my parents and through the church. I got interested in the medicinal aspect of it through the readings that I did about medical missionaries, about the caring that they did for people who normally would not get those kinds of services. I did a fair amount of volunteer work in elementary through high school, working with kids. There was a Head Start program at a school right behind our house where I did volunteer work. I also worked with the Girl Scouts and did some tutoring.

I went to Cornell and majored in biology, thinking I would be a doctor. In high school and college, I worked on and off as an aide in nursing homes, and got a lot more experience in what the medical field was about. I worked in a large nursing home outside Syracuse for a couple of summers and then in some smaller private ones that were less well maintained and managed. I spent some time as an aide in an ob-gyn clinic for poor people. Then, in my junior year, I decided that it would be helpful to see a family doctor at work because that's what I wanted to be. I had become a Quaker when I was in college. One of the Quaker men was a family practitioner in Dryden, New York. I spent time with him in the summer of 1974 to see if this was what I wanted. He had a very rural practice, with his whole family involved in it. His wife had done the nursing care and the billing. They saw patients in the downstairs of their home. Through that experience I realized that I needed to rethink how much I was willing to devote to my job and my profession, versus the rest of my life—my religious life, spiritual development, community work, sports, and family life.

It seemed harder at that point for a woman. It was one thing for a man

to ask his wife and his kids to be all a part of his profession; it's something else for a woman to say to a man, you know, "Help me out with
being a practitioner. Cover the family and cover everything while I'm out
here doing this." So I thought about making a change at that point. I still
applied to medical schools that last year, but I started looking around for
some other options. And that's when I found out about the Pace University nurse practitioner program—a program that would take people
who had a bachelor's in science, train them as nurse practitioners, and
graduate them in two years with a master's degree in nursing.

I had found what I wanted. I applied, got in, and started right away.
The university was based in Pleasantville, New York, but we worked with
New York Medical College and did our clinical work in New York City.
There were about twenty of us, almost all women. We ranged all over
the place in age and background. The group had no nurses, but we had
people with degrees in literature as well as people like myself with a science background. Most of us really didn't quite know what a nurse practitioner was and, frankly, neither did most of the people who were teaching us, because there hadn't been a lot of nurse practitioners trained. This
was 1975, and we were the second class at Pace.

It definitely was a nursing environment and very different from the
academic atmosphere that I'd been used to. It was a real shock for me
to go from Cornell, where you were expected to be the best and the bright-
est and to excel as an individual, to a place where there was still a sense
of hierarchy, of the doctor being the doctor and that nurses would still
get up and give a chair to the doctor. In the training, as well as in the
programs where we were working, we were in a system where the nurses
were to do the doctor's beckoning, period. Very few of our teachers were
nurse practitioners. They were very well educated, and had training and
experience in different areas, but this whole new role was something that
they were still trying to figure out. We were being asked to think inde-
pendently, to start to be in the role of managing medical care, and yet
the faculty was often teaching a model of hierarchy and memorization.
In the clinical area they were teaching us to obey the doctor and not question the doctor's judgment. Some of us were inclined to say, "Wait a
minute, we're independent thinkers here. We could be colleagues in this.
We could help each other. We have things to offer, too."

The program faculty taught that diagnosis was either "nursing" or
"medical." If the N.P. stayed within "nursing diagnosis," then she was
within the realm of her nursing license. If the N.P. performed a "medical diagnosis," the N.P.'s work required medical supervision or over-

sight. I'm not sure of either the clinical or the political rationale behind this distinction, but I have always found it confusing and unrealistic. So, to arrive at a diagnosis and treatment plan, we were asked, on the one hand, to use decision-making skills with all the complexity inherent in a differential diagnosis but, on the other hand, to work by protocol dictated by our supervising physician. Once we worked in the real world, especially in primary care, those earlier protocols weren't relevant. Also, even if a supervising physician wanted to develop the volumes of protocols necessary to cover all the potential diagnoses in the N.P.'s everyday work, protocols take the art, the finesse, and the intuition out of medicine and leave a dry, potentially poor substitute.

The program emphasized primary care and did a great job with it. There was a lot of emphasis on family dynamics, preventative care, patient education, counseling, as well as the medical side of the differential diagnosis. When I finished, I wanted to go to work in a health center. I knew that eventually I wanted to work in a rural area, but initially I needed to have on-the-job training because the internship that the program had provided was only three months long. I knew that I needed to spend the next couple of years learning more, so I wanted to be in a place where I could get a fair amount of feedback.

I was hired by the Anthony L. Jordan Health Center, a large clinical facility in Rochester, New York. The center had other nurse practitioners who'd been there for a while, and a good system of providing care that included social workers and outreach workers as well as N.P.s and M.D.s. They didn't have a slot for a family nurse practitioner, so I went to work in internal medicine. The center, itself, was built in the late sixties smack in the middle of the inner city in a housing project area. The population was very mixed—heavily black but also Puerto Rican and some Southeast Asians. In addition to health care, the center was intended to provide job opportunities for people in that area, because there weren't a lot of jobs there. They hired community people and put them to work as lab techs, medical assistants, and outreach workers. The entire patient population was divided among teams comprised of a physician, a nurse practitioner, and an outreach worker. We shared a social worker. It was an incredible facility, amazing. It had pediatrics, ob-gyn. It had a psychiatric center. It had dental, laboratory, pharmacy. Everything was right there. The center had funds to train people very quickly, get everybody with high school educations into training for their clinical work, lab tech, or whatever. They trained a number of people to become nurses from the community.

Since there were already nurse practitioners at the center, there were role models for me. The first year was difficult, though. There was a lot to learn. I worked by protocol—very much like a cookbook. I worked mainly with one physician, who was very, very helpful. It was a year of internship training, basically. At first the physician and I worked together, in that he would refer me cases that were routine. I'd see the call-ins and refer the tougher cases to him. Over time—I was there for three and a half years—I developed my own practice, using him as a consultant for out-of-control cases or diagnostic problems. Patients were very accepting of me and, with rare exceptions, seemed content to see whichever of us they had gotten to know.

It was very satisfying work. People in poorer neighborhoods are pretty sick and usually don't have a lot of access to someone to take them through a system—a system that can be pretty difficult. I think nurse practitioners are particularly good at helping people through the system, helping them make connections when they need to, to fit into other parts of the system when they need to. I got a lot of satisfaction out of seeing people make changes, get healthier, get care that I thought was pretty good care from the health center. We did home visits, too.

I enjoyed living in Rochester, and I succeeded in not being married to my profession. I was very active in the community at that time, and was editor of a small paper called the *Empty Closet*. It was the main paper for the Rochester group of both gay men and women. My partner at that time was also a nurse practitioner who was very involved in local politics. We set up a number of different programs trying to mediate complaints and problems between the gay community and the police. We were also active in setting up a chorus, singing groups, and organized a "Take Back the Night" campaign, promoting awareness of the problems women face on the streets. And we worked with prostitutes, a politically active group called Coyote. There were a number of gay prostitutes, both men and women, that had special problems that nobody had been paying attention to. I was also active in the Quaker Meeting in Rochester.

After a few years, 1979 or 1980, the funding at the center began to get tighter and the administration began subtly to push us to see more patients. They started printing out how many patients we saw each month, and I felt the pressure to see more. The center became much more of a mill. I felt that patient care was beginning to suffer when you asked that people be seen quickly, and there was less time to do home visits and deal with social issues that were causing the medical conditions in the first place. I was also having a hard time with the physician I was working with. He was a pleasant fellow, very nice with patients, and he had been helpful to me. But I was, I think, sprouting my own wings and beginning not to work by protocol. I was making more of my own decisions, beginning to have more of my own opinions about patients and illnesses. I needed to work with somebody who I felt would be willing to listen to an opinion I had. And so they offered that I change physicians, which I did for a year—which was a big help.

But I still wanted to leave. I loved Rochester. It has some wonderful communities, but I really am a more rural person. So I was looking for a rural job. My concern, though, was that I saw people practicing rural medicine and getting out of touch and out of date. I wanted someplace that was rural, but would still allow me to stay up to date. A friend from Pace was working in Augusta, Maine, as an N.P. in a family practice center which was the home of the Maine-Dartmouth Family Practice residency program. She called me to say they had a job opening—and I jumped at it. That was February of 1981. I've been here ever since.

At that time, the Family Medicine Institute was in an old nurses' dormitory on the grounds of the Augusta General Hospital. We were *very* crowded. The dorm rooms were converted into exam rooms, except for one that served as an office for six or seven residents and myself. It was noisy, but it was what people called funky. We were divided into two teams for seeing patients. Each team had a supervising family doc, a nurse practitioner, and a group of residents. My job was to work with the second-year residents the most. A second-year resident was in charge of managing and covering the outpatient practice, and covering our patients in the hospital next door. I would back up the residents when they weren't available, in addition to having my own practice. Every month there would be a different resident who I'd work with. It was a complicated relationship, because I was in a teaching role and a colleague role as well as a nurse role. It required a lot of flexibility on my part. I had to be able to adapt to all the different personalities and problems and quirks that the resident brought, a resident being under the most stress that they're ever going to be—and people respond differently to that stress.

Sometimes it was difficult, and other times it was pure pleasure. The residents, in general, were a very dedicated group of people who, particularly in the early eighties, were very idealistic about wanting to be family docs, out there, rural, on the front lines. They wanted to be GPs in the old tradition. We called them "the granola group," the people who were the idealists about family practice, and really were putting that first.

Those of us who have been around the program a long time look back on that as "the good old days." It seems different now, although we can't tell whether the students are changing or whether we're changing. Sometimes we think it's because we're getting older that we're seeing things differently, and other times we wonder if the groups that are coming through are different. There seemed to be a real change somewhere in the late eighties, where it seemed as if there was a much more of the "me" generation, people more interested in their own lives as primary and the profession as secondary. Maybe this was better to have a more balanced life of work, family, and pleasure. But it got harder to ask people to put out that extra effort, that before was sort of an expectation, harder to ask residents to come in more, to stay up longer, to squeeze an extra patient in here and there. There was more anger involved when they were asked to do some extra work.

The decade of the eighties was a rough one, with a lot of changes in medicine. More and more people coming out of medical school were interested in going into research and specializing. There was a concern that we weren't going to get enough applicants. We were wondering if family practice was going by the wayside as more and more specialists were being trained. And then, suddenly, all hell broke loose, good hell. The payment schedule changed so that a surgeon gets paid the same amount as a family doc does when they do the same procedure. Well, that was just totally revolutionary to me. Everybody started talking about primary care. Within a matter of two years, we swung in the opposite direction and were deluged, by comparison, with applicants. This trend continued for a number of years. The numbers, however, have started to decline again in the last two years.

There were also legal changes that affected my practice over that same time. There was a lot of battling between the state medical society and the nurses and P.A.s about independent practice for "mid-level providers" and, particularly, chart signing rules. In the end, the sign-off requirements were relaxed, making practice for rural N.P.s and P.A.s easier but, for me, the changes meant that I had to have either a third-year resident or a faculty member sign my charts. As that happened, I stopped working as closely with the second-year residents, which was too bad because they didn't really get to see what an N.P. could do. I became more of an adviser for them and less of a colleague. And, in truth, as I became more experienced and realized that the residents had so little experience, it was hard for me to go to them for advice or refer patients to them for consults. I was tending to go more and more to my supervising physician.

Part of it was the law, and, I suppose, part of it was that I was continuing to grow and learn clinically.

The other big change for me came in 1984 when I decided to take the P.A. certification exam. It was the last year that you could be "grandfathered in" as a P.A. without having gone through a P.A. training program. There were some stirrings at the time about the possibility that Medicare was going to reimburse the P.A.s but not nurse practitioners. I thought that this was a bunch of baloney since we are often in the same jobs. I took the exam and I passed in the 99th percentile. So I felt like, "There. I've done it. I'm certified. If anybody questions whether they're going to reimburse me at one level, I can be either."

There was another reason that getting certified as a P.A. appealed to me. I like the approach of the nurse practitioner in terms of the emphasis on the person, the patient education, and the counseling, and the primary care aspect. But I was not happy with nursing in general. Nurses at the national level were doing a lot of infighting. At the national level, there seemed to be a lot of emphasis on what "our role" was. People were always talking about the "role" of the nurse practitioner. We couldn't make a "medical diagnosis," we had to make it a "nursing diagnosis." As far as I'm concerned, that's rhetoric. The difference doesn't exist. I felt like we needed to take the bull by the horns and say what we are doing. We really are practicing medicine here.

You take nurses, a nurse in the emergency room. You start at a level of somebody who's basically only doing the bidding of the ordering physicians, an L.P.N. or two-year trained nurse. Then there is a person at the bachelor or master's level who can make their own judgments about a lot of situations. They anticipate what's going to be needed. They begin to make more of their own decisions. They can start to do more procedures. As a person's knowledge and experience develops, it seems silly to say that they can't do something because it's "practicing medicine." Certainly they can learn all kinds of skills that have traditionally been medicine's domain. We need to get rid of all the confusion about who can practice medicine. Let's really talk about what we're doing. Are we competent or not?

In the seventies and eighties I thought that the nursing approach to developing the nurse practitioner role was wrong. I think that instead of trying to make it a separate role from physicians and medicine, we should be collaborating and working in a way that emphasizes the strengths we have so that we can work well with physicians. We should be developing a collaborative approach, not saying that we're somehow totally different. At the state level, we were being represented and regulated by a Board of Nursing that really had no idea what nurse practitioners were, of what we really did. The P.A.s were much better politically organized. They knew what they were doing, and they went out and protected P.A.s from whatever, making sure that they were reimbursed properly, and that they had good working relationships with the physicians. In Maine, the P.A.s have gotten their message through very clearly and have been politically successful. Nurse practitioners got a late start in organizing politically. In 1991, about fifteen of us gathered in a restaurant in Augusta to discuss what we needed to do to increase the visibility and political presence of nurse practitioners. Compensation issues, particularly acceptance in the world of insurance, were of foremost importance to us. We drafted a legislative proposal and went to work on its behalf. The Maine Advanced Practice Law (Public Law 396) was eventually passed and signed by Governor King on June 30, 1995, requiring insurance companies to reimburse nurse practitioners for services provided within our scope of practice. The law also required HMOs to accept nurse practitioners as primary care providers.

The HMO influx into Maine has really made a change in providing care to families. When HMOs first came to Maine in the early 1990s, they were anxious to sign on primary care providers and were relatively accepting of nurse practitioners and physician assistants. But when national HMOs arrived in Maine, they wouldn't even consider signing us on as primary care providers. I couldn't believe that after more than twenty years of taking care of families our practice might be limited to walk-in care. The situation became increasingly confusing to patients and a bureaucratic nightmare for us. Legislation was the only answer, and we have it now, which has made our positions as nurse practitioners much stronger and clearer.

Over time I hope that the N.P. and P.A. professions will merge, much as osteopathic physicians and M.D.s have come together. They might still have some differences in terms of training and training programs, but they will function as variations on a theme. The residency program realizes that osteopaths often have a stronger training in primary care and specialty training in osteopathic treatment; the medical community has accepted them. The same thing can happen with N.P.s and P.A.s, that there are some differences in background but that basically we're talking about the same animal. I think that eventually it will happen.

I guess I've been something of a one-woman merger between professions. I am lucky to have found such a good spot here professionally and personally. We have a wonderful group of physicians, a good practice, and a stable faculty. We're growing more, but we haven't had much turnover. Augusta is a great place to live. I have enjoyed being here because it's easier for me to be a part of a community in a rural area. And I have started a family: a husband and a five-year-old daughter. I love being a mom. It's just been delightful. We live on a farm out of town. Maine is a wonderful place to live and raise a kid. I've enjoyed it over the past twenty years.

I'm still very active in politics. Through the Quaker Meeting, I joined the Council of Churches and its legislative group that watches all the legislation that comes before the state. We review the legislation from the point of view of the churches and what their interests are. This is basically for the people who have no voice—the poor, mentally ill, mentally retarded, children, and the elderly. And there's a very active gay community here in Maine. Rural active is very different, I found, than city active but still, very active. And we've had a number of gay people come through the residency program who have stayed on as physicians to become a very strong part of the community here. It has been really a nice thing to see how a fairly conservative community can deal with all that.

In 1988, I took a year off and went to Nicaragua. I went down there to do my third-world medicine, something I always wanted to do. I saw what socialized medicine in Nicaragua was like; saw how it works and how it doesn't work. Nothing works when you have no money, that's one thing I learned. But it was a very good experience for me to see what was happening and what could be made to work almost on a shoestring. You know, you talk about running health care with a bake sale, that's about what was going on. It also taught me that in order to make a change in any community, you have to stay. You can't go somewhere for two weeks, two months, or two years; you have to be in it and be a part of the process and be willing to help make a community change. And they told me that, too. Their message to me was, "Go back to your own community. You've got a lot of work to do back there. Make the changes there because that's where it needs to happen in order to help us down here." It was a year of a lot of growth for me, personally and professionally.

In 1997, I joined a local group working to provide free mediation to individuals in the community. We have now expanded to include a statewide network of groups that provide mediation services. We work in a number of areas, including landlord-tenant disagreements, human rights violations, and family and neighborhood altercations. We focus particularly on the elderly and people with disabilities, mental illness, or mental retardation.

When I look back at my younger days, my time in college, I wonder sometimes if I would have made a different career decision if I had been exposed to more role models of women in family practice, to all of the variation that people can do. Women have come into family practice and can develop a practice that is child-friendly and family-friendly. Here at the residency, we keep hoping that we are modeling different styles of practice and different kinds of residency opportunity. The faculty here is intent on demonstrating a style of practice that's healthy for the individual. Job sharing, leaves of absence, maternity leave, and paternity leave are all part of what we have done.

If I had that kind of vision back when I was in college, I think I might have continued on to medical school. Medicine really wasn't so accommodating then. But I don't regret it at all. I've actually ended up in the same place I think I would have ended up anyway. I love family practice, and I am thankful to the many people who have helped me arrive here.

CHAPTER FIVE

The System Doctors

Managed Care and Primary Care

When the idea of primary care first became topical in the 1960s and 1970s, managed care as it exists today was not part of the American health scene. The first health maintenance organizations began as pre-paid group health schemes in the 1930s and 1940s, cooperative health arrangements that were marginal in impact and generally considered subversive and off-limits by mainstream medicine. It was the Nixon administration in the early 1970s that first promoted health maintenance organizations, based on the persuasive rationale of Dr. Paul Ellwood, the Minnesota physician who coined the term HMO. The incentive structure in American medicine was wrong, Ellwood argued. Doctors should be paid to keep people well, and medical care should be organized to maintain patients' health. Although legislation was passed in 1973 that provided federal support for planning and starting HMOs, the organizations of the time were not-for-profit, heavily regulated, and generally eschewed by the medical community.

HMOs gained more prominence in the 1980s with the rapid growth of proprietary health care, which began with hospitals but quickly spread to all aspects of medical care. HMOs were natural candidates for commercial interests aiming to bring business practices to the medical care field and anxious to harvest profits from a sector judged to be disorganized and poorly managed. The rapid inflation in the cost of medical care in the late 1980s and early 1990s gave momentum to the idea that systematized, prospective management of patient care would constrain costs and benefit both individuals and populations. The business community that footed a large share of the costs of health insurance came to believe this argument, and in consequence investment capital, patients, and physicians began to flow rapidly into the managed care plans. The failure of President Clinton's health care reform effort in 1994 (a plan that itself was based on a version of managed care called "managed competition") redoubled the determination of the payer community to support managed care, and doctors and patients had little choice but to follow along.

By the late 1990s managed care—in its many, constantly evolving, and increasingly for-profit versions—had become a predominant force in American health care, with more than half the population enrolled in some form of it. Many physicians and some patient advocates judged this to be a sell-out of American medicine to crass business interests that were wringing profits out of patient care in favor of stockholders and lavishly paid executives. To others, the ascent of HMOs represented a victory for rationality in health services because managed care emphasized prevention, ambulatory medicine, coordination of care, and the efficient use of resources. Its systematic approach to patient populations contrasted with the more haphazard style of private practice. To some managed care was a lady; to others it was a tiger.

The HMO movement had always relied on primary care because the capabilities of generalist practitioners coincide with many of the values and strategies of managed care. Most managed care plans are built around primary care providers who serve as the principal givers of care as well as the arbiters of specialty referrals. In the 1990s many managed care plans went further and assigned primary care providers the job of "gatekeeping," mandating that they handle all clinical events and approve any referrals. In some systems, clinicians' incomes were tied to the number of referrals, lab tests, and hospitalizations they authorized, making the primary care physician the bearer of risk and a potential adversary of the sick patient. For a time these roles increased the power, prestige, and need for generalists, raising concerns among some specialists and the specialist-dominated medical education establishment of the country about an emergent new order. But as a backlash set in against managed care in the late 1990s, the primary care physician and the idea of primary care came under fire as well. Some patients bridled at being required to maintain close contact with their primary care provider in order to obtain any health services. Although primary care remains central to most health plans, many have relaxed their primary care requirement or are offering (more costly) arrangements that drop the primary care requirement altogether.[1]

While the rise of managed care has given primary care new currency as a clinical force, generalist physicians have also emerged as leaders, administrators, and owners of managed care enterprises. Their generalist skills have often served them well in managing health service organizations. The many accomplishments of medical generalists in the examination room and in the boardroom, however, have not immunized them from the ongoing controversies that surround managed care, as the stories in this chapter attest.

Sam Ho, M.D., has been an early, constant, and articulate advocate of the managed care "revolution." He speaks with enthusiasm for the ability of managed care to recraft the system from one dominated by inefficiency and unfairness to a highly organized, participatory undertaking. His enthusiasm is not universal, however; some physicians, including some who have played leadership roles in developing HMO systems, are critical. An early convert to managed care and a teacher of its principles, Sallyann Bowman, M.D., has had what can only be described as a rough go. The battles between managed care behemoths in Philadelphia have wounded her and given her reason to question the implementation—if not the premises—of urban managed care. Gwen Halaas, M.D., works in Minneapolis, often considered the cradle of managed care. An early proponent, teacher, and administrator of managed care systems, she is now an opponent of for-profit HMOs and a frustrated observer of the backlash against managed care. All of these stories suggest an intimate but unsettled relationship between managed care and the generalist physician.

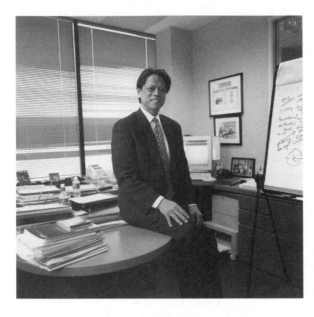

Sam Ho, charting
the future at the head-
quarters of PacifiCare
Health Systems in
Santa Ana, California.

SAM HO, M.D.

IDEALIST, INNOVATOR, ENTREPRENEUR

Los Angeles, California
Sam Ho, M.D., calls himself a practitioner of public health—private sector, market-driven, equal-opportunity, for-profit public health. Ho is vice president and corporate medical director of PacifiCare Health Systems based in Santa Ana, California. In his early fifties, he is the corporate medical director of a company that employs tens of thousands of physicians under contract to provide health care to 4.5 million people in eleven states and Guam. His domain is not the traditional public-health realm of STD tracking and restaurant checks but rather what he calls "population medicine"—outcomes management, quality measurement, physician report cards, and the company's "clinical data warehouse."

What the HMO movement has done is to privatize public health," Ho states with enthusiasm. "Managed care brings discipline to our country's generally disorganized health care system that makes health promotion and disease prevention priorities in clinical care and requires the real management of the public's health care resources. That's practicing public health."

Raised in a Chinese American family in Hawaii, the son of a general

practitioner, Ho believes his professional values are rooted in the student activism of the 1960s. "Distributive justice," "equity in medical
care," and "community health," phrases he uses frequently today, were
concepts prominent in his early career as a family medicine resident, as
a National Health Service Corps physician, and as the San Francisco
county health officer. His current conversation is also laced with such
terms as "metrics," "outcomes," "return on investment," and "entre-
preneurship." Ho believes without apology that the for-profit business
ethic is the most powerful and promising force available for the reformation and equitable management of the nation's health care system.
The "good old days" were not so good, he points out. Medical practice
was enormously variable, inefficient, and unfairly distributed. HMOs,
he argues, are improving quality and efficiency and laying the groundwork for a system that can finance the care of the entire population.

Ho estimates that he is on the road over half the time, managing and
troubleshooting, staying in touch by voice mail, e-mail, cell phone, and
pager. In Washington and elsewhere, he represents PacifiCare to industry, professional, and political groups. Despite his schedule and the tough-
ening times in the managed care industry, Ho describes his eighty-hour
workweek with ebullience and a sense of excitement suggestive of a man
half his age.

When the history of medicine in the twentieth century is written, the
arrival of managed care will surely hold a prominent place. How will
history judge managed care? Will it be viewed as overdue reform—the
emergence of new and more rational principles for the management of
health services—or will it be seen as a destructive aberration that dragged
medicine into the venal world of capitalism, debasing its Hippocratic tradition? However the story is written, it will be a complicated one. Dr.
Sam Ho—idealist, innovator, entrepreneur—will be part of that story.

WALKING WITH SOME COLLEGE FRIENDS on the North side of Chicago
on a rainy night in 1970, I came across blood on the sidewalk. Lots of
blood. A trail of blood in the pouring rain. The blood led up a stairway
into a tenement and, halfway up the stairs, to a guy with a huge gash on
the back of his head. My friends wanted to keep going, but I couldn't
leave. The man was drunk and told me to get lost: "Don't bother me.
Nobody wants to help a drunk." I walked him to his room anyway,
cleaned off his wound, and called an ambulance. Later that night I caught
up with my friends, who thought I was nuts. But I remember thinking

for the first time that this is how I could make an impact in life, that I needed to be a physician. I needed to go into medicine so that I could change society and provide services to those who couldn't afford them. This was a radical change in my thinking. The last science class I had taken was in my junior year of high school, and I had gotten a D. This was going to mean a different kind of life for me.

I was born twenty years earlier in Honolulu. My father was a third-generation Chinese American in Honolulu, and my mom was first-generation from China. We were very much a mainstream Chinese American family. My father, in retrospect, served as a role model for me. He was a modest man who worked as a general practitioner with a blue-collar practice in Honolulu's Chinatown. Many of his patients were impoverished people—Chinese, Filipinos, Samoans, and ethnic Hawaiians. He had a solo practice with two examination rooms, a ceiling fan, and rattan furniture. I spent a lot of time in his office, particularly on Sundays after church. I saw his patients as they came out, saying, "Thank you." He was very supportive of whatever their issues were. He was on call seven days a week, all hours of the night, and rarely, if ever, took vacations.

My father and mother met on a blind date in New England during World War II. They fell in love, married, and moved back to Honolulu. They were planning to go to China, where my father could practice medicine, but because of the revolution they stayed in Honolulu and started his practice there.

Some of my mom's family remained in China because they were patriots. My uncle, an engineer, stayed in Shanghai. Unfortunately, he was a victim of the repression in the fifties, and he died incarcerated. Another uncle, a physician and a medical school dean, was victimized during the Cultural Revolution but survived and is now retired.

My father and his practice were really important influences on me. Of course, I never would have admitted it at the time. I was a rebellious child of the sixties, and Dad was very strict. For many years the only thing I could talk to him about was baseball. We didn't have many points of similarity, politically or culturally.

I have two older sisters and a twin brother whom I had identified as being "Goody Two-shoes." At an early age I was determined to be different. I got involved with nuclear disarmament when I was in the eighth grade. I followed the Civil Rights Movement, the Selma and Washington, D.C., marches in 1963 and 1964. I was active against the Vietnam War from the mid-60s. In 1968 I left Hawaii for Chicago to go to Northwestern University. Being in Chicago in 1968 was a life-changing experience for many people, not just me—the Democratic Convention of that year, the urgency to change the status quo and to make an impact, to make the world a better place. I spent some time in student politics, but what got me really excited were inner-city activities: helping to start free health clinics in the Uptown and Chinatown neighborhoods, tutoring minority children, and helping the Black Panthers serve hot breakfasts to grade-schoolers.

I entered Northwestern as a sociology major, thinking I wanted to be a teacher. But after deciding to be a physician that rainy night, I had to go back and take premed courses, summer school, the whole thing. In some ways I had a big advantage over other premed and, later, medical school students, because I knew exactly what I wanted to do and why. I'm sure such motivation helped me earn Phi Beta Kappa honors.

I went to medical school at Tufts because it turned out to be the best arrangement for both me and my future wife, who was entering graduate school at the same time. Although academic medicine in Boston was relatively hostile toward primary care, not to mention family practice, Tufts allowed me to customize an elective curriculum based on all the disciplines of family medicine in both my third and fourth years. I designed my own rotations in outpatient orthopedics, outpatient ophthalmology, obstetrics, minor surgery, and so on. In the Boston academic medical community of the 1970s, students were actively discouraged from going into primary care, especially family practice, if they had any semblance of professional potential. This professional intimidation only further reaffirmed my commitment to family medicine because it convinced me that specialists were being mass-produced by the Boston medical "factories," which were not focused on the needs of the urban poor.

I was accepted in the family medicine residency at San Francisco General Hospital, and we moved to the Bay Area in the summer of 1976. I was happy to be training at a county hospital, finally doing what I had set out to do. During my residency, I helped develop an application for a National Health Service Corps site in a health manpower shortage area in a San Francisco neighborhood called Visitation Valley, an enclave of fifteen thousand Asians, Italians, and blacks with no physicians. We were formally designated a shortage area in 1980. When I had finished my residency, I volunteered for the National Health Service Corps and, with a partner, Dr. Toussaint Streat, opened the San Francisco Family Health Programs in Visitation Valley.

I loved the practice. We did real Marcus Welby medicine—obstetrics, house calls, hospice care. We truly delivered comprehensive health care "from womb to tomb." Beyond providing care for two thousand patients, I was also committed to teaching. Since we were on staff at St. Luke's Hospital, we worked with them to develop a community hospital component of the San Francisco General Hospital family practice residency.

At the same time, I was actively involved in introducing one of the first HMO contracts to St. Luke's—an activity that was to have a big impact on my future. It was a Medicaid contract through a not-for-profit health maintenance organization called Rockridge Health Plan. Since 50 percent of my practice was MediCal [Medicaid] anyway, I felt prepaid health care through an HMO was logical, since it would provide expanded benefits for patients and also help me expand my patient base. I was excited about the new opportunities where we would be accountable for the health of an entire population, well or ill, including preventive services. Prepayment really supported public health goals. In fact, I thought then that an HMO merely reflected the privatization of public health.

We affiliated with four other family docs, making up a panel of six in several parts of the city. The hospital administration was neutral about the HMO contract, but all of the medical staff were absolutely against it. They saw it as stealing their patients and as some kind of conspiracy between the HMO and the medical school. They labeled me a pariah because I was bringing in an HMO contract that would potentially undermine their finances and a residency program that agitated typical town-gown issues.

In the years following 1983, I got increasingly involved in the HMO side of the practice. Rockridge was acquired by HealthAmerica, and HealthAmerica was subsequently acquired by Maxicare. The health management systems we had developed at Visitation Valley were good systems, providing preventive services, health fairs, and the use of nurse practitioners. Support from the National Health Service Corps helped a lot. I thought we should be able to export these systems. In my practice I was making an impact on two thousand people; through the HMO, I could indirectly impact twenty thousand people. What I sacrificed in direct patient interaction and satisfaction was offset by the reward of effective policy and program development which impacted more lives.

By 1986, I felt that I couldn't keep doing everything with any degree of effectiveness. I was practicing family medicine, teaching on the clinical faculty, and administering the practice, including its HMO contract. So I gave up teaching and practice and became the medical director of Maxicare. I felt then that HMOs were absolutely the future, because they were accountable for costs, addressed health from a population perspective, and integrated clinical and financial systems. The best way to institute change in this country is through the private sector, whether not-for-profit or for-profit, using the power of the marketplace, thereby innovating and creating new programs to meet ever-expanding needs.

I didn't have any formal training in public health, but, armed with practice data, I began to see trends—for instance, in the care for high-risk moms whom we could get into special prenatal care as early as possible. I also began to look at variability in medical practice. For example, in 1987 we developed a management grid that examined the referral patterns of different doctors. Some physicians made four or five times as many referrals as their colleagues working with the same patient population. This didn't tell us which rate was right, but suggested that we needed to develop some kind of standardization, some kind of benchmark, so that we could have more consistent expectations of utilization and quality.

I enjoyed my work for Maxicare, but in 1988 I got a call from Dr. Dave Werdegar. Dave had been the chair of the family and community medicine department at UCSF during my residency, and later dean of the medical school, but when he called he was the health director of San Francisco city and county. In his own professorial way he asked, "Do you happen to know anybody, Sam, who's interested in and capable of organizing a primary care network? We're taking care of 100,000 people, but the care is really fragmented. We need somebody who can help organize our clinical activities into a primary care network." It was a setup. I told him I wanted the job.

I was hired as the health department's medical director and eventually as the county health officer. The challenge was to convert a smorgasbord of disconnected delivery, administrative, and funding systems into an integrated primary care network. Instead of receiving care from one primary care provider, patients and families often had to travel to different clinics in different neighborhoods to receive services at different times on different days. I applied the systems development approach that I'd learned in the private sector. We created common systems for staff development, quality assurance, utilization, medical records, and billing. We started to provide coordinated primary care to patients and began collecting money—from nothing to $8 million in a year! By serving as an agent for such dramatic changes, I wasn't always popular. At one point most of the twenty-five people reporting to me, as well as all of the physicians in the clinics, were in rebellion. But keeping focused and building a team made the difference. We needed to build a delivery system that could provide comprehensive care to vulnerable populations in the most efficient manner. We needed to develop a system that would be ready for a managed care risk contracting agreement scheduled by the state of California in 1992.

By 1991 I'd worked in public health, academia, private practice, and managed care. I had become firmly convinced that change was going to have to come from the system level—not the individual level. Managed care dealt in population-based health improvement, promulgating the virtues of wellness and accountability among all stakeholders. The for-profit companies had commitments to capital markets and shareholders that were forcing them to innovate in order to succeed. It seemed to me— and still does—that the American entrepreneurial system offered real hope to reform the medical system.

HealthNet, a large California-based managed care company, had been trying to recruit me for several years. HealthNet was a relatively new venture that had been converted to a for-profit company in February 1991. It had the for-profit entrepreneurial drive for innovation, but its board still had a not-for-profit attitude. In the summer of 1991, when it was clear that the objectives I had set for myself at the health department were going to succeed, I accepted HealthNet's offer.

My initial job was as Northern California medical director. The delivery system was basically irrational. There was no clear focus on preventive care; incentives hadn't been aligned to reward improved outcomes; doctors weren't given the measurement or the data tools needed to practice better medicine. I went to work building clinical systems for the plan. A year later I accepted HealthNet's invitation to move to the main office in Southern California to reorganize statewide medical operations. As health plan medical director, I created programs in diabetes, preventive services, report cards, and physician compensation. Within another year I was promoted to senior vice president for health services in charge of contracting, provider services, and medical affairs.

Then HealthNet merged with a Colorado-based HMO, QualMed. Many of the programs I had worked to develop were quickly undermined by the merger. Improving health status outcomes and physician partnership efforts became secondary to building shareholder value by driving down costs. In contrast, I personally feel that "shareholder value" can be best maximized by paying attention to customer needs, providing excellent service, and continuously improving quality. I also believe in the importance of a positive relationship with physicians.

In July 1994, I decided to leave and, fortuitously, the next month got an unsolicited call from PacifiCare, HealthNet's second-largest competitor in California, offering me a similar job. The values and culture of the company were much more aligned with my values, so I jumped at the chance. PacifiCare's model is also a network-model HMO, contracting with medical groups, which in turn contract with physicians. PacifiCare puts a premium on collaborating with physicians. Not everybody in the leadership of PacifiCare understands the concepts of clinical epidemiology, population-based health outcomes, small-area variation, provider profiling, and benchmarking. But they do understand the necessity of providing physicians with the skills, information, and tools to help them to practice better medicine.

PacifiCare currently has 4.5 million members, including 1 million Medicare HMO members, making it the largest Medicare HMO in the country. Initially I was involved in developing programs to improve physician performance and health outcomes. In 1997, I was promoted to vice president for quality initiatives and, in March 1998, to corporate medical director. I am now accountable for the strategic development of our national clinical quality initiatives, our clinical information store, national provider profiles, policy and legislative initiatives, NCQA accreditation, and medical liaison for national employer account sales. Although I average an eighty-hour, six-day week, I love my work. I believe in building an organization dedicated to improving the health and service outcomes. The way we improve outcomes is by working with physicians and members to give them the information, the metrics, and the incentives to continually improve quality.

Working in managed care means confronting controversy on a daily basis. Critics of managed care don't remember that the so-called good old days of medicine weren't so good. Old-style fee-for-service medicine produced unaffordable cost increases, less and less access to health care due to lack of affordable health insurance, and highly variable quality. Managed care has been a market response to the long-standing problem of virtually unlimited demand for services with a finite supply of resources.

For example, instead of the double-digit annual medical cost inflation of the late 1980s, managed care has helped hold medical cost inflation under 5 percent for the past several years. That amounts to a cumulative savings of over $600 billion, which has helped strengthen the general economy and the financial position of workers, employers, and investors.

Managed care has succeeded by establishing standardized performance measures and by actually improving health quality. One good example is mammography screening, which has increased from a national average of roughly 12 percent ten years ago to over 70 percent today, which means more women are having breast cancer detected earlier, when it's potentially curable. This has been a direct result of benefit coverage, minimum co-payments, patient education, physician education, and health plan accountability.

Despite its successes, managed care has been controversial for multiple reasons. The fundamental contradiction in American medicine resides in the tension between autonomy for doctors and patients to make unrestricted choices versus quality control systems which continually improve clinical, service, and cost outcomes. We in managed care haven't yet been successful in communicating and balancing these polarities. So, when infinite demand is confronted with the reality of finite resources, people become upset and "shoot the messenger" without heeding the message. The media and legislators have generally played a reactionary role regarding anecdotes. Rather than focus on population-wide statistics, individual anecdotes have been given widespread publicity and credence. For example, if PacifiCare's membership were 99 percent satisfied with its services, thirty-five thousand people would still be unsatisfied, and the press could easily find complaints among that pool of members. Second, physicians, specialists in particular, have fueled the managed care backlash because managed care has forced them to be more accountable for their performance. Many specialists have seen their incomes decrease over the past few years. This is a long-overdue marketplace correction of the gross oversupply of specialists in this country.

Corporate salaries have been another flash point for HMO criticism, and I can understand that. But this is an industry and a highly competitive one, and it needs top talent. If an executive brings shareholder value to a corporation measured in billions of dollars, then executive compensation in the few million dollar range is competitive with other industries, and a relative pittance, compared with what the executive has earned for the shareholder. It's a concept of compensating leadership based on adding market value.

Medical education of the future needs to emphasize primary care. Primary care is better positioned than it ever has been to serve as the cost-effective, quality-oriented center of medical practice. But primary care today is not even close to what it will be, given the information revolution. Right now, the technology exists for an individual primary care physician to use a wireless, palm-top, electronic medical record that feeds into a server connected to a multidimensional database—a warehouse of information—which can help provide physicians with sophisticated real-time decision support. Armed with this device, the primary care physician will be able to provide pinpoint clinical care and tailor diagnostic evaluations, treatment plans, educational information, and anticipatory guidance to the patient. Patients, too, will be linked with customized health records, including evidence-based guidelines, flow charts, and information provided through "push" technology. Information technology will take primary care to a whole different level where the generalist really becomes an orchestra conductor for a huge symphony instead of a three- or five-piece band.

I've always been driven by a vision and a passion that has translated into long hours on the job. I've been fortunate to be able to engage in work that has been exhilarating, and I suppose I have a compulsive personality. My first wife and I were married for twenty years and remain close friends. She too has been long devoted to improving policy—in the area of educational reform. Our son is twenty-four and a law student at the University of California, Berkeley, intent on public-interest law. Our daughter is twenty, a junior in college, and majoring in communication studies.

My dad passed away 1991, after a long period of debility, but my mother is vigorously active in Honolulu. She had breast cancer and a mastectomy a few years ago and, two months later, went to New England for a high school reunion. She's a wonderful, wonderful role model with a deep and sincere joie de vivre.

I love what I'm doing and, for the foreseeable future, plan to keep doing it. HMOs have the most sophisticated understanding of the customer and marketplace, and therefore serve as a conduit from the market to physicians. So, in effect, managed care is an expression of consumerism in health care. Since consumerism has prevailed over the entire economy, we've seen more accountability and better performance in airline travel, banking services, restaurants and hotels, automobile manufacturing and service, retail stores, and software, to name a few. The same has begun to occur in medicine, in spite of widespread backlash. Performance measurements, evidence-based medicine, clinical epidemiology, information technology, and the Internet are tools which are as important as the stethoscope, scalpel, and anesthesia. Engaged and informed consumers and publicly accountable physicians will be able to achieve the most significant changes ever seen. Unparalleled health outcomes will result from consumerism, which is why I am enthused about being an innovator in an HMO that in turn is a pioneer in an exciting industry.

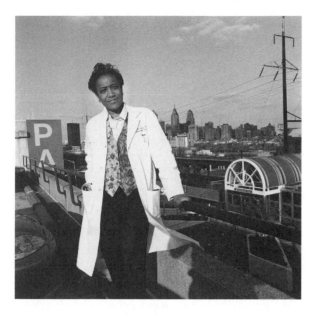

Sallyann Bowman and the city of Philadelphia.

SALLYANN BOWMAN, M.D.

A PHILADELPHIA STORY

Philadelphia, Pennsylvania
Sallyann Bowman's family has no doctors in it. Her father worked as a shipfitter, and her mother took care of research animals at the Philadelphia General Hospital, providing the youngster with her first encounter with the world of hospitals and medicine. She grew up in a neighborhood in transition from white to black, was educated at parochial schools, and had an intense teenage affair with the French horn. A series of prescient nuns and teachers pushed her toward science and medicine, a strong-arming that Dr. Bowman applauds today.

Dr. Bowman, in her early fifties, is a neat, athletic woman with tinted glasses. She is a general internist who has spent much of her career on the staff of Hahnemann Medical School, teaching primary care internal medicine to students and residents. Since the early 1990s, in several different settings, she has been involved in the practice, teaching, and administration of managed care, an approach to the delivery of medical care of which she, unlike many of her colleagues, has been supportive. "Scared, confused, and undertrained" is the way she characterizes the interaction of many physicians with managed care. The system, nonethe-

less, has not been kind to Dr. Bowman. Rapid changes in the finances
and alignment of medical institutions in Philadelphia left her briefly without a job in the prime of her medical life. That experience has frustrated
but not embittered her. "There will always be a need for compassionate,
caring, well-trained physicians who enjoy helping. There will always be
rewards in the personal relationships of mutual trust that develop over
time between patients and doctors." Dr. Bowman is a fascinating blend—
part clinician and part preacher, part businessperson and part survivor.

I DON'T LIKE TO SAY it, but I believe that the future of medicine in this
country will be quite bleak without a rational system for health care delivery and financing. The future of medicine lies in the community rather
than in a physician-led, hospital-centered delivery system. If we look
carefully, the shift has already begun. Doctors will certainly have a key
role to play in the systems of the future, but the traditional role of the
physician will change. Physicians will be sharing patient management
with others like nurse practitioners, physician assistants, and case managers. Physicians will have to adapt to the changes in communication
and information management as never before. Are we really ready to
manage via the Internet and e-mail? Some of us are still trying to acquire
skills in telephone triage! Physicians are very likely to be the agents for
micro-allocation of ever scarcer resources—a role that none of us is comfortable with.

Generalists are better prepared to make these changes than specialists.
My view is, though, that as we strive to train generalists for this future
we should be striving for a different set of skills than we have in the past.
Adjustment to change, dealing with uncertainty, applying continuous
quality improvement in patient management, responding to and giving
feedback, leadership and team-building, collecting and responding to data
are all critical skills for the generalist of the future.

I say all of this despite the fact that I have been beaten up by the system in recent years. Beaten up. I have worked in managed care settings;
I have taught managed care. Eventually for-profit managed care squeezed
the places I worked enough that I got spit out and left without a job. But
I still don't see managed care as the culprit. The real problem in this country is that we've never had a system to allocate medical resources that
worked. That vacuum has allowed the entrepreneurs and the profit takers to capture health care. There's no justification in my mind for anybody making $500,000 practicing medicine or, worse, running a health

plan. That's robbery. Managed care is going to go through its own evolution, but I still think the principles of allocation implicit in managed
care make sense and, like it or not, will be part of health care in America for the foreseeable future. There will be preauthorization and formularies and second-opinion programs. What we've got to get rid of is
the opportunists and the insurance company CEOs pulling down mil-
lion-dollar salaries and bonuses.

Despite these concerns about the future, there's nothing I enjoy more
than the practice of medicine. There still isn't anything I'd rather do with
my clothes on than make a good diagnosis. I love it. I love all aspects of
it. I've enjoyed every minute of being a general internist. I love being able
to dabble in a little of this and a little of that, read a good cardiogram
better than the cardiologist, or suggest a diagnosis and actually see it
through. Over the years I have found that inpatient practice is less and
less satisfying in large doses, in part because people are so sick. They are
desperately ill, in so many ways—physically, spiritually, economically.
By the time anybody lands in the hospital, they're desperate. And it's very
taxing and demanding. The way I do it, I don't hold back when I'm there,
and, I guess, also being a woman, people want to talk to you, so I end
up spending an awful lot of time listening to people and letting them express their concerns or tell me their stories, or try to answer their questions. I enjoy that, but it's taxing physically.

I had no idea about any of this when I was growing up. No idea! I
was born here in inner-city Philadelphia. My father was a shipfitter; my
mother was a homemaker. Dad had an eleventh-grade education, Mom
tenth-grade. I remember my childhood as a happy childhood. Growing
up in Philadelphia, you grew up on a block, so that there were ten, twenty
kids on the block. My closest friends were the neighbors from down the
street, across the street. It was almost like another community at the
other end of the block. I remember summers being long, amazing, and
lots of fun, filled with stuff to do. I was one of those kids that liked
school. I went to parochial school. It was a big deal in those days for a
black kid to go to parochial school. The neighborhood was primarily
Irish and Italian, and the Catholic church was built by the Irish settlers
in the area. There were only two or three of us who were African American at the time.

On my side of Lehigh Avenue, it was predominantly black. On the
other side, it was predominantly white. Most of the black kids in the
neighborhood went to the public schools. I was one of the few kids that
went to the Catholic school. So that was the way it started in 1955, but

that was not the way it ended up when I finished there in 1964. The neighborhood changed overnight—overnight the entire area was 90 percent black. White people moved out so fast, it made your head spin.

I remember in first grade the first time a girl called me black. I remember feeling stunned, and I got into a fight with her over it. So I went home and I told my mother, "This girl called me black." And she said, "Well, you are black." I said, "What do you mean, I'm black?" She said, "Well, you are. You're black and you're beautiful. If she calls you a nigger, then you slap the shit out of her, but otherwise, you are black."

My mom's family worked in and around hospitals, in various capacities. My grandmother worked at the University of Pennsylvania in the medical school. She had a job that doesn't exist anymore. She would help set up experiments for the med students, and she would cater lunches and things like that. She was a general, all-around kind of "gofer" lady in the Penn med school, but she loved the job, so I heard her stories about working at "The University," which is how we referred to it. You almost genuflect when you say it. My mom worked for a time at Philadelphia General Hospital as an animal caretaker. Since the animals need to be fed on the weekends, somebody needs to do that, so that was the job my mother had. I would go with her on Saturdays and Sundays to feed the animals. I can still remember the smell of the hallways of Philadelphia General Hospital. So I kind of always thought that I would end up somewhere in and around a hospital. I certainly didn't have an ambition to go to medical school. I just knew it would be something in science.

I was in parochial school all through grade school and then went to John W. Hallahan High School for Girls, the regional Catholic high school. It drew from all over Philadelphia. So there was a real mix of kids, again predominantly white. I loved the school. I loved it because I was a musician. I played French horn. I was introduced to the orchestra in the summer before my freshman year. I had never touched a French horn, but I heard a record, and I said, "What is that? It sounds really neat." "That's a French horn." I said, "Okay. Well, I'll play that." Little did I know I was picking the hardest instrument to play. The nuns were amazing with us. They took kids who had never touched an instrument, and had you doing ensemble work at the end of the year. The orchestra was the center of my life in high school. We were up at 6:30 and into school by quarter after seven, so that we could get an hour's worth of practice in before homeroom started. Then every afternoon we had orchestra practice or instrumental practice of one sort or another. I didn't have a social life in high school. I really didn't. It was school. It was the orchestra. I remember we played at the Academy of Music, so we're all sitting in our gowns and our headdresses, and our instruments poised in our lap, as the curtain goes up in the Academy, and you see 2,200 people sitting there, waiting to hear you play. It's wonderful. It was wonderful.

But the French horn wasn't my future. You can't play the French horn part-time and be successful at it. And you can't sit around playing it by yourself. I was going to go to pharmacy school. I had applied to Philadelphia College of Pharmacy and Science, and I got in. I even had a little money. But there was an Irish builder in Philadelphia at the time named McCloskey who felt that it was important for him to support minority kids in their goals and aspirations for college, and so he had set up a scholarship fund for kids going to Catholic colleges in the area. I was sitting in my history class one day, and the nun said, "Sallyann, you should write an essay for this scholarship." And I said, "But I'm going to Philadelphia College of Pharmacy and Science, and I don't want to go to one of the Catholic schools." But I wrote the essay anyway and won a four-year tuition and book scholarship at Chestnut Hill College. So I went off to Chestnut Hill, not having a clue what I was going to do.

Chestnut Hill is a women's college with about 120 in the entering class. I loved it. Absolutely loved it. Rolling campus, there's a creek that goes through. These old buildings; it's really a pretty, pretty campus. It was just what I needed. It was small. It was close enough to home that I didn't have to worry about getting to and from home, but it felt like it was away from home. I majored in chemistry, but I had no intention of going into medicine. Late in my junior year Sister Eleanor Marie—the credit is really due her—came through chem lab one day and said, "Sallyann. There's a conference at Women's Medical this weekend. I signed you up."

I said, "But Sister, I really don't want to go to medical school." "Well, you're going anyway." So I went and I got enthusiastic about it. There was a room full of girls, and there were about five or six female physicians who were really excited and enthusiastic about being doctors. They had families, they had lives, they had other interests. They weren't hard and crusty and "guyless," like you imagine lady doctors, you know, giving up everything for medicine. And that was the first time that I ever thought about it as a real possibility.

Although I didn't know it at the time, I think the other key factor was that my mother got breast cancer in 1969 when I was in my sophomore year at Chestnut Hill. Mother had a mastectomy, and three months after she got out of the hospital for the mastectomy, she had a heart attack and was in the hospital for eight weeks. During that time, my sister lived with me on campus, and the nuns never charged us a dime for room and board, in order to get me through, so I didn't have to drop out to take care of family stuff. That's how good to me they were. I remember taking care of my mom after she had the radical masectomy, followed by cobalt radiation. The burns of cobalt radiation were awesome. I was the only one to help her take care of her burns and wounds. Just touching her and helping—I'm sure that had something to do with my decision to pursue medicine.

I applied and got in to the new medical school at Penn State. We were the sixth class. But actually, it was the right decision for me, because the class size was small. The education was, I think, outstanding. Totally underrated. They really kicked our butts, but I think we got a lot out of it. The students were recruited with a push on family medicine. We had early patient contact in the first weeks of med school. I got assigned to a family my first week there, and had a preceptor my first week, and was in his office within the first month. It sort of kept you aware of why you were there, kept you in touch with why you're putting up with all the crap. So I loved it. I loved it at Hershey.

I know exactly the minute I chose internal medicine. I was on a neurology rotation and there was a gentleman there who was quadriplegic. He had a fracture of a cervical vertebra. Everybody else was going off about the neurologic lesion, and how the neurologic lesion did this and that, and what he couldn't do. And I wanted to know *why* he fell. It turned out, nobody had asked the question. He fell because he had a TIA [transient ischemic attack], a drop attack. Well, once I knew why he fell and what I needed to do about it, I could get excited about his neurologic lesion. That's what internists do—look at the big picture. That is when I decided on internal medicine. Never thought twice about it. But I knew I wanted to come back to the city. It was hard to be anonymous as an African American in Hershey at that time. I mean, just going to the grocery store, people would say, "Oh, you must be from the medical school." You go to the movies, "Oh, you're from the medical center?" During medical school, I did two rotations at Martin Luther King Hospital in Watts in Los Angeles. It was wonderful. It was the first time that the only thing that distinguished me from others was how well I did what I did, and not because I was different because of the color of my skin, which is usually how you stand out. It was the first time I had worked among predominantly minority physicians. I was flabbergasted for the first couple weeks I was there. So I knew that after medical school I wanted to come back to Philly and I wanted to blend in.

I did come back to Philly—to the Albert Einstein Medical Center Northern Division as an intern in internal medicine. They put you through the internship, I believe, so the rest of your life pales in comparison in terms of the stress and sleep deprivation. It was okay. I got through it. The teachers were the specialists. Our perspective in those days was totally that of the hospital. We saw the community physicians as the dreaded "LMDs" [local medical doctors] who would drop in and interfere with what you and your teaching attending were trying to do. So I didn't have much of a relationship with community doctors at the hospital. And the expectation was that you do a specialty fellowship of some sort after the basic residency. I did a rheumatology rotation, liked it, and started a rheumatology fellowship. But I soon became frustrated functioning as a specialist, frustrated at not being able to treat uncontrolled hypertension when I found it, at diagnosing hypothyroidism in a young man with a wrist problem and having to send him back to the referring doc to get it treated. I wanted a more holistic or global approach to care. I wanted to be able to take care of people. Soon I knew I wasn't going to stay in rheumatology, but it was a good place to hide out for two years.

And then a job opened up in general internal medicine at Hahnemann. It was in town; I wanted to stay in town. I applied for it; I got it. And then I started getting excited about medical education. It was a whole new field, and I found out I loved teaching. The job was a staff position in general internal medicine. I was the internal medicine course director for the junior year of medical school—for seven years. It was just a whole new world of stuff. I still enjoy it. I'm one of those people that used to love getting dressed for graduation and sitting on the stage and watching the students go by as doctors. You've got a story for each and every one, as junior course director. They all came through your office, one way or another. I was very active clinically as well. I had four or five patient sessions a week, and made rounds twice a week. I was in the hospital seeing patients fifty weeks out of the year.

In 1985, I switched my clinical work from the university faculty practice to an HMO—HealthAmerica. I continued to teach half-time at the medical school, but I went to work for the rest of my time in a staff-model HMO. The HMO practice was structured; it wasn't happenstance. The HMO physician group was on the medical staff of the hospital that was two blocks away. They were good docs. Board certification was one of the requirements to be eligible for the position. I liked that. It was a multispecialty group. You had pediatricians and obstetricians in the office. But when I started I realized I didn't have a clue about managed care. For example, I had to put pregnancy back in my differential diagnosis of abdominal pain, because that's just not the kind of patient you'd see at that time in a university faculty practice. A guy walks in from work and says, "My face doesn't move." It was Bell's palsy—something you never saw in internal medicine at the university because it was screened out and sent to the neurologists before it ever got to you. We did peer review of our consults. On Friday afternoons, we would all meet and say, "Why do you really need this bone scan?" And if you defended it well to your peers, you got it. If you didn't, then you'd have to come up with another strategy, because we all sat at the table together and went through the referrals.

Once I got over my own personal culture shock, I said, "This is cool stuff, and we're not teaching it. We need to teach it." It was 1986 or 1987 that we developed a managed care teaching module for sophomore students. I had a lot of fun with it, I really did. We developed patient problems, mostly around choosing health insurance. I took the same materials that we gave employees to make their choices about health insurance. It included a commercial Blue Cross option and one or two HMOs. One was a staff model, one was an independent practice association [IPA]. There were two different families. We'd say, "Here's family A, here's family B. You've got thirty minutes to choose a health insurance plan." It was always amazing how students made their choices. They had their consumer hats on, of course, because that's all they have at that point. It was very interesting that the relationship with the doctor was at the bottom of the list of the things that medical students used to make decisions about insurance coverage. The first was affordability.

Most of what I learned about managed care, I learned through the newspapers, through the *Wall Street Journal,* through the *New York Times,* what was happening around the country, what was happening in Congress, what employers were saying about the cost of health care. That's where the debate was. The debate still isn't in the medical literature. The driving forces are coming from society as a whole.

In 1989, Hahnemann got a grant to set up a primary care internal medicine residency program—a program dedicated to training true internal medicine generalists. They asked me to come back full-time to direct it. I said, "Absolutely," because it was the first time that my experience clinically, academically, and pedagogically came together. This was a sea change in mentality from traditional training to a generalist focus. The first year, I spent most of my time talking to specialists about primary care—explaining that just giving the resident the dermatology syllabus doesn't mean that this is good training for the primary care setting. And to allergists, "No, I don't really want them to know about every bizarre immunodeficiency in the world, but could you please spend some time on making rational choices among antihistamines?" The first two years were really spent doing the legwork with the specialist faculty to tailor a primary care curriculum for the residents, working to build the culture of generalism. Primary care is not synonymous with ambulatory care, something a lot of people misunderstand. It took a real battle to make sure that the psychosocial issues were included; to make sure that the curricular content included generalist-focus topics. To fight the tide of the specialist bent, you've got to have somebody that is constantly looking to bring generalist relevance to the curriculum that's presented, to go out and to find quality training experiences, and not just a place to stick a student or a resident.

There *was* a change in the culture. More residents were choosing general internal medicine out of the program, and it wasn't because they didn't get fellowships. They decided they wanted to be primary care internists in their second year, and they stuck with it. But to really succeed at teaching primary care in a medical center, you've got to have leadership that is committed to a generalist focus. The leadership in the department was not committed to a generalist focus. Also I realized that the fact that I had not been involved in research and had not published much was catching up to me. I was going to need to make a professional career change because I would not have viability as a chair, or as a division director, or section chief, just because my CV was "too light" by traditional academic standards. So I knew that I would probably be looking at a managed care company, or hospital administration, or group medical directorship, as my next step.

I left the university and moved to Health Partners in November 1994. Health Partners was a not-for-profit IPA-type HMO with seven Philadelphia teaching hospitals as owners and seventeen or so other affiliated institutions with various degrees of risk. It was the third or fourth largest managed-care operation in the Philadelphia area and had a contract with the Department of Welfare to run a Medicaid managed-care program. The vast majority of the patients were Medicaid recipients.

I was the medical director for quality improvement, working on quality improvement and credentialing. The several thousand physicians in

the system saw our clients in their private offices or hospital-based practices along with other patients of theirs. At that point, the doctors were
generally scared, confused, and undertrained. A few years before, most
physicians had been outright opposed to managed care. By the mid 1990s,
they were resigned to managed care but hardly prepared for its demands.
A lot of the practices were in desperate communities and had been walk-
in practices forever. We'd come in and say that one of our standards was
that patients had to have the availability of appointments. This was a
business requirement because it's a care requirement, because it's good
care. Charts. Organized medical records. Just trying to reinforce to docs
that it was not acceptable to use three-by-five cards for medical records
anymore. You would think you shouldn't have to do that in 1996, but
we did. Doctors would walk away from their offices on weekends or at
night and leave patients to the emergency room. That was not acceptable. We required them to have an answering service and coverage. "No,"
we told them, "you can't just shut the door and go home to the suburbs
over the weekend."

I don't believe that managed care is a separate discipline. I believe that
managed care is a layer of clinical practice that you do simultaneously
with your care of the patient. To practice good managed care is good medical care. It's not too much and it's not too little. In the right managed
care environment, you're doing it with more information than you ever
had before. You have information on your prescribing patterns, on your
financial utilization, on your hospital bed days, on the quality of care
that you practice compared to your peers, on how many immunizations—
age-appropriate and disease-appropriate immunizations—in your practice versus someone in a practice just like yours. I think that enhances
your ability to practice good medicine.

There were critics of Medicaid managed care who claimed that we
didn't provide the social service and community backup that, say, community health centers tried to provide. But the good part about the managed care system was that there was a battery of people available behind
the company. We had expanded benefits that were not available under
routine or fee-for-service medical assistance that even the community
health centers didn't have. When the guy at the community health center saw a baby with fleabites, he told the parents to take the cat out of
the house. But the kid came back three times with fleabites because the
house needed to be fumigated and Medicaid and welfare did not pay for
fumigation. But it made common sense for a Medicaid managed care plan
to pay the bill for the exterminator—and we did.

Overall, I think managed care has a lot to offer the Medicaid population because basically care for poor people sucks. And I basically think
that—I'm sorry—some of the medical brethren and sistren think that poor
people deserve crappy medical care. It was not hard back then to see that
what was coming down the road would be ugly. Unless the country got
honest about health care delivery and made health care a right, the system was heading toward a debacle—HIV, geriatric care, underfunding,
commercialism. This handwriting was on the wall. Unless we addressed
those issues, the whole system would slip into crisis. There wouldn't be
enough money to take care of anybody. Salaries obviously would drop,
and care would get sketchier. I did think the generalist would be in a better position to survive, because the generalist has a different armamen-
tarium of skills that would help pull a rabbit out of a hat when it comes
to taking care of a patient. The clinician who is able to multitask, I always thought, would do better.

I stayed at Health Partners for about a year and a half, but it became
clear that there were some cultural differences developing between me
and the corporate environment. So in the fall of 1996 I moved to the Institute for Women's Health at the newly merged MCP-Hahnemann Medical School. The Institute included a Women's Health Education program,
a Women's Executive Leadership in Medical Education program, and a
clinical Center for Women's Health, where I went to work. I loved the
work right from the start. I saw patients half-time and worked with other
agencies around the university half-time to promote women's health and
to try to develop women's health educational and clinical programs. We
planned continuing medical education conferences around women's
health. We set up a quality assurance system and revamped the budget
of the office in an effort to bring it into closer line with the financial realities of clinical practice.

I loved my work, but trouble was coming. MCP-Hahnemann and the
Institute for Women's Health were both owned and managed by a huge
umbrella organization called Allegheny Health Education and Research
Foundation [AHERF]. Unbeknownst to me and most everyone in Philadelphia, AHERF was failing financially. When a health care system im-
plodes, it happens slowly and subtly. There weren't many warning signs
along the way, but the organization was collapsing. I can see that now,
but at the time it just appeared to be a series of setbacks that you
couldn't quite explain or that you didn't get a good explanation from
the administration.

I know exactly when the light came on for me. We were at a meeting

concerning a new community-based women's health facility with the
AHERF CEO and mastermind Sharif Abdelhak in April of 1998. A community representative asked Sharif Abdelhak point-blank about rumored
financial trouble and whether or not the funding for the facility was going to be available. Mr. Abdelhak responded that the funds would come
from grants, which I knew was a lie, since there were no grants or grant
applications pending. Things went downhill from there. The program
director was moved out, we started getting shuffled around from one department to another, and everybody was scrambling just to keep their
jobs. We took 15 percent pay cuts, we didn't have supplies, we didn't
know from one day to the next if the door was going to be padlocked
when we showed up. We read the newspaper to keep track of what was
happening to us.

AHERF declared bankruptcy in July of 1998, and eventually Tenet,
a for-profit hospital corporation, took over and kept our lights turned
on. More recently, Drexel University took over the academic side of
things. We were lucky that there was a great deal of university support
for us to continue in our patient care mission, although we were threatened the whole time because our primary care practice could never quite
seem to break even. In the months that followed, faculty were laid off,
contracts were not renewed, we were constantly being scrutinized and
second-guessed. I think the word is *devastating*. It was a devastating time.
I stayed because I still had residents and students, I still had patients, and
I still had hope that things were going to turn around. My greatest concern was to salvage the practice that I had been building since 1981.

Then, just before Thanksgiving 1999, we were given six months' notice. They told us that if we didn't meet certain financial targets we would
not be reappointed on July 1, 2000. Our "financials" did improve, but
the administration seemed determined to close us. I felt used by the medical school—and I was not alone. There were four primary care physicians not given reappointments, and all four were women. Now that might
be coincidence, but it didn't seem like it to us. Two of the women were
part-time, which made them particularly vulnerable. Racism is a harder
call. I looked around the institution for which I had worked for eighteen
years and wondered. Where were the African American physicians behind me at the medical school who would be able to carry on the mission
of diversity and commitment to the minority community? I didn't see any.

It was certainly the finances of primary care that were at the heart of
our problem. The practice itself wasn't worth a lot by medical market
standards. Nobody was going to buy us or invest in us. Over the years,

insufficient work was put into managing the practice to make the most of the compensation potential we had. Just working harder, seeing more patients didn't work anymore. Just opening up early and closing up late didn't get the bills paid. That is how the system is rigged. Technology gets the big dollars and pure doctoring—what we were doing in primary care for women—just wasn't being paid at a fair rate.

The practice did not do a financial turnaround, and on July 1, 2000, the university terminated my contract. The hardest part of the last two months in the practice was having to say good-bye to the patients. Many were as devastated and unbelieving. They appealed to me to open a private practice, and when I couldn't, I felt like I was letting them down. I was furious that the administration seemed to care little for the relationships that my patients and I had built over the years. It was impossible not to take that personally. At the end I went to see the dean to let him know what I thought—that the loss of the Women's Health program, the other primary care internists, and me was a travesty. Before I left his office, he put his arm around me and told me that I had done a good job. It was patronizing as hell and sexist to boot. But, I hate to admit it, that little validation felt good.

I had no job. The whole ordeal had been a huge blow to my self-esteem. I had never been without a job since I was a teenager, when I'd worked at Gino's and McDonald's. But now nothing. I simply didn't have the money or the longevity to invest in starting a private practice. I had the credentials to get an administrative job in a managed care company, but my heart wasn't in that. I only enjoyed the corporate stuff to the extent that it related to advancing clinical practice. I always felt like I was an infiltrator in managed care—I learned the language, I learned the styles and the methodology so that I could bring it back, somehow, to primary care and make primary care viable. But I didn't want to do it again. I really like putting hands on patients and interacting with people's lives. I just couldn't see myself *not* practicing somehow.

So I went to the unemployment office and applied for benefits. I figured out too late that I needed to go in earlier than I did, so I lost a couple of weeks of checks—$374 a week. It helped. And I started looking for a job. I went to the usual places—the *New England Journal of Medicine,* the *Annals of Internal Medicine,* the Internet. But it was an ad in the *Philadelphia Inquirer* that did the trick—the *Philadelphia Inquirer!* I answered an ad for a Student Health Services physician at the University of Pennsylvania. They looked at me, and I looked at them, and it was a take. It was exactly what I needed. We take care of everybody on campus—some in a total health plan and others for episodic care. I see the whole range of problems of young people in the course of the day, but it's very different from my previous work. I'm very unlikely to see anyone over the age of forty. I'm sure I'm not going to write another prescription for hormone replacement therapy anytime soon. I need to learn a lot more about international medicine now than I ever did before because so many of the students are from abroad. I don't have to manage anything, but I will be teaching. We have residents from Penn and other programs who rotate through our program, and I'll have the opportunity to attend on other services in the Penn system.

I like being at Penn. I like the ambience and the energy that the students bring. It is actually a bit of a homecoming for me, since I was born in the University of Pennsylvania Hospital. Many members of my family, including my influential grandmother, worked here in a variety of low-tech, service jobs. I feel very connected to their spirits as I walk across campus.

Looking back over the past few years, I'm not bitter. I am sad, and I am disappointed. This is not what I had envisioned for myself ten years ago. It's not what I thought would happen. I wish I could get angry, but it's hard to get angry at anybody. Sharif and his crew are all gone, and the people who are still there are just struggling to survive. And I don't see managed care as my nemesis. It has brought principles and change to health care that are positive and overdue. It's the lack of a decent system to manage health care overall that gets to me. That and greed. And we have plenty of that.

Through my ups and downs, my home life has provided me safe haven and a great deal of joy. An important aspect of who I am in life and in medicine is that I'm gay. My partner Donna and I have been together since 1984. She's a pediatric OR nurse. I came out late in life. I was thirty-one. I had strictly heterosexual relationships throughout my twenties, which I enjoyed. But when I discovered that I was gay, I was comfortable with it and, being thirty-one, I was already in my career at that point. I didn't have the threats of exposure that younger gays and lesbians think about in medical school and in college and high school. I didn't have to go through that.

Donna has two children from her marriage who are in their twenties now. For many years we had them with us every other weekend and for two weeks in the summer. They were great kids, and now I think they're exceptionally nice men, even if I say so myself. I think they're caring, sensitive people, and they're finding their way in the world.

In 1988 when Donna and I had been together for four years, I had a retroperitoneal bleed from an angioma in my right kidney. It ruptured acutely, and I never knew I had it. I went into shock, got rushed to the hospital, and had five units of blood and a nephrectomy. But that night, that experience, and the look in my partner's eyes as I got wheeled into the operating room, I mean, if she could've yanked me back from hell, she would have. After that, it was, "I don't care. This is my family. This is the woman I love, and I don't care what other people think." And so that politicized me, too. I was never really closeted. I think Rita Mae Brown had a term, "The closet door is open for anyone who wants to see." I never denied being gay at work, but that event made it clear to everyone I worked with that my partner was conducting business for me. She was my support person. She was my significant other. And I had only positive experiences around that. So it was very heartening, that people came forward to help her and to help me who I never expected would have.

I became more radical when my best friend was diagnosed with HIV. John is as close to a soulmate as I've ever had. He felt bad about himself as a gay man. And I think because he felt bad about himself, he took risks that he shouldn't have taken. I was just so angry, and I'm still angry, at whatever it was that made him feel bad about himself, and not proud of himself. It's homophobia. I don't know another word to describe it. I mean, John was the most monogamous man in his heart and mind. That was his desire, but he would never have thought to have brought a male partner home to his family. That would have crushed them. So instead he took chances, and there was an epidemic out there that happened to get him. But I was so angry at that. His disease politicized me as a lesbian.

Then I got really political because of my affiliation with the lesbian doctors' group, the Gay and Lesbian Medical Association, an organization founded by a friend of mine from medical school in the early 1980s. I went to the meetings most years, and I ran the 1993 meeting in Washington, D.C. That brought me out a little bit more, too, because the American College of Physicians *Observer* published an interview on me. So every internist in town, homophobe or not, read it. So it was like, "Hi. I'm the same gal you've always known and loved. There's no problem. What's different about me now?" Sometimes it's hard to be sure how people are reacting, but I certainly know of opportunities where other women have won out when my CV, in many areas, was stronger than theirs. There was only one person who was blatant enough to tell me to my face. I was considering joining his private practice. I said, "By the way, you need to know that I'm gay, and my lover's white." He pushed back from the table, and he said, as far as he was concerned, I had died. That ended our negotiations.

I still don't think that there's anything more satisfying than taking care of patients. It's the one thing that's always at the forefront of my mind. When I haven't been sure of what will happen next or how I'm going to pay my bills, I'm sure I want to practice and teach medicine. I've been a teacher all these years. I will die a teacher. Someone asked me recently what I was most proud of professionally. My answer was . . . Bernie White. Bernie was a medical student of mine a few years ago. I first met him when he was applying to medical school. He was on the weak side, but there was something about him that I thought had promise as a physician. I pushed for his admission and worked with him as he struggled in school. It took me six years to get that boy through, including telephone calls at one o'clock in the morning for panic attacks before tests and countless dinners Sunday night at my house. But he made it. I had tears in my eyes at graduation when we hooded him—when *I* hooded him. He went out to the Wadsworth VA to do a medical internship—and he was Intern of the Year for his year. I'm most proud of him.

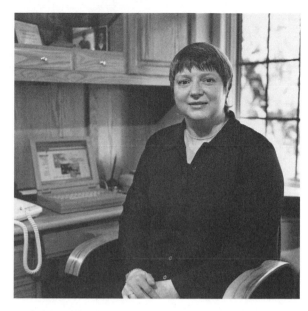

Gwen Halaas with her
ever-present computer.

GWEN WAGSTROM HALAAS, M.D., M.B.A.

EVIDENCE-BASED DOCTORING

Minneapolis, Minnesota
Gwen Halaas says that managed care has always made sense to her. The
cooperative and frugal principles that undergird the theory of managed
care resonate well with her Swedish-Norwegian roots and the values of
her social worker father and her minister husband. After medical school
at Harvard, she returned to Minnesota to train in family medicine and,
after time spent in private practice, took an academic job and enrolled
in an M.B.A. program. Her growing interest in health systems led her to
HealthPartners, a large not-for-profit HMO, where she became associate medical director in charge of medical policy in 1994. "It was a great
job. I saw myself as a family physician helping to care for 800,000
people." She felt she contributed to improved patient care, public health
practice, and the careful use of the health care dollar.

But the backlash against managed care has affected Halaas. "I was
spending too many of my days dealing with doctors' complaints about
limits on their decision making, about having to take extra steps, whether
it's just to look something up in a formulary or to get a preapproval."
In 1999 she left her administrative job and took up teaching full-time,

directing the HealthPartners family medicine residency. "I believe that systems of managing care are the way of the future," she says, "systems in which sensible people decide on rules and guidelines and trade-offs. It takes physicians to make good medical care work. We need all of the energy that physicians are currently using to get around the system redirected into evidence-based medicine and cost effectiveness. Then we will have a truly good system."

⤺

MANAGED CARE. MANAGED CARE, MANAGED care. For almost my entire life in medicine, managed care has been *the* topic. I have learned it, practiced it, taught it, and managed, yes, managed it. More and more, it has become the subject of discussions and debates—not only in my work but also outside of my medical practice. How does it work? Does it deny people needed care, or is it, in fact, providing better and more comprehensive health care? Is it containing costs and making care more affordable or just making stockholders rich? Is it driving doctors out of medicine, or is it the blueprint for the rational and best practice of medicine in the future?

While some physicians have steadily resisted it, the transition to managed care here in Minnesota has been slow and steady. Even though things have been happening dramatically in the past few years, the stage was set for all of this to occur because prepaid group health insurance has been present in Minnesota since 1957. Minnesota state law requires all HMOs to be not-for-profit. Minnesota is a fight-for-the-underserved, be-nice, do-the-right-thing kind of culture. It's a very different environment for managed care here than elsewhere in the country.

As a young physician starting into practice, I wasn't particularly happy with managed care, having to deal with lots of rules and limitations and different formularies for different payers, and having my patients frustrated by being limited in their choices. But I was familiar with all of that even during residency, and I had found that part of learning how to take care of patients was learning something about their insurance. Doing so made the lives of both physician and patient easier. You just become accustomed to that as a way of life.

The more I got into it and chose to advocate for my patients with the medical directors of the plans, the more I realized that there were reasons for managed care plans doing what they do. The formularies didn't limit me from giving drugs I wanted, they just cut out some of the more expensive ones or some of the newer relatives of the drugs that were already in place.

The medical directors I have dealt with over the years have understood about advocating for a particular patient. Most of the time they agreed with me and covered whatever it was that I thought appropriate, so I didn't really find it so terrible. What was most frustrating were patients who would insist that they needed to have a CAT scan because they had a headache, or a treatment for Lyme disease even though they didn't have any diagnosed Lyme disease. It's frustrating, because you want to meet their needs and make them happy, and explain to them some rationale for the decisions that you make, but they don't always leave happy in those circumstances.

Managed care has always made sense to me. Maybe it's my roots. I was born in and have lived almost my whole life in Minnesota—the Democrat-farm-labor state. My ancestry is a mix of Swedish and Norwegian. I was born in 1954 and grew up in Fargo-Moorhead, a border city with Fargo in North Dakota and Moorhead in Minnesota. My parents lived in Moorhead because they went to school at Concordia College and then stayed on. My dad was a social worker, and my mother became a school psychologist. Both are retired now. Fargo-Moorhead has a population of about 150,000 and is rich in colleges. There are three of them: Concordia College, North Dakota State University, and Moorhead State University. Growing up, there were a lot of cultural opportunities, rich in music, academic interests, and sports, but there weren't many professional women role models then.

I also went to Concordia College and majored in psychology and social work and minored in music. Medicine wasn't in my mind then. I met Mark Halaas, a handsome religion major and college student body president. We were married after my sophomore year, when I was nineteen. When he graduated from college he went to work as a college administrator, but he had always planned to go to the seminary. His father was a Lutheran pastor. He postponed the seminary to work when we were married. He worked in development, fundraising, and alumni relations at Concordia College. He went to seminary down the road a bit, when I was a medical resident.

We stayed in the area when I graduated. I took a job as a biofeedback therapist at the Neuropsychiatric Institute in Fargo and began working closely with a neurologist in the area of amyotrophic lateral sclerosis [Lou Gehrig's disease] and multiple sclerosis. I helped him write a book on neurology for the primary care physician. The neurologist told me one day that if I was going to consider graduate school, I really should think about medical school. I told him he was crazy. No one in my family was a physician, and physicians weren't held in particularly high esteem by my family. Minnesota is a Scandinavian culture where people don't go to doctors unless they are dying. My roots are all from Norway and Sweden, and intuitively I understand the culture. People simply don't think of the GP as their friend. Moorhead Scandinavians don't look for help from anybody, including physicians. They are folks with a strong work ethic and a streak of independence and self-reliance. Doctors are not a big deal for them.

But, in truth, I liked science, and I came to like the idea of medicine. I only had Biology 101, so, while I kept working, I started my premed studies. When I finally applied in 1978, I got into the University of Minnesota and, much to my surprise and delight, Harvard Medical School. Going to Harvard was great but a little frightening because I had lived all my life in Moorhead. My husband came with me, but I didn't feel that I had the full support of my family, who were concerned that medical school was going to be too difficult for me and possibly end my marriage. Mark, in fact, considered attending seminary, but, in the process of interviewing there, was offered a job as a development officer for Boston University's School of Theology, which worked out very well for us both.

Early in medical school, I discovered that I really wasn't interested in the pursuit of science to the nth degree. I was more interested in people of all ages and what I could do to help them, which did not fit my previous ambitions in neurology. Slowly family practice emerged as my interest. I was familiar with family practice because Minnesota is a strong state for training family physicians, but there were only two family physicians in the city of Boston in the late 1970s, so I had little in the way of local mentors. I was, in fact, discouraged by the faculty, who were generally disappointed that I chose family medicine, which they deemed nonacademic and unrealistic. They tried to talk me out of it, but I had made up my mind. I knew that I wanted to work with the whole human span of life and I wanted to do prenatal care and obstetrics. I actually got more support from classmates than from the faculty. We had a great class that turned out one of the highest percentages of family practitioners ever from Harvard—twelve or so in a class of a hundred and thirty.

When I gave birth to my son, Per, in Boston during my second year of medical school and I didn't have any family there, it was a little lonely.

I was eight months pregnant with my daughter, Liv, when I graduated. Minnesota was full of excellent family practice residencies, so it made the decision to go home easy. I started residency at Bethesda Lutheran Hospital, next to the state capitol in downtown St. Paul, in 1982. I loved it. Bethesda Lutheran was a family practice hospital, and the family practice program was the only residency there. It was really like a family. We were trained by family physicians with consultants available at the invitation of the family physicians. It was a wonderful learning environment, and I really enjoyed the community of it.

In my second year of residency, the administrators at Bethesda asked the residents if any of us were interested in setting up a practice in affiliation with the hospital. I was interested and so was Reid Gilbertson, one of my partners in the residency. We talked to the administration and they agreed to set us up in practice when we had finished the program.

We started from scratch in my second year of residency, picking out a practice location, designing the clinic, hiring staff, going through all the legal work and all the things required to hang out a shingle. The hospital talked us into practicing downtown in a high-rise office building on the skyway, which is an enclosed bridge across Jackson Street in the center of St. Paul. This had never been done before. There were no family practice clinics downtown until St. Paul Family Physicians. I had the fun of being a pioneer without going rural. We opened our doors in September of 1985, one week after my third child, Erik, was born.

We designed the contract with the hospital so that we could opt out at the end of three years, because we didn't know what kind of practice we'd build downtown. But, in fact, we built a rather interesting practice that included young working people who enjoyed the clinic and brought their families, as well as the elderly and the handicapped who lived downtown. It turned out to be a wonderful, interesting place to practice, and ended up being a full-service family practice, with just the two of us. We had a lot of fun. We were good friends and enjoyed each other and each other's patients. We admitted to Bethesda Lutheran Hospital, where we had done our residency.

In our second year in practice, however, we realized that the finances weren't as promising as we had hoped. Eventually we hired a financial consultant to help analyze the situation. We were not well trained in business, but we did know that we had a pretty busy clinic with a pretty good revenue stream. We weren't savvy enough to understand why business wasn't better for the work we were doing. The consultant concluded that the problem didn't have to do with the practice but, rather, with overhead expenses, given the downtown location and the amount of money that the hospital had spent on the improvements to create the clinic in the first place. Given our payback commitments, it was going to take a long time to get into the black.

In the end we concluded that we had to get out of the contract. This required us getting a lawyer and going through an unpleasant negotiation with the hospital. We already had been searching out other opportunities for where we could move our practice, because we had a good sense that we would take a lot of patients with us. We chose to join a larger group that had three sites, and in 1988 we moved our practice to a northern suburb of St. Paul, Vadnais Heights. It was a good practice, and we were gratified that most of our patients followed us.

I worked very hard, as did my partner. I had two other women partners initially, but they left, so I inherited many of their patients. I burned out with the OB, doing all my own deliveries, as I was up many nights out of the month, in addition to practicing in the clinic. It just got to be too much. The senior partners of the practice were all older men who were basically trying to work less, earn more, and eventually cash out, working the new partners hard until we could earn our way in. This was not unexpected, but there was a level of disrespect—some of it was toward me as a woman, some of it was just toward me as a younger partner—that I found difficult. Between working so hard and having to deal with some of that, I began to get frustrated and looked around to see what else I could do.

I had taught the whole time. I had started teaching part-time for the residency program at Bethesda Family Practice Clinic in 1986, in addition to my full-time practice. On my day off, I precepted the residents. My partner kept saying, "Give up the teaching. You're crazy," but I couldn't because I liked it so much. So finally a little light bulb went on that said, "Maybe you ought to teach. Try that full-time." I'd always thought I would teach eventually, but the time came sooner than I expected. In 1992, I left the practice and became the assistant director at my old program, the Bethesda Family Practice Residency Program.

Life was hectic with three active children. The reason I could do it was because of my husband's support and his willingness to be the primary parent for the children. He was a student at Luther Seminary when I was in residency, which gave him a little more flexibility in his schedule and the ability to do most of the childcare. When the children got a little older we had day care, but he has always been responsible for the daily needs of the kids. Once he graduated from seminary, he took a call in a church in St. Paul, where for seven years he was the associate pastor. His working hours remained quite flexible. There were times when it was frustrating for me, being a mother fully engaged in medical practice. My husband was always willing and happy to do the child raising, but I would feel at times that I wasn't the best mother I could be. There were times when I wasn't available, or I was exhausted and crabby. Fortunately, I always felt confident that my kids were getting good care. Well-meaning friends or family members would sometimes make remarks about "poor Mark," you know, having to do this kind of work, or "what kind of a mother are you?" for whatever the incident was at the moment. These comments didn't make me feel good about myself, but I knew they were more a reflection of these people's expectations than of any justified concern.

My experience as a woman in medicine has been good. I didn't think too much about it when I went to college. I thought I could be whatever I wanted to be. My parents instilled that in me. They expected me to go to graduate school, and they expected me to do whatever I wanted to do. My class at Harvard was about a third women, and I made some very good female friends there who were great role models. I can't say that I met very many good role models as women faculty. There were some who were too tough and not nice people, not sympathetic. Incidentally, there were no women's bathrooms in Harvard Medical School, only a powder room. It's probably still that way, for all I know. When I was pregnant, taking the physiology exam, I had to go to the bathroom and didn't want to walk for two blocks to the powder room, so I went in the faculty bathroom and thought I locked the door. The professor came in while I was there; he was a little embarrassed.

During residency, there were two women in our group of eight, and more women in other years, so we had a pretty good representation of women in family medicine. Training in family medicine was easier in that regard, because there was special respect for the family. Being a woman during medical training wasn't nearly as big an issue as when I got into the business of medicine. Once in the business of medicine, I suddenly experienced a change in approach and a lack of respect related to gender. When I had to negotiate contracts and issues with lawyers and hospital administrators, the traditional old boys' network became quite evident, and I had to become much more aggressive than was my natural style.

Having decided to teach, it was easy for me to go back to the residency where I was trained. Due to hospital mergers at that time, Bethesda

Hospital had closed, so when I came back to teach full-time, it was at the same program which was affiliated with the Department of Family Practice and Community Medicine at the University of Minnesota. My principal job was as the medical director for the Bethesda Family Practice Clinic. I discovered I didn't understand much about the business of running a clinic, even though I had managed my own practice downtown. Running a large academic clinic raised some problems that required more business understanding to handle. So my training in business management began with a course in management for physicians at the University of St. Thomas in Minneapolis, which I took in the fall of 1992. It was a thirteen-week evening program, offering some broad concepts in finance and accounting, managed care, and practice management. I had sworn I'd never go back to school again, but it was a lot of fun and very useful.

As it developed, I loved teaching, and I tried to develop new curricula in practice management and understanding managed care for the residents. The trouble was that the faculty who had been there for a long time didn't necessarily agree with some of my ideas for improving the clinic services, and they weren't very supportive of teaching the residents practice management or managed care. So I began to feel a level of discomfort again working in an environment where the kinds of things that I wanted to do weren't necessarily welcomed. I think a big part of it was that most of the faculty at the time hadn't practiced in a community setting for many years. They hadn't worked in a managed care environment, and they really didn't understand it. They were a little threatened by it, so they just weren't very supportive. It was as if they thought that managed care was going to vanish, so learning about it would be a waste of time. What I was proposing was hardly radical. Managed care has been on the scene in Minnesota for twenty-five years. When I trained it was already well under way. HMOs were in place, and we had to deal with many different managed care contracts, so we understood a lot of the details about how to deal with managed care just from having to do it.

In 1993 I was asked by the chairman of family practice at the university to become the medical director for UCare, the Medicaid managed care program that the department had developed. The job allowed me to continue to teach half-time in the residency program. On the management side at UCare, I learned a lot. I made decisions about coverage for the 35,000 Medicaid members in the program at the time. It was my responsibility to deal with issues about how those members were receiving services or care in certain clinics. Eighty-five clinics saw members of our program, but most of our patients were in the six residency clinic sites. I chaired the quality assurance committee that monitored quality for those patients and was involved in the development of a number of unique projects. For instance, we had an incentive program for prenatal patients because many of them never came in for prenatal care. We developed a program where we gave them a $5 coupon for groceries every time they came in for their prenatal visit, and if they made a certain number of those visits, they got a $75 Target coupon when they came back for their postpartum visit, to purchase supplies for the baby.

I developed a UCare 2000 Plan with preventive service goals, trying to maximize the rates of mammography, Pap smears, and other preventive services. Convincing this population to get preventive care services was difficult and required a lot of creative thinking. Although in the academic setting there was still some resistance to teaching about managed care and practice management, my work was being better received. I wanted to be able to teach at all six sites, rather than just the one, and have better opportunities for communicating with physicians.

I had been in the UCare medical director job for a year when I got a call from HealthPartners. HealthPartners is a family of the largest nonprofit Minnesota health care organizations focused on improving the health of its members and the community. HealthPartners provides health care services, insurance, and HMO coverage to nearly 700,000 members. The job offer was for associate medical director of data management and quality and utilization management while maintaining a certain percentage of clinical time. I told them I wasn't much of a number cruncher, but I was interested in policy issues, in medical education, and in mental health coverage. So I was offered the job as associate medical director in charge of medical policy, and involved with developing medical education opportunities. I hadn't intended to change jobs, but this one was too good to refuse, so I took it. This was in September 1994.

HealthPartners is the merger of a staff-model HMO, Group Health, which dates from the 1950s; a group-model HMO formerly called Med-Centers; and, most recently, the Ramsey [now Regions] Hospital and Ramsey Faculty Associates, which is an academic teaching hospital that serves the underserved and the faculty practice. It's an interesting blend, with a very strong mission that is present everywhere you look. That mission is to improve the health of our members and our community.

That job was great. Twenty-five percent of the time I continued to see patients and precept the residents. That was important because in addition to being fun, it kept me in touch with the real issues of patient care and medical practice. In my administrative role I had two jobs. I ran a department that helps develop the policies that go to all of our clinics, explaining what services are covered. The other part of the work was reviewing and deciding on coverage for cases that require prior authorization; these are cases that are experimental, extremely expensive, cosmetic, or controversial. I saw myself as a family physician helping to care for 800,000 members. I was intrigued by the courses I had taken at the University of St. Thomas, so much so that when I heard about a new M.B.A. program in medical group management for working professionals, I applied and started in the first class in 1993. It was an exciting three years, learning from the experts in health care and from my classmates—physicians, nurses, managers, salesmen, computer experts, and more. That education developed my confidence and leadership skills and prepared me for my position at HealthPartners.

I've been through managed care from the beginning. I learned about it, grew into it, and understand how it works clinically and administratively. I think most physicians my age are comfortable with the concept of managed care and understand the rules and how to play by them. At times, they may be frustrated for themselves or their patients, but on the whole the mental health of providers here has been pretty good, because managed care has been a rather gradual transition. I think it's been much harder in areas of the country where the changes have been more rapid and adjustments have not been nearly as easy.

In Minnesota we have grown beyond what others understand is the concept of managing the cost of care to understanding and improving population health, and that has made a tremendous difference for me and helps me sell managed care to physicians. It's exciting to be part of an organization that has developed practice guidelines that are very effective, that has set out public goals such as decreasing the rate of heart disease, diabetes, maternal-child complications, domestic violence, and dental caries. Our work goes beyond the usual managing cost to improving health.

A lot of the larger contracted care groups have been partners from the beginning in the development of the guidelines and are very active in patient education and health promotion activities. Does every physician buy into these goals? No. Salaried physicians, working in the staff-model HMO, may buy into these goals more easily, but so do many of our contracted physicians. I spent a lot of time working with the latter. I visited five of those clinical sites on a quarterly basis to work with the physicians on their utilization and how it could be improved and on the goals and how to work together to reach them.

Public health goals should not be controversial. Everybody wants to increase early detection of breast cancer, decrease the rate of heart disease, and decrease the complications of diabetes. HealthPartners offers them resources that they wouldn't otherwise have. We give all of our clinics an updated list, on a quarterly basis, of all their women who haven't had mammography who should have, and of others needing preventive services. We try to make it easier for them to implement their own ways of improving their outreach and their ability to provide preventive services.

During my time as medical director for medical policy at HealthPartners, I was challenged to put my business education to work to help the health plan make difficult decisions about coverage. I developed principles for making exceptions to benefits—guidelines for medical directors to make exceptions based on the individual situations. I also developed a process for making coverage decisions about therapies that are new—beyond the experimental stage but not yet standard-of-care. This process involved reviewing the available scientific evidence and expert opinion about such therapies and coming to a decision about coverage.

These last years have not been an easy time for managed care. Despite the work of HealthPartners and other health plans in the United States in improving health and managing cost, the expectations of the public for health care services remain high, and the tolerance for managing cost and quality is almost nonexistent. I think that managed care has often made physicians better physicians because the demand for evidence, the demand for quality, has really helped them stay on their toes and do a better job. Managed care has also made physicians more cost-aware— something they didn't learn in medical school and haven't had the incentive to learn in practice. You can practice good medicine and still be cost-conscious.

But physicians are also feeling what they consider to be the loss of their autonomy. There's frustration with limits on decision making, about having to take extra steps, whether it's just to look something up in a formulary or to get a preapproval. The political campaign for a patients' bill of rights has come from these sentiments and, although I know that our practices at HealthPartners are well within any proposed legislation, it is very difficult to listen to all of this managed care bashing. And it comes from everywhere.

These attitudes literally drove me out of the work of being a medical

director for a managed care organization. I got tired of having to respond
to all the negativity all the time. In my day-to-day work as a medical director, I was the one that had to make the final decisions about whether
or not certain services would be covered. But even when I was doing good
things in the organization, the negative pressure from the media, from
lawyers, from the public was so strong that it was hard to take pride or
pleasure from my work. In 1999, the position of program director for
the HealthPartners Family Medicine program became vacant. I interviewed and was chosen for the job, and it has been great. Residents are
enthusiastic learners, and the faculty is committed to teaching evidence-
based, high-quality medicine in communities of need. We treat patients
in the hospital, clinic, homes, schools, nursing homes, jails, homeless shelters, and teenage drop-in centers. I continue to see my own patients and
teach residents, but I am also responsible for the financial success and
daily operation of the residency program and the clinic—Ramsey Family Physicians.

Resistance to managed care has remained fairly strong in academia.
At the university there are still faculty who oppose managed care or who
do not understand what it is. As a result, residents aren't necessarily understanding or supportive of managed care. This has resulted in Health-
Partners' developing an Institute for Medical Education, designed to impact the curriculum and to train medical students and residents in the
fundamental changes in funding and practice that are taking place. We
want to teach managed care from the beginning, rather than having to
reeducate physicians when they are hired. The university has been very
receptive and has partnered with us in the development and work of the
institute.

Specialist physicians are in a fight for their lives, here as elsewhere.
Just as there have been too many hospital beds, there continue to be too
many specialists. Within managed care, the specialists have had to play
by the rules and have learned how to manage care, how to relate to primary care physicians, and what it means to be part of a gatekeeper system. But now their incomes are coming down, and they're not replacing
the partners who are leaving. Competition has increased between groups,
the potential loss of contracts with payers or hospitals has grown, and
much more attention is being paid to the quality of specialists' outcomes
and the cost of their care.

There is plenty of uncertainty in the system. Roles for primary care
physicians continue to evolve. The concept of hospitalists is being developed. Delivery systems continue to struggle with the right balance of

generalists and specialists, nonphysician providers and physicians. Costs continue to rise, especially in the area of drugs and technology, and the prices of insurance premiums are not keeping up. Physicians' salaries are stable or decreasing, and compensation plans are becoming more complex and potentially more punitive for inadequate productivity or utilization.

My perspective these days is a bit discouraged. Like many administrators in managed care organizations, I have tabled my ambitious goals for reform, and I'm just waiting it out. I think managed care organizations in general are sitting back and watching while prices rise, while premiums go up—waiting to see where this managed care backlash will go. Ultimately, I think we will see a financial crisis or an access crisis—or both. It will take tragic stories and a lot of angry people to get any kind of response.

I believe that systems of managing care are the way of the future. The systems will get better. They may not look just like the systems we are building today, but they will have to be systems in which sensible people decide on rules and guidelines and trade-offs. There is certainly a limit to the resources that we have available to pay for health care. If we really want to provide universal access and maintain or improve the quality of care, we have to have a systems approach. We have to think along the lines of population health and not just individual health. As a physician I haven't given up because I can still practice good medicine and I can still teach the principles of managed care to my students. It takes physicians to make good medical care work. We need all of the energy that physicians are currently using to get around the system redirected into evidence-based medicine and cost effectiveness. Then we will have a truly good system.

As for my own future, I've become much more involved in the ethics of health care related to policy and to the concept of providing fair and equitable health care benefits. So I'll continue to learn, although I'm trying to stay out of school. I may pursue more learning in the area of ethics and will continue to be a resource for other organizations that are trying to develop opportunities.

I will continue to be an advocate for informed and ethical decisions in health care. I have worked hard. I have also been able to enjoy my family. My husband, Mark, has combined his work in Lutheran ministry with fundraising and development work and is called by the bishops in Minneapolis and St. Paul to be a resource to congregations on giving gifts to the church and church-related charities and organizations. We have been very happily married for twenty-seven years. My children are healthy and becoming very independent. My oldest son, Per, is at Luther College in Decorah, Iowa, and is interested in music, drama, and English literature. My daughter, Liv, is at Concordia College, my alma mater. She is fluent in Spanish and interested in art and international business. My youngest son, Erik, is a teenager having great fun in high school and is active in soccer and basketball. The children have each come to work with me and have special memories about those experiences.

I see myself as a caregiver and a person who is committed to leaving the world a better place. My Lutheran faith has always been a strong part of my family upbringing, and my religion supports me in my work. I get my reward from being able to make people's lives better.

CHAPTER SIX

The Quixote Factor

Generalists Doing Special Battle

The medical generalist is really a "clinician for all seasons." Broadly educated and given to big-picture concerns, generalists find their way into unusual areas of the medical enterprise. Add a sense of cause or moral purpose that motivates and nourishes many generalists, and some truly remarkable stories emerge—stories of medical Don Quixotes.

In the late 1970s, William Kapla, M.D., was a family physician concerned with the health issues of the gay community in San Francisco. Then AIDS erupted underneath him. The past twenty years of his life have been spent on the front lines of this new epidemic, grappling with its changing clinical and social personae and providing care to thousands of HIV/AIDS patients. Barbara Ross-Lee, D.O., has been a one-woman civil rights movement, coming from modest roots in Detroit to become the first African American woman to serve as dean of an American medical school. Along the way she has broken many color and gender barriers. Janelle Goetcheus, M.D., has been guided by her religious faith in providing almost three decades of leadership to inner-city primary care and community causes in the District of Columbia. The homeless, immigrants, mothers and children, and pretty much anyone down and out have been Goetcheus's patients and partners through her years of work. Primary care provides an avenue to take on virtually all of the challenges of the medical care system.

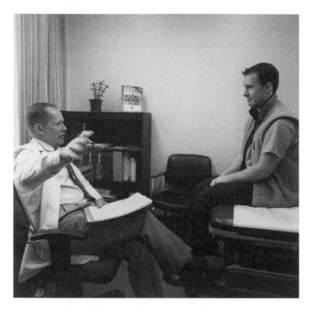

William Kapla
instructs a patient.

WILLIAM KAPLA, M.D.

LIFE AND DEATH IN SAN FRANCISCO

San Francisco, California
Bill Kapla was a medical pioneer when he opened his office in San Francisco's Castro district in 1977 specializing in gay medicine. His predominantly male, homosexual patient population was troubled mostly by eminently treatable problems such as sexually transmitted diseases and hepatitis. As it turned out, he was at ground zero for the oncoming AIDS epidemic, and his doctoring was soon consumed by the care of the critically ill and the dying. Working with patients, public health officials, students, and researchers, Kapla has practiced his way through the epidemic, losing his lover as well as hundreds of patients and friends to the disease. Recalling these years, Kapla sits at a handsome mahogany desk amid statues, artwork, and neat piles of patient records and medical journals. Behind him is a bookcase containing Grant's *Atlas of Anatomy,* Osler's *Principles of Internal Medicine,* and the *Physician's Desk Reference* as well as an open case displaying a set of turn-of-the-century surgical instruments belonging to a long-deceased Colorado general practitioner. Kapla has a well-developed sense of history. He is an articulate, tidy man with a blond mustache who speaks with modesty about his ac-

complishments. "I always have done primary care," he recalls, "but that meant everything, including a great deal of thanatology."

⟜

I FIRST BEGAN TO REALIZE I was gay when I was twelve or thirteen years old and I discovered that I was attracted to other boys. That made for a huge struggle within me. Could I really be bad, evil, sinful, perverted? I denied my instincts, and I fought to be "normal." Being gay didn't fit with what I was being taught either by society or the church. How could God make such a despicable person as me when he was such an all-loving, omnipotent entity? I had no idea then that being gay would provide the overriding definition of my personal life as well, ultimately, of my professional life.

I was a good midwestern boy from a very modest background, born in Duluth, Minnesota, in March 1943. My father was an automobile mechanic who later worked overseeing quality control at construction projects. My mother worked in a grocery store checkout line. My parents were very loving, and I'm sure their goal in life was to raise their two sons as successfully as they could. Our family was Lutheran. We went to church and Sunday school regularly, and I said my prayers every night until, my God, I must have been in my second year in college.

We moved to a suburb of Denver when I was five or six, which is basically where I was reared and educated. The move from Minnesota to Colorado was very exciting. I loved cowboys and Indians, and here we were moving out West where the real Indians lived. My father used to rent a horse for me and walk alongside when I was too small to ride on my own. Then I began to ride seriously on my own, and to this day riding is my great passion.

My first recollection of an interest in medicine dates from when I was about eight years old. My mother, brother, and I were playing a board game, and I asked my mother what she would have chosen if she could have married anyone. She said, "Oh, sweetheart, every young girl wants to marry a doctor." From that point on, I planned on medical school. By junior high, whenever I was asked, "What are you going to be?" the answer was always, "I'm going to be a doctor." All my courses from high school on were directed toward premed.

I went to college at the University of Colorado, a gorgeous campus in Boulder with beautiful flagstone buildings. My years there were among the most positive of my life. I worked very hard, enjoyed the school, earned a B.A. in psychology, and was accepted at the University of Colorado Medical School in Denver. In college, being gay provided a tremendous motivation for achievement and success. I felt that, if I were such a despicable person, at least it would be much harder to step on me if I was a doctor than if I was a janitor. Instinctively, it seemed to me that I would be more accepted in society if I had a respectable position. I don't think I ever stopped and thought about it out loud, it was just always there.

At the same time, it was a tremendous struggle. I felt extreme isolation and fear that something would happen to me physically. Disease was not the issue then, it was physical harm. To this day, when a gay man of my generation walks along the street, all he needs to hear is "Hey, faggot," somewhere in the background, and he'll think, "Oh, dear, my time to die!" Straight people may not be aware of it, but queers still get bashed for the sport of it. So growing up in the 1950s and 60s was terrifying.

I was dealing with these issues with the help of a counselor in college. Then, on the first day of medical school, we were all in the auditorium being asked to sign a bunch of papers, and one paper came by that was an attestation to "moral character." It asked if we were free of any character disorders, and said that any knowledge to the contrary would be grounds for immediate expulsion. Well, I knew what *they* meant by a character disorder, and I said to myself, "Oh, my God. Sign that puppy and move it along." That was the kind of anxiety that was ever present in medical school. In the second year of medical school, the top student in the class was gay. His mother and father knew it and were promising him a Corvette if he changed his sexuality. The stress of being gay led him to commit suicide in the fraternity house. The school was in an uproar; no one could understand why he had killed himself. I knew. So I went to the dean of students wanting to inform him but not to incriminate myself, and he was actually understanding and sympathetic. I told him about the stresses on gay students and reminded him about the "moral character" paper we had had to sign the first day. He seemed understanding, and there were no repercussions from our talk. I felt that maybe the conversation had accomplished something.

Dating was also stressful. In the second year of medical school, I was going out with a nursing student for the sake of having a girlfriend, and we tried having sex. It was dark and it was a struggle, an absolute struggle, but I finally had an orgasm in my clothes on the floor of her apartment. When it was all over, I got up, said I had to go, and walked home. Then I got in my car, went down to a gay bar in Denver, and went home with some nice guy. Then and there I decided that I wasn't going to play the straight guy any more. I was gay, and that was the way I was going to be.

My next crisis came in the fourth year, on a psychiatric rotation. A hospitalized psychiatric patient recognized me from a gay bar and told his attending psychiatrist that the medical student was a faggot. I was called in to the attending's office and told, "Well, this is pretty serious. We're going to have to take you off the rotation and tell the other students why this is happening." First I denied it. Then I said, "Well, there was a time when I probably was considering it, but I'm going with a nursing student." I still had contact with Nancy, thank God, so I could use her as an alibi. Eventually the attending physician decided that his response had been too harsh and that he would treat the issue as a problem of the patient. I think his dilemma then (it was the mid sixties) was, "Is this student gay and, if so, what are our procedures for dealing with him?" But since I denied it, it let him off the hook. Had I admitted being gay, I'm not sure what would have happened. My fear was that it would have meant expulsion. The incident left me panicky—I was within six months of becoming a doctor, and I thought I was going to lose it all. I went to talk to a psychiatrist friend on the faculty who brought me back down to earth. He just said, "Calm down, don't do anything, don't say anything, and don't admit to anything. Everything will be all right." And in fact, it was. I graduated and went on through.

In 1969, I moved to San Francisco to start residency training in internal medicine at Presbyterian Hospital. Originally I'd planned to go east for my residency, since I'd spent all of my life west of the Mississippi. But a girlfriend pushed me to consider San Francisco. She claimed that it was a wonderful city, but my impression at the time was that it was a city full of kooks. In the third year of medical school, a friend and I took a trip to California with the idea of looking at residency programs. We arrived in San Francisco for an interview, stayed at the YMCA, which was a notorious gay hangout, and we just went crazy. We spent the entire week in San Francisco, never going on to Los Angeles, because we loved the city so much. When I applied for internships, all of them were within a hundred miles of San Francisco, and I was matched with Presbyterian.

After two years of residency, I joined the Navy. It was 1971, the war in Vietnam was raging, and all doctors had to serve in the military. I chose the Navy because, in my mind, it had more gay people than any other service. I did worry that I'd be shipped to Vietnam and die, but instead I spent six months in Pensacola, Florida, being trained as a flight surgeon, and then was assigned to the Marine Corps Air Station in North Carolina.

The Marines and the Marine Corps were wonderful. The image of the Marines appealed to my own personal values and to my sexual fantasies. Presumptions aside, if you are a neat, clean, squared-away person, they'll ask you to wear their uniform. Well, I wore a Marine Corps uniform the entire time I was in the service. I'm adaptable and try to be an engaging person, so I had no problem with the military. It was easier for me because I knew I wasn't going to stay there. I like orderliness well enough, but it was still hard. I knew that I couldn't stay in the military twenty years and be gay—although, to my great surprise, I met a lot of gay people and realized that the Marine Corps attracted many, many gay men. Of course the word "men" wasn't quite right since many of the Marines were actually still adolescent boys with questions about their sexuality. The camaraderie and all the buddy business appealed to the homosexual tendencies in many young men. Unfortunately the Marines were also viciously brutal if they caught a gay guy in the Corps; they would humiliate him and destroy his career. Homosexuality exists in the Marine Corps, but it's dealt with harshly when it's discovered.

I enjoyed my time in the military because, first, I wasn't going to be there forever and, second, I was always a doctor first and a military officer second. I had tremendous rapport with the troops and the officers. People knew I wasn't a "lifer," so they could come to me if they had problems. Within the underground it was known that I was gay, so that gay troops tended to come to me when there was a problem or issue.

I spent six months aboard a helicopter aircraft carrier in the Mediterranean. People got very gay aboard a ship. In the ship's setting, where there's no other outlet, sexual contact with a man wasn't viewed as badly as it was off the ship, when the standard roles reassert themselves again. I think that we probably respond to each other first as human beings, irrespective of gender, on a big bell-shaped curve. There are probably a few pure homosexuals among us, a few pure heterosexuals, and most of us are bisexual. When you add the influence of society, history, and religion, it skews that curve markedly toward heterosexuality. It's interesting to note that 25 percent of gay men have children and that many men "come out" only after a marriage. On board a ship, you could see that curve move back toward the middle.

I got out of the Marines without destroying the moral fiber and character of the military and headed back to San Francisco, where I worked as an ER doctor for four years, taking lots of side courses. I found that it was a great joy to take care of a person in the emergency room and then have him come back again and get to know him as a person. Over time, I became skilled at primary care medicine, and in 1978 I challenged the family practice board examination, passed, and became a certified family physician.

During my four years working in the ER, many friends had wanted me to care for them, but the only thing I could do was to bring them through the emergency room and deal with them there. In the process, I was actually creating a very nice gay practice. It finally reached a critical mass, and psychologically I was ready to really deal with people that I liked. So in 1978 I started a primary care practice and forthrightly called it a gay practice in the Nob Hill neighborhood near St. Francis Hospital. I immediately became one of the few doctors in the city specializing in gay health. Herb Caen, the famous columnist for the *San Francisco Chronicle,* picked up on it immediately. His comment in the paper on gay medicine was that, "I thought you had to be sad, hurt, or in pain to go to the doctor, and here you can be gay and go to the doctor."

The practice was probably 90 percent gay men and 10 percent lesbians. The patients loved it because, in general, medicine had had no time for gay and lesbian patients. Their sexual preference was seen as a disease itself. Doctors wanted to send homosexual patients for shock therapy. For the most part gay patients had to keep that aspect of themselves secret from the medical profession. In my practice I saw the whole gamut of health problems that affect twenty- to forty-year-olds. On top of that, I saw a horrendous incidence of sexually transmitted disease. This was the sexual free-for-all time when the gay male was becoming a person unto himself, with a new attitude: "No one's going to tell me what to do; I'm going to have sex with whomever, whenever, wherever, I want to." So I dealt with the STDs quietly. I also became the community's expert on ambulatory proctology because no proctologist wanted to deal with a faggot and his problems.

I reported the STDs to the Health Department, of course. They were obviously concerned about the STD rate, and a wonderful assistant director of the Health Department named Selma Dritz reached out in a motherly way to the gay community. She wanted to know why there were so many cases of parasites in San Francisco, and she thought that maybe it was originating in the gay community. So a rapport was established, and we fastidiously reported all of the odd parasites we discovered to Selma. She started characterizing enteric parasites on a public health basis and producing papers and epidemiological studies. The rapport we established with the STD clinic, based on the contact tracing that we did, was helpful when AIDS struck in 1981.

The practice was successful. I didn't know much about how to run a business, but it all seemed to work out. I was all alone until 1984, when I moved to Davies Medical Center in the heart of the Castro, ground zero of the gay community in the world, and two of us joined together to form one practice. I enjoyed being on the crest of the wave of gay issues and gay medicine. I became an expert in caring for the gay patient and was asked to give talks on the subject to interns and residents and medical societies. It became steadily more topical because physicians began to ask, "Oh, my God, you mean I've got faggots in my practice?" And my answer was, "You'd better believe you do—now, here's the way to deal with it." So that was fun.

Around the same time the gay physicians in San Francisco got together to create a gay physicians' support group, the first in the country. These groups now exist in other major areas, and there's a national organization. We couldn't use the name "gay" or anything like it so, to this day, it's called Bay Area Physicians for Human Rights. The fear was always state reprisals—that the medical board of California would take our licenses away. The medical society of the city of San Francisco would not even allow the gay physicians' association to meet in its building until 1980; they were not going to let faggot doctors in the building. The attitude of organized medicine has been conservative, prejudicial, and slow to change. The American Psychological Association listed homosexuality as a disease until 1974. The following year the AMA finally agreed that homosexuality was not a disease category. The AIDS epidemic has helped a great deal in sensitizing people to the rights of gays.

As soon as I became board-certified in family medicine I was appointed to the clinical faculty at the University of California at San Francisco Medical School. Being gay was not an issue there. At first, gay students heard about my practice through the underground, and started taking electives with me. The rotation became so popular that we started getting straight students as well. I do feel a special obligation, however, to help gay students. It's important to show them a role model that says, "Hey, you can be as gay as you want to and still be successful."

After the gay physicians got permission to go into the medical society's building, we held a continuing medical education course there on gay medicine. No one else was going to teach us, so we made our own course. In August 1981, Dr. Friedman Keene from New York City came to San Francisco to present a talk on a strange cancer—Kaposi's sarcoma—that he was seeing exclusively in gay men. He said he was terrified of what it might mean. I remember thinking, "Oh, God, this is too hard to believe. We're having a wonderful, gay old time; we're curing our STDs and doing what we want. There can't be anything to stop this now." It was that same summer of 1981 that Michael Gottlieb published the first reports of deaths of gay men dying from *Pneumocystis carinii* pneumonia. That was the beginning of our knowledge of AIDS—right under us, right in our community.

We had no name for it. It was just a disease complex that was happening—and it was happening in homosexuals. A few bad apples, but not us. Then in 1982 one of our physicians developed a Kaposi's lesion in the back of his throat, and he was dead in two years. In terms of my own practice, it was unbelievable. I remember a horrifying case. I had to tell a nice young man I had taken care of, maybe twenty-three or twenty-four, that his HIV test result was positive. He seemed devastated, but after we talked about it he seemed okay. The following morning I got a call from the coroner: "Could you come down, Dr. Kapla, and identify a body that we cut from a tree in Golden Gate Park?" I couldn't do a thing about it. Some of the finest, most talented, educated, successful people were dying—and no one cared. When you're seventy or eighty, with diabetes and heart failure, and you die, everybody says, "Oh God, wasn't it a blessing." If you're thirty-two and die, they say, "Good, he was a faggot. . . . It was God's revenge. . . . It was deserved."

Early on, we started to have struggles with bathhouses here in San Francisco. Bathhouses were viewed as the bed of this disease, so there was a movement to close them. But we couldn't just close our sanctuaries, our palaces. The debate was emotional, passionate, vociferous—it was terrible. There was a sense of entitlement: "You can't tell us what to do and put moral restrictions on us." We knew that when a guy checked into a bathhouse, he got a towel and key, put his clothes into a locker, and then went around and did whatever he wanted to with consenting males. We knew from exit surveys that someone who went to a bathhouse had an orgasm on average two and a half times each trip. Epidemiologically, he came in contact with about twenty people for each orgasm. So he essentially had sex with fifty people each visit. We have on record people with three and four thousand one-on-one contacts in the early days of the epidemic. This became the staggering geometric progression of the active gay male in San Francisco in the seventies. And no one wanted to stop.

In retrospect, it's easy to see how AIDS just exploded in the gay community. In response, society wanted to close the bathhouses because they thought that that would stop the sex. But we knew it wouldn't. Closing bathhouses was not going to stop sex. We concluded that the only way to control the disease was to educate. So we, as gay physicians, created our own approach to AIDS: the establishment can't stop this disease, but we'll educate people and tell them how to avoid it. In late 1982, six or eight of us got together in an office over on Fillmore Street to create the first safe sex guidelines. They've been modified and become more sophisticated, but the basics are still with us.

Clinically there were slow but important steps in dealing with AIDS, and by 1984 we were able to test for the disease. But testing could lead to a loss of job and health insurance and make a bad situation terrible. The advent of anonymous testing was a godsend, because we could test people without destroying their lives. But we didn't really do a lot of screening; we were making most of the diagnoses when people walked in manifesting the disease. Now, in retrospect, from hepatitis studies that were underway through the 1970s, we know that as early as 1978 5 percent of gay men in San Francisco were HIV-positive. By 1980 it had reached a critical mass of 20 percent, and from that point on it exploded. It stayed steady for a long time at about 70 percent of the gay men in the city, but that generation is now dying off from AIDS.

Our safe-sex education efforts since then have been so successful that we have now wiped out over 90 percent of STDs in the gay community. It was astounding that sexual behavior could be changed to such a dramatic degree after such uncontrollable activity. If you take the gay white population alone, new cases of AIDS have dropped to almost zero in the last three or four years. Now the great concern is reaching subgroups like Hispanics, blacks, and youth. That's probably the most difficult problem we have—how to reach gay youth. They've grown up in the era of safe sex, and their guard is down. You can't get into the schools very easily to talk about sex, and now the religious folks are saying, "You can't encourage them to have sex. Tell them no." I don't care what you tell them, that method is not working. The religious types just can't deal with giving a kid a condom. They see it as encouraging, giving them implicit permission to have sex. But if I don't give them the condom, they're still going to do it anyway. Kids view AIDS as the old man's disease, the thirty- and forty-year-old's disease. They see themselves as omnipotent, invulnerable. It's very hard to reach them.

In 1985 the first drug against HIV—AZT—came on to the market. People struggled to take the drug at virtually three times the dose we give today. Rapidly, desperately, we tried to get some parameters of what to do. We had a tough time with AZT, but at least people were living longer. It was 1991 before the second drug, DDI, was approved for use. Then there was an onslaught of new drugs in the mid-1990s. But it was the appearance of protease inhibitors in the summer of 1996 that has changed things dramatically. We have seen a precipitous decline in the number of acutely sick patients requiring hospitalization and a marked decline in the number of deaths and death rate of the AIDS patients. This has made life different and better from a clinical point of view not only for the patient but for the doctor. I just don't have to cope with as many critically ill patients and dying patients day in and day out. This consumed a tremendous amount of emotional energy and intellectual energy in the past—working with not only the patients but with their families as well.

My practice—like many HIV/AIDS practices—has become more out-patient-oriented, probably a little easier, although still very demanding because these patients continue to be very complex and time-consuming. They're a lot more stable, so there's less change from visit to visit as compared to times past. In addition, unfortunately, we still are seeing people seroconvert, so we're still having to deal with new patients, some of whom suspect they're HIV-positive and some who don't. For people who don't suspect, the diagnosis remains as devastating as ever, requiring a great deal of support from me.

Gay physicians became medicine's experts at dealing with AIDS. We were called upon incessantly for help, guidance, and education, because we were already running annual updates and education courses for ourselves. It just got larger and larger. We were our own educators and the educators of others.

Since the beginning of the epidemic, all the diseases occurring in association with AIDS were known diseases, but they just happened to be occurring in God-awful unexpected situations and combinations. Even though some of them were unusual and difficult to treat, at least we knew what we had to deal with—pneumocystis, fungal diseases, lymphomas, and the like. AIDS really needs to be treated by a primary care physician because so many organ systems and medications are involved. The patient needs a single doctor with an overview to guide him through the incredible quagmire of care. Most care today is managed on an outpatient basis, and primary care for the person with AIDS is often a team affair that includes the patient. Doctors don't usually deal with patients who know about their diseases, let alone patients that arrive at the office armed with the world's literature on the disease. But the AIDS patient often does. So we learned that it was all right to tell the patient, "I don't know, but we'll find out together." AIDS patients don't expect the doctor to know everything because treatments are changing so fast that nobody knows everything about AIDS. So we really had to forge a new kind of partnership with our patients.

We have become compassionate experts in death and dying. Medicine has always dealt with death and dying—oncologists with cancer patients, for instance, and internists with the elderly. But what do you do with a strapping thirty-two-year-old male who's dying on you? What kind of effort do you make medically? Do you give him every single thing medicine has to offer and make him suffer terribly in the process? Fortunately, we have gotten better at dealing with death, and we now have some very good legal instruments with which to modify the all-out approach that can be so punishing. We learned the art of how to care for dying patients and make them comfortable. We tell them to let us know when they have had it because we won't do anything to prolong the suffering. We let Mother Nature take her course. That has now become the standard of care, reflected in our directives.

In my practice today, I continue to work with an associate. We see about 1,200 to 1,500 people, some 85 percent of them gay, and some 90 percent of those are male and 60 percent are HIV-positive. We're on the Davies campus of California Pacific Medical Center, in the Castro area of the city. Since the gay community moved into this area over the past three decades or so, we've had to address their issues and needs, and this is now the premier private AIDS hospital in San Francisco. When AZT first came out in the early 1980s, this medical center was prescribing 10 percent of Burroughs Wellcome's entire production of the drug. There was a time when there were about twenty primary care practices that served the gay community of San Francisco, and fourteen of them right here at Davies. Gay patients are a little more spread out now because there are more physicians who will treat them, and insurance company reassignments have distributed the community a bit farther into other medical practices. The white gay community is a very successful segment of the San Francisco society, both professionally and financially, and therefore they usually have great health care benefits. The Hispanic and black gay populations are not as financially successful overall, they don't have the same benefits, and they're much harder to reach with educational programs.

In recent years it has become increasingly difficult to practice medicine in California because of financial downturns and financial constraints dictated by managed care and the third-party payers. I think it would be fair to say that many physicians' personal incomes have decreased a lot over the last five to six years. It's very frustrating and demoralizing to experience a standard of living that continually goes down, and in many cases physicians are unable to contribute to any kind of retirement program. My practice has been very, very satisfying over the years, and I've always said that if I died suddenly, my overwhelming sadness would be that I didn't get to do it longer. But I guess today I would have to think about that a little bit. The benefit of a premature death would be that I would not have to fill out any more preauthorization forms or deal with any more insurance companies.

In 1979, I met a wonderful man, an architect named Jack. We lived together in a beautiful home overlooking the city. In 1984, a good friend who was living with us developed AIDS, and that's when Jack and I decided to get tested. He was positive and I was negative, an agonizing situation. Although initially I thought nothing would actually happen to him, in 1987 Jack developed AIDS and started on a very difficult, three-year downhill course ending in his death in 1990. I spent ten years without a partner, and that was very difficult. Physical beauty is highly prized in the gay community. Gyms are filled with gay men taking care of themselves and working to stay young. But because of this, a gay man in his forties and fifties goes through a lot of adjustment because he's no longer as physically desirable. Often it is difficult to socialize and to find another partner as one ages. I'm still hoping to live to be 101, and I'd love to be able to celebrate a thirty-year wedding anniversary. Happily, in August of 1999 I met a wonderfully loyal and devoted man named Mark and we're off and running on our thirty years.

My gayness was very hard for my parents in the beginning, but the last fifteen or more years have been wonderful. They don't talk about my sexual preference to their friends and family, but I think it's generally understood that I am gay. They adored Jack from the start, and that helps me to know that they are fully accepting of me. My brother has a hard time with my being gay, as does his wife, and I'm not as close to them as I would like to be. They have four wonderful, successful children that I've always felt were kind of kept distant from their funny uncle in San Francisco. I have become involved in an exciting program here in the city involving mentoring of gay youth. I think the youth are our most valuable commodity in this country, and I'll probably devote the rest of my life to making growing up gay easier than I had it.

Today you can hardly find anybody in society who hasn't been touched by AIDS. Awful and tragic as it has been, the epidemic has done a great deal to educate the community in general about sexual preference, sexuality, and goodness knows, HIV disease. There's far more acceptance of gays now than there was twenty-five years ago. For someone my age, I'm just astounded by the changes. I thought I would live to see the day that maybe it was okay to be gay and yet, now, we've got such incredible political power here in San Francisco and elsewhere. And I'm blown away by the talk about gay marriage—I just never expected it. Changes are coming so fast it's amazing. I guess that's part of getting old. Life's going so fast; it's going to be over here soon.

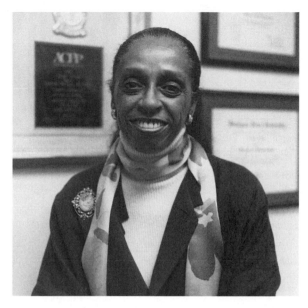

Barbara Ross-Lee
and her wall of
academic achievement.

BARBARA ROSS-LEE, D.O.

GROUND BREAKER

Athens, Ohio
Barbara Ross-Lee is well-versed in minority issues. She is the first African
American woman to be appointed dean of an American medical school—
an osteopathic medical school. The daughter of a union organizer and
the eldest sister of singer Diana Ross, Ross-Lee grew up in Detroit in a
family rich in values but short on money and amenities. She had worked
her way through college, begun teaching, and started her own family
when she had the opportunity to go to medical school at a new osteopathic program at Michigan State University. She took it, trained in family medicine, and ran her own private practice in Detroit for ten years
before returning to academia to become a leader in medical education
and dean of the Ohio University College of Osteopathic Medicine. Ross-
Lee is an athletic woman with a striking smile and elegant hair. She is a
forceful presence at the podium, in the classroom, and at the policy table.
"To a patient," she tells her students, "you are not white or black or
green—you're a doctor. They assume you care, regardless of your race.
In fact, they expect you to care. And as long as they know you care, they'll
help you understand them."

⌒⟶

I'VE LIVED IN OHIO FOR ten years now, and I'm dean of a state-supported osteopathic medical school. But my first recollection of Ohio was in 1952, when I was ten years old and my mother came down with tuberculosis. She went into the hospital and had part of a lung taken out. Our family of five children, the youngest at that time being only about a year old, was shipped off from Detroit, where we lived, to Alabama to stay with my mother's sister. The most vivid memory I have of the trip was that Cincinnati was the place where we had to get up out of our seats and go to the back of the bus. We were an African American family, and Cincinnati was the turning point from north to south. That's what I first knew about Ohio.

I was born at Women's Hospital in Detroit ten years earlier, the first of my parents' six children. Shortly after my birth my father joined the Army as an MP. When he came out of the service he wanted to be a policeman, but he couldn't because of the racial situation in Detroit at the time. So he went to work at a factory, Anaconda American Brass, where he stayed until he retired. He spent most of his time in the plant and became a union man in the United Auto Workers union, which later became part of the AFL-CIO. When the labor movement really gained momentum, probably the early 1950s, he became very active in the union. His union involvement was a big help to the family because being a union representative allowed him to have a job in the late fifties when everybody else got laid off. While my father never preached union ethics, his concept of working together as a team for the underdog and looking out for everybody pervaded the family. Helping and sharing were very much a part of our family upbringing. All of the issues of workplace fairness were very much a part of our growing up.

My mother was a homemaker who made all of our clothes. She had a year or two of college and had taught in community organizations before she and my father married. That was a time, though, when women usually didn't work outside of the home, but she had to work from time to time, because we were poor and frequently unable to make ends meet. My mother's family was a huge help to us, with aunts who jumped in and took care of us when we needed the help. In fact, one of my mother's sisters lived with us and was always there for us.

My mother was the one who inspired the family to believe that they could do anything they wanted to if they worked hard enough. I sometimes joke that my mother felt it was a sign of maturity to be able to delay gratification for a better reward. I remember she wanted some new living room furniture, but we couldn't afford it. She would not settle for cheap furniture, so for five years we had an empty living room with the best cocktail tables that she could find. We had no chairs, but she saved and bought one item at a time when she could afford it. She taught us that you don't give up, you just keep on going. You've got to work and plan, but you'll get there. I think she probably had more of an influence on the kids than my father did.

Being the oldest of six children, though, taught me a thing or two about parenting as well. At times I served as a surrogate parent. I remember when my brothers and sisters were teenagers, my mother would call me and say, "Let me tell you what your son did." I'd have to remind her that they were not *my* children.

When my mother developed tuberculosis in 1952, we went south to live with my aunt in Bessemer, Alabama, a relatively small city then and very segregated. I was an avid reader at that time, but I was not allowed access to the public library or many other places in Bessemer. I got to see the Ku Klux Klan parading down main street, which made a big impression on me. We had to get adjusted to going to school in a segregated and hostile environment that was very different. I think as a family we all became much closer during that year. I couldn't wait to come back to a bigger world—one in which we didn't have to feel so cramped. When we got back to Detroit, though, I realized that the street we lived on was a little narrow street, and it wasn't quite the big thoroughfare that I remembered.

I remember the years after that as a happy time. We lived in the inner city in a large apartment building. There were a lot of children around, the playground was less than a block away, and our school was right across the street. It was really a community where people had lived forever. You could go blocks away, and if you did something wrong, people would tell your Mom. I didn't even know I was poor until I left that community to attend junior high school outside of our district. My mother sent me there so that I could get a better education, and it was wonderful because it got me back into reading. I worked as a library aide and challenged myself to read every single book in the library before I graduated.

At that time my family was forced to move from our home into the projects because my father got laid off. Eventually he went back to work, but we never really recovered from that. From that point on it was always a struggle. I can remember the battles over this. My mother insisted that we take public assistance, and my father did not feel that he should ever take aid. I can remember a year of not having heat or electricity because we just couldn't afford to pay. My father was bringing home $26 a week, and the rent was $75 a month. There were six kids by then; my youngest brother was a baby at the time. This was within a few years of my mother getting out of the hospital.

I lived in the projects with my family until I was twenty-one. Although my father was working, he could never make enough money to move the family out because the rent was increased as his salary increased. It wasn't until my next-oldest sister, Diana, started singing and made some money that the family was able to leave the projects and move into a house that she bought.

I attended a college preparatory school, Cass Technical High School, which had a special emphasis on science, much like a magnet school. When I went there it was probably about 5 percent black and the rest white. Today it is probably 98 percent black, and its college-bound rate and scholarship rate set national records. It's a wonderful school. It just so happened that the projects were close to downtown so I could walk to Cass Tech every day, while most of the other kids took public transportation from all over the city.

At the time, the expectations for black students were not very high. But you learn to live with bias. By senior year, most of us had been lost through some sort of attrition, and we felt relatively isolated. The music instructor, for instance, would never let Diana sing because she claimed Diana didn't have "the voice." After Diana's group, the Primettes [later the Supremes], made their first record when Diana was a senior, some of the teachers insisted that she be given an opportunity to try out for the senior production. I can remember the music teacher predicting that Diana would never be successful singing—Diana Ross! The Primettes were the sister group to the Primes, who later became the Temptations. I didn't see her perform for years because they were on the road, but when they came to Detroit to perform I remember telling her, "I can't believe it, you really are professionals." They had changed from little girls that used to sing at the drop of a hat into a really poised group.

I had begun thinking about medicine then and expecting to go to college, not fully realizing the money needed to do that. I was admitted to three colleges after graduation, but couldn't attend my first choice—Michigan State—because my father couldn't afford it. Likewise, the scholarship to Albion didn't pay for room and board, so I went to Wayne State University, commuting on a daily basis. I really liked Wayne. It probably was much more comfortable from a diversity perspective. I majored in chemistry and biology, but after two years I decided that maybe I wasn't going to go to medical school after all. My marks were average at a time when I knew it was really difficult for minorities to get into medical school. So I decided to be a bit more realistic and get a degree in the sciences instead.

Meanwhile, I fell in love and got married, really ending my medical school dreams, I thought. I graduated in 1965 with a bachelor's degree in chemistry and biology, only to realize that it was not a very useful degree. Parke-Davis offered me a job weighing rats. That's what my bachelor's degree in science was going to get me. Instead I took a job working at an osteopathic hospital in a Detroit suburb, the Martin Place Hospital in Madison Heights, Michigan. That was my first contact with osteopathic medicine.

Laboratory services were just starting to become more mechanized then, with autoanalyzers and coltercounters. They needed somebody with a science background to troubleshoot the new machinery. It was wonderful because it was a small hospital and I got to learn to use everything in the lab, but once I had mastered everything, I became a little bit frustrated with what appeared to be a dead end. Then in 1965 I got an opportunity to join the National Teacher Corps. It was an ideal choice because my first husband was also a teacher—and I took it. The Teacher Corps was a domestic version of the Peace Corps. The program was structured so that with a college degree and some practical experience teaching in poor and minority communities, you could earn a master's degree in education. We were placed in a teaching environment and took graduate courses in the evening at the College of Education at Wayne State. I was placed at the very school that was next door to the projects I had lived in. These kids were the difficult students—discipline problems assigned to us by the other teachers. There were five of us on the teaching team with a team leader, in a class with fifty students.

If you went into these kids' homes, you would never look at them the same way again. As much as my class may not have taken advantage of what a school could offer, at least the school was safe. This was just after the riots of 1967. It was an interesting time. I had one child, Stephen; Monica wasn't born until January 1969. I lived on the northwest side of Detroit, which was the safest area, but my family—in the home Diana had purchased—was right in the riot area. The National Guard was all over the community. All the stores were burned down and nobody could get food, so we were trying to bring food in to my family from the northwest side. It was really touchy because the National Guard was so trigger-happy. My oldest brother, who was nineteen, was arrested during that time for driving our sister Diana's expensive foreign car, and was badly beaten by the police.

After the riots, the *Detroit News* did a survey of the entire Detroit community, and they hired black college students to do the work. I took the job on a part-time basis while I was teaching. My job was to visit all of the houses in a section of the East Side of Detroit and complete a questionnaire about what the people there did during the riots. I went into homes that if a child of mine visited today, I'd probably have a heart attack. I don't think my mother knew what I was doing. I'd go and sit in homes trying to get answers to a long questionnaire. People in the black community were very supportive of us, so it wasn't as dangerous as it might have been. Many times I heard, "Leave that girl alone, she's a school girl." Education was revered.

I grew up in a family that didn't really have a doctor. We used emergency rooms when we had to, so that my interest in medicine wasn't based on any role models. Rather it came from seeing a need that was just not being met. It was the Civil Rights Movement that really opened up medical school for me. A friend in the National Teacher Corps told me in the spring of 1970 that Michigan State was opening an osteopathic school in Pontiac and suggested that I apply. I was teaching school at the time and raising two babies. It was the year after I finished the National Teacher Corps, and my first marriage had failed. I was trying to decide what was I going to do with the rest of my life. The school was taking students for their second class and, despite the fact that I didn't have enough hours in physics, I made the decision, took a summer physics course, and was admitted.

In Detroit the Civil Rights Movement was quite visible, and political empowerment was a direct result. But economic empowerment was lost after the 1967 riots. After Martin Luther King's death, when the new osteopathic medical school was opening, there was a clear commitment to affirmative action; the classes would be diverse. That was impressive in light of the fact that the classes were so small in the first couple of years. A lot of that can be attributed to Mike Megan, the dean of the new school. He was committed to diversity. In the first class there were two blacks and one woman in a class of seventeen. And in the next class, my class, there were two women and two blacks in a class of twenty-one. That was significant at the time.

This was a three-year program in which we got very little time off.

After two years in Pontiac, I spent a little over a year in clerkships all over the state. We weren't based at one hospital as in most medical schools but went to many osteopathic hospitals in the state for our clinical rotations. Osteopathic physicians were extremely committed to making this school successful. They were willing to volunteer a lot of their time both lecturing at the college and precepting us in their practices. It was a good program and a perfect match for me. I did feel guilty the whole time I was in medical school about not giving my two babies a fair shake. I felt that I could be working and making real money and not struggling, and the kids would not have to be without their mom. My mother and my aunt and my sister made it possible for me. They kept my kids for me in a two-family house in Detroit. Family was there all the time, so I could go to school. The only problem was that neither my mother nor my aunt drove. I had to teach my mother how to drive, and my aunt never learned.

When I finished my degree, I did a rotating internship back at Martin Place Hospital in Detroit. I thought about doing a residency in pediatrics but decided that since I was an "old lady" of thirty-two, divorced with two children, I shouldn't wait any longer to get started. The osteopathic tradition was to begin a general practice following a rotating internship. First I signed on with an older doctor in Detroit who, it turned out, passed out a lot of codeine, amphetamines, and Valium. I left him after three months and went to work on the East Side for a physicians' group that ran clinics all around the Detroit area that turned out to be Medicaid mills. They could see 250 patients in a seven-hour day without one scheduled appointment. They were doing more triage than actual treatment, and I didn't want to practice that way. After six months I left them, and on July 1, 1974, I opened my own practice in a freestanding, modified dental office on the west side of Detroit. It was hard to compete with the group practice I had left, though. I resented them for the first three years of my practice because I couldn't figure out why patients went to them in droves when I was dispensing good care while struggling to build a practice.

The name of my practice was Community Family Practice, which I think came before its time. It was a solo practice for the nearly ten years I worked in Detroit, both family- and community-focused. I moved into a part of the city that was undergoing dynamic change, a lot of white flight. Physicians were moving out as well, so it was possible to build a really good practice with lots of young families new to the community. It was great. I treated all kinds of medical problems. My approach was to diagnose the problem and then refer the patient to the appropriate specialist only if necessary. Most of the workup had been done by the time the patient saw the specialist. But I didn't do much inpatient hospital care. I made social rounds on all of my patients who were in hospitals, but I didn't really treat them there.

My decision to enter academia was actually reactionary. By 1982 I'd been in a solo practice for eight years, and I really wanted more stimulation. I found myself becoming excited about finding some terrible disease process and disappointed if it wasn't present. I was also unhappy with the changes taking place in health care delivery. I spent more time trying to get paid than I spent seeing patients. I'd reached a point where I was talking to third-party computers more than real people. That's when I started looking around for other things to do.

At about the same time, I got a call from my alma mater, Michigan State College of Osteopathic Medicine, asking if I would be interested in being considered for the position of chair of the Department of Family Medicine. I asked if I would be considered as a serious candidate or did they just need some affirmative action representation. I was told that I would, indeed, be a competitive candidate, so I went ahead and submitted my application. Ultimately, I was offered the job, although it was not an easy process. Early in the interview process, the dean himself, my old mentor, Mike Megan, told me that I was not qualified to be a chair because I didn't have research and academic experience and that I was wasting my time. At that point I had nothing to lose, and so I completed the interviews. Others thought differently of my credentials, and subsequently the university provost said they couldn't give the position to anybody else until I turned it down. So I started my academic career working for a dean who really did not want me to have the position. One of the things I liked least about my time at Michigan State was the politics of the profession. It truly was an "old boys'" club. It's changing now, but it's not all the way there yet.

While I was learning some lessons about faculty politics, we did wonderful things in the Department of Family Medicine. I thoroughly enjoyed including students more effectively in the department, designing a new curriculum, and bringing a more scholarly focus to the department. A special problem for osteopathic medicine was that, even at Michigan State, osteopathy was seen in the shadow of allopathic medicine, a minority profession with a minority mentality. This perspective limited the vision of the participants and made them very defensive. People in osteopathic academic medicine have found it harder to change because they've secured a space and are afraid to step out of it for fear it will be taken from them. There is security in a majority mentality that doesn't come easily when you are a minority. In my experience, this is true in race relations as well as in medical relations. So I found it was a little bit harder to make changes in the department than it should have been.

But Michigan State also had exceptional circumstances. It was the first public osteopathic school and, despite our differences, Mike Megan was dynamic, hard-driving, and a very bright dean. He took the school where he wanted it to go and brought the rest of the profession along with him. Deans at private schools, because they report to very political boards, do not have the flexibility that Mike Megan had. The whole profession was willing to allow the school a lot more latitude in developing because it was the first public school. Many of those trained at Michigan State moved into leadership positions at many other osteopathic medical schools.

Health policy—the issues, forces, and players that shape the health system—was another area that became increasingly important to me in my role as a department chair. I had been involved in policy at the state level, particularly with state public health reports on children, perinatal centers, perinatal regionalization, and minority health issues. When I left practice, I thought that in academia I would have an impact on minority health or the health of youngsters. Although I learned that a policy role is not a given for an academic, I worked with the public health department at the state level, eventually teaching policy formulation. In 1990, I learned about the Robert Wood Johnson Health Policy Fellowships, a year-long Washington-based fellowship program designed to give academics a firsthand policy experience. Ultimately I was selected and, truly, it was an experience that changed my life.

The fellowship expanded my vision of what's possible. After an orientation phase during which the six of us visited all over Washington learning about national health policy, we selected a member of Congress for whom we would work as a health staffer for the rest of the year. I chose Senator Bill Bradley of New Jersey. Over the year I learned how to position a member of Congress around an issue, how to evaluate a situation based on who is on your side and who is not, and understanding why they're not on your side.

Bill Bradley offered me the opportunity to play politics with the big boys and to champion the kinds of issues I was interested in. I worked on a lot of Medicaid reform, the Family Medical Leave Act, veterans' issues, and children's health programs such as immunization. The senator was not very informed about AIDS, which was a rapidly emerging policy issue in 1990. So it became part of my job to orient him on AIDS so he would know how to vote on the floor. The senator was also very committed to improving race relations, and we worked on that. I was there for the Thomas hearings, and was able to give him my perspective on his vote on Clarence Thomas. He voted against Mr. Thomas's appointment, a position and vote that I supported. It was a fascinating and valuable experience.

Coming back to academia was a little deflating because it was difficult to explain my fellowship experience and what it was like. Nobody quite understood what it was all about except that I had worked in a senator's office. To capitalize on the experience, I negotiated with the new dean at Michigan State to become the associate dean for health policy. I wanted to work on issues on which I thought the profession needed to take some positions. When I was in Washington, most people on the Senate health staffs had never heard of or had understanding of osteopathic medicine. The profession ran into crises like being left out of the Medicaid regulations, or having bills drafted that openly said a doctor had to be board-certified by the American Board of Medical Specialties. And so we structured the associate dean position to allow me to continue to work on the national and state levels and with groups such as the American Association of Colleges of Osteopathic Medicine and American Osteopathic Association.

The fellowship also opened another door for me, although it was not apparent at the time. Based on my work in Washington, I received an invitation from a group of students to speak at Ohio University College of Osteopathic Medicine in Athens, Ohio—a relatively new (1975) and growing public school that was part of Ohio's higher education system. I went and spoke in early 1992. I had no intention of leaving Michigan State and no aspirations to become a dean, but when the deanship in Athens became available in summer of 1992, the students at OU begged me to apply. The students actually recruited me for the position and even started looking for jobs for my husband. It was very flattering, and they were really an interesting class.

I did talk to a former dean of the school, Gerald Faverman, about the position. He told me there was no way that Ohio University, in the middle of Appalachia in southeast Ohio, would be able to accept a black female dean. My reaction to that was, "Well, maybe that's true, but I'm not taking your word for it. I'm going to have to go down there, I'm going to have to see it, and I'm going to have to be uncomfortable." I enjoyed the interview process. Faculty and staff wanted "change." Clearly a black female dean was a change from the current white male. I was offered the position and started in August 1993.

One of my first jobs was to position the college for whatever was going to happen in the changing health care environment, which meant that we had to build a stronger practice base for training locally. Ohio University is located in a grossly underserved area. One of our residents just went to join a doctor in the next county who was the sole physician for the entire county. For that reason, my strategy when I began was to build up a clinical base right in our area. If every hospital in the state closed, I would still have an obligation to train a hundred students per year. The school has the luxury of being in an area that can expand, whereas many of the other medical schools around the state have to downsize. At the two community hospitals in Athens, we have nearly doubled the number of physicians since I arrived in 1993. And at our clinics we are building a stronger ambulatory base. We have a clinic on campus and satellite clinics in all the surrounding counties. We also have contractual relationships with the Chillicothe County Veterans' Administration for inpatient/outpatient services. We still need more ambulatory training sites as we change our curriculum.

We have seen some successes. We have doubled our patient load and our patient visits so we can provide early clinical contact on site, without having to farm out our medical students. In this way we avoid having a large number of adjunct faculties, and we are instead able to provide that ambulatory training to our students here. Meanwhile, we restructured our clinical training base and developed what we call a CORE system, which stands for Centers of Osteopathic Research and Education. It is a statewide integrated system for pre- and postdoctoral students. There have been frustration and morale problems among the faculty due to the changes, but they were ultimately completely successful.

One of the objectives I have had as dean is to build an academic cadre of osteopathic physicians. This is a concern I have with new osteopathic medical schools opening up with insufficient faculty with academic background. They're going to need deans and department chairs and faculty for these institutions. It's not that it can't be done, but I think the profession hasn't done a good job of creating a pipeline for academicians and academic administrators. I wasn't prepared; I was lucky.

Another area in which the college has made a contribution to osteopathic medicine is in the training of minority students. We estimate that 15 percent of our students are from underrepresented minority groups as compared to 7 percent in osteopathy in general. We have also done a good job of educating doctors for Ohio with an emphasis on primary care. For each class of one hundred graduates, at least 75 percent choose postgraduate programs in Ohio, and of those about 70 percent enter osteopathic training programs with the rest selecting allopathic family practice programs. Fifty-five percent of our alumni are in primary care, mostly in family medicine.

As I look toward the future, I see the similarities between osteopathic and allopathic medicine as far greater than the differences. Osteopathic and allopathic medical education are almost identical, the practices of the two professions have been merging all along anyway, and as osteopathic and allopathic hospitals come together—as they are—the barriers against joint and combined training will erode. When this occurs, the distinctiveness of the two professions may disappear. I think that ultimately we're not going to need two professions.

I do think that what osteopathic medicine has done from its minority position for health care and primary care in America has been unbelievable. I'm not sure that history is appreciated by the allopathic world because they are still coming from a specialty perspective. They don't yet see the value of primary care or the fact that you can do a wonderful job in a different kind of environment and come out with an excellent outcome.

Just as family support made medical school and graduation possible for me, my professional and academic successes are the direct result of family support. I married my second husband, Edmond Beverly, in 1976 during my time at Michigan State and created a blended family of children. We have what I call a "Brady Bunch" family—his, mine, and ours. I have two children from my first marriage, I raised two children from my husband's first marriage, and then we had one child together. Interestingly, our older two children are both male and named Stephen, although they have completely different personalities. When I assumed the deanship in Ohio, our youngest child was a senior in high school. I had to leave her in Okemos, Michigan. Today the geographic separation from family continues as the kids leave the nest and my husband's career as superintendent of K–12 school districts keeps him professionally in Michigan. The older of the two Stephens is an engineer with an M.B.A., and he's in San Francisco now. The second oldest Stephen is in education; he's teaching in a boys' school in Muskegon, Michigan. Monica, the third oldest, just completed her allopathic training in ob-gyn and is employed by Ford Hospital in Detroit. Our youngest son, Kevin, is a policeman in Ann Arbor, Michigan, and our youngest daughter, Alaina, is starting her senior year at the University of Michigan law school. I am currently enjoying role reversal—they all worry about me.

When I speak to students or residents about medicine and some of my personal concerns about the underserved, I often tell some of my personal history. Although I don't perceive it as a bad health history, it is not a simple one. I lost my very first child to rubella during the rubella epidemic of 1964–65, even though I never knew I had it. The child was born with transposition of the great vessels. During my later pregnancies I suffered from an incompetent cervix. My youngest daughter, Alaina, was born prematurely at twenty-three weeks and barely made it, and I lost two more pregnancies after that. I learned a lot of lessons along the way about how people are treated in hospitals—how assumptions are made based on what you look like versus what you come in with, and how doctors don't listen. It doesn't matter who you are, doctors don't listen; it's a power position. When I lost the baby with the transposition, I was not in medicine, and they misled me to think that this was a minor problem. They didn't realize how much I needed to know the truth to prepare for the baby's death three days later.

Being African American has given me insight into the debate regarding the advantages of having minority physicians working in minority communities. What I have to offer is not just who I am, but what I do. I could and should be able to practice medicine anywhere. I knew from a service perspective that my skills could benefit many people, yet I chose to work in an underserved community because they needed me. I felt compelled to work with people who had been ignored and poorly served by the medical system. This was my choice. In truth, though, as a minority physician, I didn't have people knocking down my door to come practice in Beverly Hills. In many ways there is an expectation that a minority physician will practice in a minority community, and that limits opportunities for minority physicians.

Patients in need don't care what color you are. You're not white, black, or green—you're a doctor. They expect you to care about them and care for them. The problem is that minority communities want and expect quality care from doctors, and they frequently don't get it. If we depend only upon black physicians to treat black patients, for instance, there simply aren't enough to go around. We'll end up with an awful lot of premature and preventable deaths of black patients. To me this is "Jim Crow with a twist," and I resent it.

The real issue is providing better service to minority communities with the doctors available to us—minority and majority. Patients who need medical help expect that if you're a doctor you will help them, irrespective of who you are and who they are. The system hasn't gotten there yet. Quite frankly I think both the patient and the physician are victims when they don't understand that the barriers between them don't need to be there. That's what cultural competence is, and that's what a lot of my work in medicine has been about.

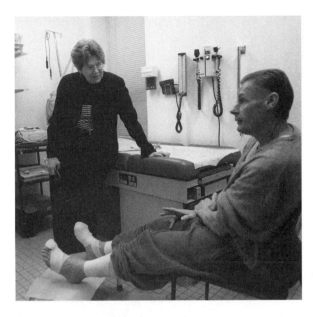

Janelle Goetcheus
worries about her
patient's feet.

JANELLE GOETCHEUS, M.D.

DOCTOR SUCCOR

Washington, D.C.
Blankets, vitamins, condoms, and mittens: these are items that Janelle
Goetcheus dispenses while visiting homeless patients. One part Saint Joan
and two parts Mother Teresa, Goetcheus has been an omnipresent force
in the care of the indigent, the impoverished, and the homeless in Washington, D.C., since the mid-1970s. During this time she has treated thousands of the city's most down-and-out patients and founded or helped
in the founding of an extraordinary series of service programs—Columbia
Road Health Service, Christ House, Mary's Center, and Joseph's House,
to name a few. Religion and spiritual commitment have always been important to her. She and her Methodist minister husband intended a life
of missionary work abroad when a chance trip brought them to the nation's capital in 1975, and they discovered and took on a lifetime of challenges. Since 1995, she has served as the medical director of Unity Health
Care, an amalgam of Washington's Healthcare for the Homeless program
and the city's two community health centers. She and her husband have
raised their family living in Christ House, sharing their home and their
meals with patients and colleagues alike.

Goetcheus is soft-spoken and straightforward, with a perpetual aura of kindness. She speaks with great satisfaction about her calling, which she defines in terms of service and healing. But she is not altogether content with her quarter-century of giving succor to the vulnerable. "I still feel a sadness from seeing so much unnecessary suffering. There are younger people out on the street today, many of them crack-addicted, lining up for the soup kitchen, and clearly feeling hopeless. This country needs to make a much more fundamental commitment to care for all of its people."

I'VE WORKED AND LIVED IN the inner city of Washington, D.C., for almost a quarter of a century, but Indiana and my faith in God are my real roots. That's where my life and where my vocation began.

My father grew up in Indiana and Illinois, where my grandfather, who was a United Methodist minister, had several parishes. My mother grew up in North Manchester, Indiana, where she was a member of the Church of the Brethren. The Brethren are one of the Anabaptist groups of German origin related to the Mennonites and the Quakers. Marrying outside the church was a difficult decision for my mother, even though she was marrying a minister's son. I was born in Indianapolis in 1940 but grew up in Muncie, Indiana, where my father worked as an auditor for the state of Indiana. My mother taught school all of her life, first in public schools, then in a parochial school, and finally as a tutor for homeless adults who were learning to read.

My parents belonged to the High Street United Methodist Church, a large downtown church in Muncie. Going to Sunday service and Sunday school each week was very much a part of my childhood. Prayer was always important to me, even as a child. It was during time spent in prayer that I think I began to think about where I was headed in life. Within the church, it was assumed that some people would go into full-time Christian service, as we called it. In our Protestant tradition, that usually meant that men would become ministers and women would become missionaries. I never really wrestled with whether or not to go to the seminary because very few women became ministers at that time. My primary goal was to live with and help the underserved.

I also decided at an early age that I wanted to be a physician, but that specific vocational goal was less important. First I knew who I wanted to serve—the poor. The question of how best to manifest that service was secondary. I was a shy person on the surface and not the type people

expected to go to medical school. In fact, the career counselor in high
school suggested that I consider alternatives to college, such as secretarial work. A few years ago, an article on me appeared in a medical school
alumni magazine, and that same counselor, then in her nineties, saw the
article. She actually remembered me and called me here in Washington.
She said she never thought I'd become a physician, and we both had a
good laugh about it over the phone.

I finished high school in 1958 and went to Ball State Teachers' College,
now University, in Muncie on a three-year premed program. I lived at
home and continued to worship at our family church. A number of overseas missionaries came to speak at the church, and I expected that, eventually, my work as a doctor would take me overseas because I assumed
that was where the greatest need was; I simply didn't think in terms of
major medical problems here in this country.

I went to Indiana University Medical School from 1961 to 1965.
Eleven women started out in my class of two hundred, but only eight of
us graduated. Other women I've spoken with from my class seem to have
more memories than I do of feeling intimidated and squelched at various points in medical school. I was very focused on why I was there, so
I just didn't pay much attention to sexism. Of course there were off-color
jokes and things like that, but I was a quiet person and just didn't let it
bother me. One unpleasant experience that probably wouldn't happen
now was being selected as a research subject in a physiology class. The
teacher wanted women subjects for an experiment on basal metabolic
rates. Another woman and I drew straws; she got the hot room and I got
the cold room. I had to put on a bathing suit and sit in there, monitoring my temperature with a rectal thermometer. My lab partners were
watching, and the whole thing was very cold and very degrading.

The faculty physicians were supportive in general, but I didn't receive
much encouragement from them about my interest in general practice.
Most people went into specialties at that time, and the local family doctor was always considered the low person on the totem pole in terms of
intellect. When I was a senior, I had my first real experience with family
practice because I was one of two people in our class allowed to spend a
semester working with a family physician. That internship really opened
my eyes to a different way of looking at medicine. I lived with the family physician and his wife in a small town in northern Indiana. The doctor was in private practice and made house calls. Everything he did, I
did; it was really wonderful.

In my third year of medical school, I went to work in the Congo for several months with a group of Indiana doctors. A war was on, and the Belgians and others were pulling out, so the hospitals were very short-staffed. We lived in the bush area and worked in a two-hundred-bed hospital with TB wards and a leprosy camp. I was very naïve at the time, but I could still see how U.S. policy had been bungled there and the far from positive role that America can play in other people's history. During a subsequent conflict between tribes, the physician that I worked with there, Glen Eschtruth, was taken out to the bush and killed. Everything about this four-month experience was very significant for me. The people of Congo taught me a lot and brought me a deeper understanding of my own faith. When I left, I fully expected to go back one day. I never thought I'd end up in Washington, D.C.

In an amazing twenty-four hours in June of 1965, my husband to be, Allen, was ordained a United Methodist minister in the afternoon, we were married in the evening, and I graduated from medical school the next morning. Allen and I had actually grown up together in Muncie, but we didn't really date until my junior year of medical school, when he was in his first year at the Garrett Theological Seminary in Chicago, part of Northwestern University.

After we were married, I moved to Chicago to be with him, and I did a one-year rotating internship at Evanston Hospital, affiliated with Northwestern. It was a wealthy hospital, and so there was a lot of observing rather than hands-on experience. We spent the next several years moving back and forth between Chicago and Indiana as my husband continued his postgraduate training and I did various short-time medical jobs to help pay the bills. My first son was born in Indianapolis in 1967. In 1969 we moved to Upland, Indiana, where we stayed until 1976. My husband was head of the speech and drama department at a small Christian college and worked with a religious drama group. I practiced medicine in nearby Marion, Indiana, where I worked at the Marion Hospital as the first dedicated emergency room doctor. Some physicians were afraid they were going to lose their patients to me, but, as I continued my work there, acceptance grew, and finally we had a group of five ER physicians. The hospital, the only one in the county, was very busy and turned out to be a great educational experience for me. It's really where I got my residency training. When I needed a cardiologist, a cardiologist came in; when I needed an OB consult, an obstetrician came by, and so on.

After that, I worked for a year with a group of family physicians. We had two more children by then, and I wanted to work set hours so I could be home when the children were little. The experiences in Marion led me to feel fairly comfortable with most medical situations, which was extremely helpful to me later. When we moved to Washington, D.C., I could walk into an inner-city health service and handle a good deal of the problems on my own.

While we were living in Marion, we were looking for ways to go overseas, but nothing seemed to work out. One of the last ideas we explored, in about 1974, was heading to Pakistan, where my husband was going to teach and I would work in a hospital. We waited months for a visa, but there were so many obstacles being American Christians applying to go to a Muslim country. In the process of waiting for that visa, we came out here to Washington, D.C., for a visit that proved life-changing.

Before the trip to Washington, my awareness of racial inequities and health care needs in this country was very limited. When we lived in Chicago in the mid-sixties, I had had a bird's-eye view of the riots when Martin Luther King Jr. was killed. I remember seeing the fires and the deserted subways in downtown Chicago. But even after that experience I had little direct understanding of suffering and racism in America. In Marion, the African American community lived primarily in just one section of town; I don't remember thinking this was unjust or wondering where these people got health care. In fact, I later learned that Marion had been the northernmost city where a black was hung, back in the 1930s. But my own awareness of this oppressive history just wasn't there; I was very focused on the needs of people overseas and not in this country.

We came to Washington for a weekend to visit a small ecumenical community called Church of the Savior. Members of this community had begun a series of ministries in the Adams Morgan neighborhood. When we arrived, the church had just acquired its first apartment building, called the Ritz. Jim Rouse, a well-known local developer, had an interest in low-income housing and had helped the Church of the Savior buy the apartment building. Before renovation the Ritz was a terrible, run-down, inner-city building, with a leaky roof and garbage all through the basement. It had a terrible smell, and people jammed into every apartment. We were introduced to the tenants in the building, and somehow it came out that I was a physician. Several of the people began telling me how hard it was for them to get health care here; it was an eye-opening experience for me.

After that weekend, we were never quite the same. Although we went back to Upland and kept waiting for the Pakistan visas, we also began to explore the idea of moving to Washington instead. There was no particular health service going on in D.C., and there were already many

United Methodist ministers in the area. But we became more and more certain that we needed to move to Washington. Although we were very certain that God was directing this, we worried about the risks involved— we had three little children, and neither one of us had jobs lined up. In the end, we decided to accept the risks. We felt loony trying to explain our idea to our friends, but we retired the missionary idea and decided to go to Washington to find out what we were all about.

We moved in August 1976 to suburban Columbia, Maryland, where the family would be comfortable but we were close enough to work in inner-city Washington. I took a job as a part-time physician in the emergency room in Howard County Hospital. In Columbia, there was a religious community patterned after Church of the Savior. The Church of the Savior talks about a person's inward journey and outward journey. These journeys involve spending an hour each day alone in prayer and participating in a small mission group in which everyone works toward a common goal. I joined a mission group that focused on health issues, and we soon began working with the Church of the Savior in D.C., opening a part-time health service in the Ritz apartment building. We put up dividers and exam tables in a small community room and went to work.

In 1978 I was asked to help begin a health service in another low-income apartment building that had been purchased by Community of Hope—an organization which provided housing and social services for the neighbors around Belmont Street. The building, unbelievably, was in worse condition than the Ritz. As my practice began to grow with patients from both the Ritz and the Community of Hope, I needed to be on a hospital staff so I could admit and refer patients for specialty care. I checked with Georgetown University Hospital, but they didn't have general practitioners on staff at that time, and they certainly didn't want my uninsured patients. They referred me to Providence Hospital, a community hospital in northeast D.C. with a mission of serving people from the inner city, regardless of insurance status, and I met Sister Irene, a saint of a hospital administrator who made things work at Providence. She welcomed me on to their staff, initiating a wonderful relationship with Providence Hospital that has endured to the present. This, however, didn't solve my problems with diagnostic testing and specialty referrals, so I next appealed to the public hospital, D.C. General. But in 1977 they would make no special arrangements for us, so we had no choice but to send our patients who needed diagnostic tests to the emergency room with a slip of paper and hope for the best. Sometimes this worked, and occasionally—very occasionally—I would get a note back from the hospital with information on the test results. It was extremely frustrating.

In those days, I got into trouble with D.C. General because I preached a "sermon" about these issues during a worship service at a nearby coffeehouse, one of the outreaches of Church of the Savior. I shared my experiences trying to get patients through that D.C. General system, and someone sent a copy to Bob Johnson, the chief administrator at D.C. General at the time. He was madder than a snort at me and sent me a nasty letter. But as the years went on, he became a friend and worked to help community clinics with their referral needs. We tried through interfaith groups and through the D.C. medical society to get a group of specialist physicians to see our patients in their offices, but we never could really get it going. Eventually, with the help of the Catholic archdiocese, we were able to address this problem. Dr. Ed Pelligrino, a Georgetown physician and noted ethicist who was on our Columbia Road board, went to the archbishop of Washington, Archbishop [now Cardinal] Hickey and explained the trouble we were having. Cardinal Hickey wrote all the Catholic physicians in the Washington metropolitan area and invited them to a beautiful dinner at his residence. During dinner, he got up and spoke in terms of the need and connecting it with one's faith journey. Out of that came a small group of physicians who helped set up the Volunteer Health Care Network, which now—twelve years later—consists of about 350 specialists who volunteer their time to see uninsured patients from inner-city clinics. As helpful as it is, the network is swamped with requests. There are simply never enough of certain kinds of specialists.

In 1979, our family moved from our home in Columbia to the Adams Morgan neighborhood where I was working. The decision to move to the city was a major one. We worried about safety issues for the children. What's more, the children thought Columbia was heaven; it had every recreational thing a child could ever want. There have been times since then when we have asked ourselves, "What have we done?" There have been times when the children were frightened, or had things stolen, or were mugged. But if you talked to them now, I think 90 percent of what you would hear would be very positive, a real appreciation of the gift it was for them to live here. Their lives in Maryland had been so separate from the daily suffering we see here. It didn't work for us to just bring the kids by once or twice a week. My patients and the people I

work with are like family to me, and I'm grateful for them. We wanted
the kids to have those kinds of experiences and to really know the richness of the people that we knew. That's one of the joys of being here.

The year 1979 was eventful in another way too. With support from
the W. K. Kellogg Foundation, our small health service expanded and
became the Columbia Road Health Service, and we moved from our original room at the Ritz into a two-bedroom apartment down the street.
Our patient population grew rapidly. I worked as the physician and Allen
as the pastoral counselor. In addition to the Ritz, eight other low-income
apartment buildings in the area were purchased by the Church of the
Savior group called Jubilee Housing for the purpose of renovation and
community building. Our population also changed dramatically. There
was a huge influx of poor Latinos into Washington in the early 1980s
because of the war in El Salvador, so we had to make sure that our staff
could speak Spanish. Later a large number of people from Vietnam also
moved into the nearby Mount Pleasant area.

By 1989, the Columbia Road Health Service had outgrown the two-
bedroom apartment and moved to a new space on Columbia Road in
the heart of Adams Morgan that we still occupy. We continue to this
day providing services to any poor neighborhood resident with no other
resources.

In 1982 two other physicians joined us at Columbia Road Health Ser-
vice, Don Martin and David Hilfiker. David began going with me to
Community of Hope, and Don joined me in going to So Others May Eat
[SOME]. SOME was feeding over a thousand homeless each day, and
Father John Adams invited us to help with the health service.

But it was frustrating because, after seeing these homeless, sick patients, we had to turn them right back into the street. In 1984, Washington, D.C., applied for and received a grant from the Robert Wood
Johnson Foundation and the Pew Charitable Trusts. Thus Washington's
Health Care for the Homeless project was begun and allowed us to begin placing health services directly into the homeless shelters. The first
shelter we went into was Pierce Shelter in an old school building. We did
exams in the coatroom. Eventually we built another little room onto it,
and that was our first on-site health service under the Health Care for
the Homeless grant. At that time the shelters were quite an experience.
There were rats, and sometimes no running water. We carried in water
to wash our hands. The medical teams would see patients at the shelters
but bring their charts to our back-room administrative office at Columbia Road.

Since that time, our activities have expanded, as have the needs. The federal government began support of health care for the homeless with the McKinney Act of 1987 and has provided us funding since that time. The numbers of homeless people increased through the 1980s as the cheap, long-term boarding houses disappeared and more and more people were left out on the street. Drugs were coming in and adding to the problem. Fortunately there were people in Washington like the homeless activist and advocate Mitch Snyder, who wouldn't let anybody forget what was happening here.

The next step was to fulfill the clear need for a place where homeless people we cared for could come to recover from their illnesses. This led to the creation of Christ House, a twenty-four-hour medical facility for homeless men and women with debilitating illnesses. Christ House, a thirty-four-bed, four-story building on Columbia Road, bought and renovated through the generosity of one woman, opened on December 24, 1985. Christ House has been a learning experience for me and part of my faith journey. We thought we knew pretty well who would be coming, but the people were much sicker than we anticipated. I think that situation has worsened as the years have gone by because people are kept in hospitals a much shorter period of time and then put back out on the street. Christ House was not meant to be a permanent residence. The men and women typically stayed a few weeks to a year, and then we tried to help them find apartments. We found, however, that we needed to provide longer-term care to certain of the chronically ill who had multiple health problems like strokes. In January 1996, we opened a permanent housing facility nearby with thirty-seven apartments for chronically ill homeless people. It's called Kairos, which means a special time in someone's life, a time of change.

Christ House was very much a place where we as physicians and staff also wanted to live, since we wanted to be with the people we served. All of the physicians already lived in the neighborhood. David lived just a few blocks away, Don lived down the alley, and our family lived a block away. The decision to move our family to the neighborhood in 1979 had been a major transition in our lives, but when we made the decision to move into Christ House about seven years later, it was a relatively easy transition for everybody. Here, again, we wanted to be closer to the people we were working with.

There are many gathering times at Christ House. The residential community gathers for a meal and sharing each Monday evening. Every Thursday evening everyone joins together for a candlelit dinner where there is a simple liturgy, a good meal, and frequently an African American gospel singing group comes in. The healing that occurs at Christ House is often much deeper than just the physical healing. Persons are encouraged to see themselves as special and gifted. A small group of former Christ House patients now provide leadership for the Kairos program and are on the boards of Columbia Road Health Service and Christ House. On Sunday mornings there is a more formal ecumenical service involving Catholics and Protestants. We use a black Catholic hymnal that has all the old Protestant hymns sung in African American churches. The service is often like an AA meeting with the Eucharist at the end.

One project seemed to lead to another. In addition to the growing numbers of homeless, we also began to see many more patients with HIV. In 1990, three of the men with HIV moved into guest rooms at Christ House and later, with David Hilficker and his family, moved into a house close by to begin Joseph's House, a home for terminally ill persons with HIV. Services for prenatal care were almost nonexistent in this part of town. In 1983 the city approached Columbia Road Health Service with an offer of $50,000 to start a prenatal program. We hired two nurse midwives who were given staff privileges at Providence Hospital and allowed to admit uninsured patients; but the need continued to grow. A few years later we were offered funding by the city to combine our prenatal program at Columbia Road Health Service with a city-funded program. A place for a health service was located a few blocks away on Columbia Road, became a separate nonprofit, and was named Mary's Center. Maria Gomez became the administrator. Today Mary's Center is a beautifully renovated factory building a few blocks away, serving a largely Latino population of mothers, children, and teenagers.

The work of the Healthcare for the Homeless organization grew through the late 1980s and the 1990s. We set up a permanent clinic at the gigantic, 800-bed shelter originally founded by Mitch Snyder and the Community for Creative Non-Violence [CCNV]. We also worked in horrendous emergency family shelters like the Capital City Inn and the Pitts Hotel, in multiple small neighborhood shelters, and at a public housing complex devoid of health services.

During this same period, the city's two large, federally supported community health centers were dying. Their finances were in shambles, and they weren't making payroll. In 1995, in an effort to keep them open, the federal government asked us—Health Care for the Homeless—to take over these two huge centers. This was a tough decision for the Health Care for the Homeless board, for Vince Keane, our executive director, and for me. We knew that the size and problems of the community health centers had the potential to overwhelm the program for the homeless. There was a lot of soul-searching, but we ultimately made the decision to do it. Our hope was that we would enhance our services, not only to the homeless, but also to very poor people. Funded programs label and compartmentalize the poor for the purpose of services, but homeless people and the health center's patients were really all a part of the same larger community.

It was hard initially bringing the two staffs together. The homeless staff felt that they were going to be swallowed up in the new organization, and the health center staff wondered who all these new folks were and whether they really knew anything about community health. But as people began to work together they grew together. In 1997, we changed the name of the whole operation to Unity Health Care, reflecting our larger mission. In 1998, we set up a managed care company called Health Right and competed successfully for a Medicaid managed care contract. Only a little over 10 percent of our patients have Medicaid. So keeping them with us is important to staying open.

These days I spend at least two-thirds of my time doing administrative work and only a day or two a week seeing patients. Administration is not one of my gifts, but it is what needs to be done. We have about twenty-five physicians, nurse practitioners, and physician assistants working for Unity and a total staff of 160. They are wonderful people. They speak half a dozen languages. They come from inner-city D.C., all over the world, and everywhere in between. They do a wonderful job of caring for people despite many obstacles.

I think it's part of a physician's duty to think about the community's health, and part of that involves advocacy work. But invariably that work puts you in conflict with people you have to work with. That's always been a struggle for me. I know I need to work with D.C. General, so how much do I go after them in terms of quality-of-care issues? How much do you go after a TB clinic that at times has no X rays or no developing fluid? A man in the elderly unit at the CCNV shelter, for instance, had abnormal chest X rays. We told the city TB officials, and they dismissed it as "just a little TB." Then we got a sputum positive test result for TB on him, but they still insisted that we keep him in the shelter.

We have always relied on city funding and city programs. We need to be able to work with the health department people and the city politicians. They are our allies in much of what we do. But the city programs have real problems—problems that we know better than anyone. When the situation deteriorated at city shelters, we testified as expert witnesses against the city. That sort of activity is necessary. We couldn't allow people to continue to suffer. We couldn't endanger other people because of bad city policy or programs.

The last straw was the mishandling of a patient in the city prison who was told he had simple pneumonia when he actually had multiple drug resistant [MDR] TB. He was released, became homeless, and was eventually admitted to a local hospital. Then he checked out, used drugs, and was readmitted. Eventually the hospital called the city's public health department. I was working at the CCNV shelter when the health department called wanting to bring the man to the shelter infirmary. I knew he was a sputum-positive, MDR TB patient and I said no, since we could not isolate him and he would be a lethal threat to everyone in the shelter. I was told that there was no other place to put him. We went to the press—and got good coverage on the story. We didn't get the patient, but Christ House, which had received city grants, permanently lost all of its funding—40 percent of the budget. So advocacy work is tricky.

As I think back over the more than twenty years I've worked in this community, there is happiness on several levels. Being part of a supportive community of people has been wonderful and, on a daily basis, just being with people at Christ House has been enriching and brought me lots of joy. A group of us at Christ House has met together regularly year in and year out to talk and to pray. That's my community in terms of discerning new things. I'm never alone in discerning things. It's sitting down with others, seeing that there are other people who have the same dream, who believe that this is something that we are being asked to do. I pray every day on my own, but reflection with others is very important to me, too.

When we first thought about Joseph's House, for example, we realized we would have to go out and borrow money, something we had never done. We were skeptical. I remember Don Martin, one of the physicians who lives at Christ House, reading to us from the Old Testament about looking at things in new ways. We sat there all together, and he told us to go out and find the money. So that's what we did. We had a terrible time borrowing money to open an HIV home. A prominent bank here in the city just outright told us that they did not lend to "the AIDS industry." But we eventually got a loan, and Joseph's House is open and doing wonderful work ten years later.

Christ House has been good for my family as well. My husband oversees the management of both Columbia Road Health Service and Christ

House. He was initially on staff at Potter's House—a ministry of Church of the Savior—and he also developed religious drama. He works as a pastoral counselor at Columbia Road Health Service and provides leadership for the faith community at Christ House. Our oldest son, John, went to law school at Catholic University and is now an attorney with the office of the Senate legislative counsel, working in Medicare areas. He and his wife live nearby, and we have two grandchildren. Mark, our second son, is part of a ministry in Seattle. He is a case manager for homeless persons who stay on the streets of Seattle. He is definitely in the family tradition, but then so is our youngest, Ann. She was an emergency room nurse at D.C. General Hospital but now is in medical school at Howard University. They can all tell some pretty horrendous childhood war stories about living in the city, but I think they all believe it was a good place to grow up.

I feel a sadness in the sense of seeing so much unnecessary suffering. There has definitely been deterioration in terms of health care access. I think it's worse now than at any time I can remember. There are younger people out on the street, many of them crack-addicted, lining up at the soup trucks and kitchens, and clearly feeling hopeless. There are also more people with HIV and substance abuse problems. Even the hospitals, which have often been very generous in the past, are being forced to cut back. We know what it means for someone not to get health care. We know the ravages of sickness on the human body. We know all of that. We've got all the studies we need. Everything is so much worse when you don't have health care—people will end up in ICU who don't need to, babies will be born deformed, people will die. We know all of this, and yet we don't really do anything about it. Morally, we're on a downward path and we will not survive unless something changes.

But I continue to dream. I know that many things that I haven't thought possible in the past have happened. That makes me hopeful for the future.

CHAPTER SEVEN

Building a Better Future

The Case for Primary Care

The stories of the men and women of *Big Doctoring* paint a portrait of primary care as it has been practiced in the latter part of the twentieth century. They are a committed group, partisans of generalism, practitioners of a revitalized, redefined field of medicine. Their work and their lives throw down the gauntlet for the twenty-first century.

Where is primary care headed? Where, indeed, is the health system—which represents one-seventh of the nation's economy—headed? Fifty years from now, would the speakers in this book look back with a sense of satisfaction that their legacy had been valued and built firmly into the country's systems of care and healing, or would they find their tracks erased by an onslaught of technology, specialism, and individualism?

There is, of course, an infinite variety of possibilities as to what shape the future may take. Forces that are not entirely predictable, such as the economy and the advance of science, will have important influences, as will totally imponderable factors, such as war or global calamity. But ten years or fifty years from now, both specialism and generalism are certain to be present in health care because both philosophies are inherent in the ways humans solve problems and manage business. The uncertainty is in what proportion these tendencies will be represented. Will health care be an aggregation of multiple, segmented, specialty services, or will it be a system built around a human healer, a giver and integrator of care? The answer to this question will tell a good deal about the nature of health and well-being in our society.

We have the opportunity to influence the course of events through the principles we enunciate and the investments we make today in areas such as education and public institutions. The rationale for building the base of primary care in this country is compelling. While many Americans like their doctors and are proud of the scientific prowess of the medical system, there is concurrent dissatisfaction with the system as a whole and a realization that its considerable cost does not match up with its more modest outcomes. Many realize that our system is exceedingly expensive, lavish in its use of technology, and undistinguished in its results. The quality of medical care, as measured by everything from consumer satisfaction to iatrogenic deaths, is not high. Fifteen percent of our population does not even have health insurance. By most measures, we have an enormously top-heavy, procedure-prone system dominated by a specialty model of care with relatively little investment in primary care. This system consumes an ever-expanding portion of our gross domestic product, increasingly competing with every other economic interest, personal and public. The health care reform movement of the early 1990s took on this set of problems but failed. The offensive of the late 1990s, touted as a "market solution" to this same conundrum, has not worked either, affronting patients and physicians alike and controlling costs only briefly. And innovation—new pharmaceuticals, diagnostic devices, and treatments—seems only to complicate the decisions that are necessary to craft a system that uses our science effectively, satisfies patients, and is fair.

Primary care built on the broad base of generalism, as practiced by the big doctors profiled in this book, offers the basis for a reconceptualized, rebalanced system of health care in America that will move us beyond the expensive and dispiriting medical swamp in which we have found ourselves in recent years. Toward that end, I offer the following thoughts on the future, a gentle manifesto for the role that primary care can play in improving American health.

TECHNOLOGY AND PRIMARY CARE

Two characteristics of our health care future seem predictable, since they are obvious extrapolations of powerful current trends: continued technological innovation and the ubiquity of information. Together they are going to affect medicine in ways that will underscore the importance of the generalist approach to health care.

Scientific innovation is a permanent feature of the health care system. In the twentieth century biology has given us antibiotics, physics has led to the CAT scan and nuclear magnetic resonance imaging, and exquisite engineering has produced smaller and more effective endoscopes, pacemakers, and insulin pumps. In the twenty-first century, developments in genomics, molecular biology, and computer science will lead to wonderful new diagnostic and treatment tools. The intertwined development of many medical specialties and medical technologies (radiology and the X ray, cardiology and the electrocardiogram, genetics and chromosome mapping) suggests that specialism is the inevitable result of scientific advances. Official and unofficial medical subspecialties continue to proliferate, and the interest of young people in medicine in pursuing these clinically stimulating and financially rewarding opportunities remains high. The scientific and clinical efficiency of specialization is a durable feature of medical care.

Will the continued application of science to health care lead inexorably to more and more specialization and the extinction of the generalist? Intuitive as a positive response to the question may seem, the history of technology does not, in fact, support it. All technologies tend toward simplification and adoption by a larger and less technically trained set of practitioners. Two of the most successful twentieth-century technologies are prime examples of simplification and dissemination: computers and vaccines. The well-known but instructive story of electronic computation starts with the mainframe, a large and complex piece of equipment entirely managed by computer specialists. Improvements in processing technology and miniaturization transformed the mainframe into the now ubiquitous personal computer. The PC is no longer the domain of the specialist but is available to the public at large.

Through the first half of the century, paralytic polio was treated with progressively complex respiratory support mechanisms, of which the "iron lung" was the most complicated and highly developed. It required substantial resources and specialized personnel to deliver its life-sustaining service. The introduction of the polio vaccine in 1953 eliminated the need for the iron lung and moved the management of polio from a high-tech, specialty environment to the pediatrician's office and the public health clinic. Technology radically simplified the "treatment" and delivered it into the hands of generalists.

It is the natural tendency of innovations to move from an exclusive specialty environment to generalists and, sometimes, on to public usage.[1] Medicine is replete with examples of this progression, including blood pressure monitoring, pregnancy tests, and blood glucose checks. Many technologies that were once the domain of specialists are used effectively today by generalist practitioners including the electrocardiogram, the X ray, and the ultrasound. A variety of analyses once performed in specialized labs are now carried out in the primary care office, including rapid tests on blood, urine, and bacterial specimens. Procedures such as flexible sigmoidoscopy and echocardiography, once the exclusive domain of medical subspecialists, are now performed by internists and family physicians. Many medical technologies move from the research lab to the specialist practitioner to the primary care setting with increasing effectiveness and utility.

This natural migration is being complemented by the upgrading of training and competence in primary care. The minimally schooled GP of the early twentieth century has become the residency-trained and board-certified family physician of today. Primary care internal medicine and pediatric residencies are devoting more time to training new physicians for the technological and systems management aspects of medical practice. The advent of the nurse practitioner and physician assistant represents a dramatic example of educational upgrading, with the training of nurses, military medics, paramedics, and college science graduates as advanced-level clinical practitioners. Programs of continuing education and in-service training, now far more developed than in the past, allow primary care practitioners to modify and improve their competencies as science offers more clinical innovations.

Together, the migration of technology to less specialized settings and the progressive upgrading of the primary care workforce will produce a generalist sector prepared to deal effectively and prudently with many illnesses and conditions that were once the domain of specialty practitioners. This process will be accelerated by the growth of evidence-based medicine, the rapid aggregation of information on clinical processes and outcomes that is bringing greater precision to medical practice. Typically, clinical conditions that are poorly understood tend to be dealt with by specialists who work in a problem-solving mode. As a disease is better understood, however, patterns of pathology are discerned, and diagnosis and treatment can be carried out by individuals with less specialized knowledge. Eventually, when the characteristics of the condition are clearly delineated, the diagnosis and treatment can proceed on the basis of guidelines and protocols. This progression means that illnesses previously in the realm of specialists can move "downstream," with generalists assuming a larger role in their management. HIV/AIDS is a good example, as is the management of diabetes and ear infections by nurse practitioners and physician assistants. And the process does not stop with clinicians. The natural downstreaming of technology is meeting an ever more informed public that increasingly will want to take over-the-counter drugs that once required prescriptions, use home tests for strep throat and pregnancy, and make treatment decisions based on information gleaned from the Internet.

Despite the early, natural linkage between technology and specialism, the natural history of innovation is simplification and migration to lower-tech, more regularized settings, which make its benefits less expensive and more broadly available. Certainly some technologies—surgical intervention, for instance—will remain the realm of specialists, but many will evolve in a way that will make them natural elements of primary care practices. These trends suggest that the primary care clinician of the future will provide skilled, scientific care for a broader array of conditions promoting integration, continuity, and perspective in the management of human health. Quality, satisfaction, and costs should all be well served.

INFORMATION, INFORMATION, INFORMATION

In the past, scientific information has been available to the medical community in a relatively rarefied and limited form, used largely by researchers and, to some extent, clinicians. Scientific investigation and new clinical knowledge were entirely paper-dependent, with medical journals and professional meetings serving as the principal vehicles of information dissemination. Specialty medicine benefited the most from the information that science yielded, forming clinical disciplines built around specific domains of information. Among the most constant allegations against the old GPs was that they "weren't up-to-date" and "didn't practice scientific medicine." Scarce, cumbersome, and arcane, scientific information in medicine barely trickled out to the general public. The electronic revolution, however, means that the information landscape is changing rapidly and permanently. Physicians, patients, insurance companies, and governments will all have access to data in ways that would have been unimaginable in the past. Data on individuals, groups, and populations will make possible all manner of ratings and projections which, in turn, will stimulate the further development of evidence-based guidelines for the management of health and disease. All of this will be readily accessible to health professionals and the public, research scientists and clinicians, specialists and generalists.

Information, indeed, is a vital asset for the future of primary care.

While the adage that no one can know everything in any field grows more pertinent every day, the tools for managing information are developing more quickly than knowledge itself. The computerized medical record, electronic databases, and powerful programs for decision analysis are being matched by the omnipresence of the personal computer and of compact, portable information management devices. The primary care clinician of the future will be able to retrieve information, manage it, and bring detail to bear on diagnosis and treatment in ways far more precise and profound than ever before. Well-managed information will empower the generalist to speak with clinical insight and authority and address the chronic challenge to primary care practice, that no one can possibly "keep up" except in limited, specialty areas. The ready availability of information will enhance both the quality and the span of the generalist's counsel to patients. The primary care clinician, for instance, will be able to discuss personalized prevention with patients, equipped with complete information about the individual's health history but also armed with cohort and population data that will allow doctor and patient to review hazards and options based on current, community-wide trends.

These emerging capabilities suggest a further role for the generalist of the future. The generalist, broadly trained and powered by new information systems, is in a key position to practice population medicine— the intersection between personal care and public health. Generalists working in managed care organizations have been exploring this role, but the long-term commitment of these organizations to patient populations in the current competitive environment has been limited. The prudent use of resources is always important to an organization (private or public, for-profit or not-for-profit), but the investment made in long-term prevention depends on the organization's perception of its long-term responsibility to its members. Whatever the fate of managed care as it has been practiced in the past, the future will surely have systems that care for patients over time, systems that will inevitably value both prudent resource use in the present and good prevention strategies for the long term. Primary care clinicians are well placed to play central roles in these organizations, both by taking primary clinical responsibility for panels of current patients and by playing a leading role in the management and strategic thinking for the long haul.

Genetics is probably the best current example of the intersection of technology, information, and primary care. The success of the Human Genome Project has raised the possibility of genetically driven breakthroughs in the diagnosis and treatment of conditions that lie buried in our genetic makeup. We are confronted with the likelihood of waves of new genetic information becoming available, pertinent at times to the population as a whole and, at other times, to individuals with specific conditions. Until recently medical genetics had relatively little to offer to patients because its clinical applicability was strictly limited. What happens now, as vast quantities of information become available, raising varieties of testing questions and the potential for new treatment choices? Does this call for a rapid expansion of the clinical specialty of genetics? Will every concerned citizen have to have a geneticist to advise her what tests to take and what to make of the results?

The answer is no—unless we are seeking to construct a system of endless fragmentation and cost. There is a better solution. Clearly it will take a firm scientific base for a clinician to advise patients on how and when to proceed with expensive and difficult decisions about genetic testing and treatments. But this is a field in which emerging information can move readily from the research setting to clinical protocols and be made available electronically to both doctor and patient. Primary care practitioners are naturally positioned to discuss issues in genetic testing and treatment and should be the first line of counsel and education for patients. Clinical genetics will need to be given clear emphasis in the future training of generalist practitioners to keep them abreast of emerging developments. The alternative notion—that every family would have a geneticist the way they have, say, a dentist—is implausible, and so, by extension, is the notion's application to other emerging areas of human biology that will require similar anticipatory and preventive deliberations. Rather, these situations call for the well-trained generalist who knows the individual well and can help him navigate a system that will surely grow more complicated.

THE BATTLE FOR THE FUTURE

More technology and more and better information are certain to be features of health care in the future. Other probable trends include increased consumer involvement in health care, a strong focus on wellness, and a heightened concern about the quality of care. We are looking at an inexorable demographic shift toward an older population and, since the cost of health care is again on the rise, we can expect constant tensions (personal and public) over health care expenses. In this environment patients are going to continue to need care—smart, able, responsive, affordable healing and succor. New importance, though, will inevitably be placed on the ability of doctors to interpret and coordinate information and services. Patients faced with quantities of data and multiple therapeutic choices will value clinicians who can help them weigh options and choose courses of action. Referrals will be a key to success in this world. Knowing where to go, and when, is a challenge that will only get more difficult as information and options proliferate. The doctor who can help her patients navigate the system by referring prudently but well will be critical in managing satisfaction, cost, and quality.

Imagine for a moment a world without primary care, a future that devalues and marginalizes primary care, a projection from today that builds on the most centrifugal and most individualistic tendencies of our present system. Increasing numbers of highly trained but narrow specialists would pursue their crafts in relative isolation. Innovations would be rampant, expensive, poorly validated, and inequitably distributed. Direct-to-consumer advertising would drive much of the system with TV, newsletters, websites, and chat rooms offering a cacophony of information and advice. Patients would shop in a kind of medical food court, choosing providers or interventions based on data acquired from scientific references randomly mixed with exhortations from commercial and self-serving sources. Whatever the appeal of this world might be to the libertarians among us, it is a formula for rapid escalation in costs, maximum discontinuity of care, bad outcomes, and continued barriers to universal coverage.

There is an alternative. The abiding and, in many ways, the most important quality of primary care is that it provides a centering force for both individuals and systems. It offers coordination, integration, and perspective. Primary care provides the human touch—the relationship that will pull the system together and add value for the patient. The future might best be constructed around the empowered generalist model, in which the principal responsibility for patient management resides with primary care practitioners. In this model the generalist and the patient together serve as thoughtful consumers of technology, calling on specialists for advanced or invasive treatments but not for regular care. This is really the general contractor model of health care, borrowed from the construction industry. The general contractor is a broad expert who, working with the client, coordinates specialized activities. Working with the patient, the generalist will decide when to call on a cardiologist, when a psychiatrist is necessary for the treatment of depression, or which of the available cancer centers would be best to work up a newly diagnosed mass in the colon. The generalist will be the human magnet who holds the increasingly centrifugal world of medicine together for the individual. This role, of course, is not a new one for the generalist, but the challenges of a highly technological and potentially fragmented system are greater than ever. Specialists tend to see the world through the prism of their specialty, and that view may lack perspective, balance, and in some cases good judgment. Decisions in areas such as end-of-life treatment, the initiation of life-long medications, and surgical interventions for benign prostatic hyperplasia or strategies for breast cancer treatment all deal with areas of specialized skills but call for a generalist perspective. It is big doctoring, the smart clinician who knows the patient and, ideally, the family, who can help patients with the many complex life decisions they will face. The generalist of the future will be part pilot and part air traffic controller. He will be committed to the care of the individual, but he will also help the patient steer through the complicated and risky system.

The aging of our society presents a particular challenge to primary care. Good public health practice and advancing science together are keeping people alive longer, rapidly increasing the size and age of the elderly population. As a result, geriatric care and geriatric medicine will become ever more prominent parts of health care in the United States. These are quintessentially generalist challenges that meld clinical science with issues of quality-of-life and palliative care. It is the generalist who holds the promise of charting a sensible course for patients through the thickets of age-related illness, where the potential for costly, wasteful, painful, and degrading interventions abound. Perspective, perspective, and perspective will be the running rules of this work, and this is the currency of primary care. The integrative, supportive, educational, and, at times, pastoral role of the generalist will be vital to the future care of the elderly in America.

Despite the impact of technology and informatics, human birth, growth, maturity, debility, and death will continue. Fifty years from now parents will still be tenaciously involved with the health of their children, the elderly will still want to die with dignity, and mental health, birth control, and infectious disease will still be important medical topics. Medical knowledge and medical possibilities will increase, but monitoring and managing the human life cycle is an enterprise that is generalist to the core. This is not a romantic idea but a practical one. We will need the generalist in the future not because we know so little but because we know so much. Balance, navigation, and ombudsmanship will simultaneously become more important to keeping the system effective and human.

PROMOTING PRIMARY CARE

Rescuing American health care from progressive fragmentation and expense will require this country to make some plans. This is the realm of health policy, where values, data, and intellect come together in decisions about the ground rules and funding of our health system. Sometimes these decisions are enabling (funds for biomedical research or the National Health Service Corps), and sometimes they are restrictive (licensure laws and limits on tobacco advertising). Forces outside health care, such as technology and the economy, influence the character of the system, but it is the policy process that offers the most palpable and objective opportunity for shaping health care in America. It is here that primary care must wage battle.

Primary care is peculiarly dependent on health policy. The technological commercialism that drives much of the medical sector today is a natural engine for specialty medicine. The capital investments behind many medical innovations and new pharmaceuticals directly and indirectly promote specialty medicine through such mechanisms as direct-to-consumer advertising and subsidized training for medical specialists in the use of new technologies. The cognitive and nonprocedural work—the talking and deliberating—that comprises much of primary care can claim no such benefactors. Primary care, therefore, is far more sensitive to and dependent on the policies governing health care (laws, regulations, and compensation formulas) than is specialty medicine. If those policies are supportive of primary care and create an environment in which generalism can thrive, the future role of primary care in the system will be a substantial one. If, to the contrary, those policies do not nurture and support the idea of primary care, highly fractionated systems of specialty care will prevail. The nature, therefore, of health policy, in realms from education and reimbursement through the priorities of private purchasers and insurance intermediaries, will be crucial for the success of primary care.

There are six broad areas of policy in which the primary care agenda needs to be articulated and pursued to build a better system. They are: systems reform; compensation; education; professional structure; communication; and leadership.

Systems Reform: Putting Primary Care at the Center

A generalist system needs to be built on a generalist base. Every patient should have a designated primary care clinician who will serve as their doctor of *first* resort and their source of referral for specialized needs. This concept is essential to constructing care that is accountable and coordinated.

This principle has been at the core of health maintenance organizations since their inception and is also the basis on which systems in many other countries, including Canada and Great Britain, are constructed. The use of the "primary care gatekeeper" by the burgeoning commercial managed care movement of the mid-1990s has created a negative patient reaction to "gatekeeping" and, in some cases, to primary care itself. Patient frustration has been fueled by the unstable commercial health insurance market, in which many businesses switch health plans yearly, requiring their employees to change doctors each time. Continuity, the doctor-patient relationship, and health maintenance are all casualties of the vicissitudes of a situation that has been created not by health policy but by the commercial insurance market. Primary care is going to have to stand firm on the centrality of the generalist to the care of all patients. Despite the churning of managed care plans and patients' objections to heavy-handed gatekeeping, the principle that every citizen have and use a primary care clinician is of paramount importance. The enactment of a single-payer form of national health insurance would facilitate the creation of a primary care–based system, but the same goal can be attained through the pluralistic system that exists now. Financial incentives and benefit packages need to be structured to promote patient selection of primary care services and a specific primary care clinician. A broad campaign of patient education needs to be undertaken to provide encouragement and support for primary care selection, and patients must be able to keep their primary care providers regardless of the vicissitudes of the insurance world. The route to full implementation of a primary care–based system will depend heavily on creating incentives in health plans for both patients and doctors to make the primary care provider the pivotal player in the system. Public (Medicaid and Medicare) and private insurance plans need to embrace this standard fully, and primary care proponents need to speak firmly in advocating it.

Among the innovations that managed care has brought to primary care practice is capitation, a monthly payment from insurance companies to physicians based on the number of patients enrolled in a practice, regardless of whether the patients are seen. This system has the benefit of giving the physician and the insurance company predictable monthly cash transfers. What it does not cover is "risk": the likelihood that the patient will need special tests, referrals, or hospitalizations. In many plans today, the physician is asked to assume the risk in return for a higher capitation payment, meaning that the cost of tests, referrals, or hospitalizations effectively comes out of the doctor's pocket. This creates a conflict of interest: what is best for the patient's health may be at odds with what is best for the doctor's finances. The generalist has to be the unequivocal advocate of the patient. This by no means suggests that she will agree to every referral or test that the patient might want, but it does mean that she cannot have a personal financial stake in these decisions. Capitation itself is not the problem. Risk allocation is, and the primary care system of the future needs to pay the generalist without resorting to compromising incentives. The generalist cannot be a trusted counselor and an agent of the insurance carrier at the same time.

Entering the twenty-first century, more than 40 million Americans are without health insurance. Quantities of evidence confirm that the lack of health insurance is associated with disproportionate debility and death—an enormous inequity in a wealthy country. The barriers to care inherent in the lack of health insurance cause problems all along the spectrum of service delivery, but they are at their most unfair with regard to primary care. The United States is today the only country in the developed world that does not have a system in place to assure primary care services to all of its citizens. Universal coverage must be at the top of any policy agenda and an integral part of a primary care–based system.

Compensation: Pay Parity for Primary Care

Payment policy is of critical importance to any field. Over the years primary care has been systematically underpaid. As specialty medicine emerged in the first part of the twentieth century, its practitioners were able to charge paying patients "usual and customary" fees for their services that were well in excess (on an absolute and on a per-hour-worked basis) of those charged by primary care physicians. In the latter part of the twentieth century, with the emergence of systematized billing and the universal adoption of relative value scales, the differential between primary care pay per hour and specialty pay per hour became entrenched in the system. Diagnostic and therapeutic procedures can be billed at rates far in excess of what nonprocedural physicians can expect to be paid for their time. This differential has played a central role in attracting physicians into specialty medicine and promoting a system that is heavily subspecialty-based. We must pay our generalists on a par with our specialists, or they will forever work at a disadvantage, and the system will remain forever tilted toward specialty care.

Health care legislation in recent years has been incremental rather than omnibus. The failure of the Clinton health reform effort and the subsequent passage of legislation such as the 1996 Health Insurance Portability and Accountability Act (the Kennedy-Kassebaum Act) and the 1997 State Child Health Insurance Program suggest that the efforts to expand health insurance coverage will develop piece by piece. Whatever the shape of the increment (for children, for mothers and children, expanded Medicaid eligibility, lowering the age of Medicare eligibility, etc.), primary care will surely be covered, creating both a better financial environment for primary care providers and an increased demand for their services. Both developments will have positive implications for generalist practice, making some clinical settings such as safety-net providers more financially viable and increasing the demand for primary care clinicians.

Compensation policy in the future must be rebalanced to increase the pay for the noninterventional treatment, counseling, and education that generalists provide. Policies designed to do this will have the double benefit of supplying a relative incentive for young clinicians to choose primary care careers and a relative disincentive to procedural overuse in the specialty sector. Both outcomes would provide important stability and cost containment for the system as a whole.

Education: What Are They Learning in School?

If primary care is to be central to the delivery system, it must be central to the missions and curricula of medical, nursing, and other health science schools. The selection of students, course offerings, faculty role modeling, and institutional values all exert powerful influences on the career choices and attitudes of future clinicians. Medical education is particularly challenged in this regard because medical schools double as research centers, with faculty salaries, promotion, and prestige often tied to research achievements. In this environment, primary care is easily marginalized and discounted. Few generalists serve as department chairs in internal medicine or pediatrics; many of the best-known medical schools have been reluctant to develop family medicine departments; and everywhere faculty members challenge students interested in generalist careers with disparaging comments about primary care. Medical education at all of these institutions is nonetheless built on a primary care base, with generalist physicians teaching the foundation courses in physical diagnosis and clinical medicine. They are advisers, teachers, and role models, yet the importance of their generalist work to education and service is frequently discounted.

Health professions schools, and particularly medical schools and teaching hospitals, need to put a high priority on the task of educating the generalist. The size and quality of the primary care workforce needs to be seen as one of their core responsibilities and measures of their success—not as an afterthought to training specialists or creating new biomedical technologies. This is not an easy mission, and it cannot be relegated—as it often has been—to rural or state-supported schools. It needs to be manifest at all of our educational institutions, including those that are private, urban, and research-oriented. Currently there is no commonly defined "core curriculum" for primary care. Departments of pediatrics, internal medicine, and family medicine rarely collaborate on educational substance, even though there is considerable overlap in the clinical principles they are charged with teaching. Bridges—causeways, really—need to be constructed between admissions strategy, the preclinical and clinical curriculum, and residency instruction in the primary care disciplines. Many of these principles and much of this instruction pertain to the training of physician assistants and nurse practitioners as well, inviting the creation of a modular, interdisciplinary curriculum. Streamlining and coordinating the core generalist curriculum would provide welcome efficiency and collegiality for all students of primary care.

Training for the generalist must include not only clinical medicine but also instruction in systems and systems management, informatics, decision science, and communications. Courses normally taught in graduate schools of business, social work, and communications need to be incorporated into the health sciences curriculum. These are skills that will produce a practitioner with a more diverse set of capabilities and position these clinicians to work effectively and centrally in the health care environment of the future. Adapting the findings and implications of genetic information to the primary care curriculum will be another important challenge, as will developing better and more extensive teaching in geriatrics. The many issues entailed in the development of a primary care–based system in the United States, in fact, call for new knowledge not only in clinical areas but also in epidemiology, health services research, economics, and sociology. These are tasks for academic health centers.

Government funding provides important levers in educational policymaking, and all levers should be pulled on behalf of primary care. State governments are principal players in the funding of medical schools and training programs for nurse practitioners and physician assistants, and state health policymakers will have an important role to play in steering the priorities and educational strategies of these institutions. The federal government plays a much more important role with regard to graduate medical education where, through Medicare direct and indirect graduate medical education funding, important funding is provided to training hospitals. Graduate medical education (GME) is a governing part of the educational continuum since it is an absolute requirement for obtaining a medical license and entering practice in the United States. Many efforts during the last decade have been directed at modifying policies governing GME funding to encourage more training in primary care. Although most of these proposals (legislative and otherwise) have failed, the continued expenditure of large sums of money (over $6 billion in 2000) makes federal GME policy a particularly important arena for future primary care strategists.

Targeted subsidies for training in primary care medicine, nurse practice, and physician assistant programs have been part of Titles VII and VIII of the Public Health Service Act since the 1960s. The support for these programs is relatively modest compared to Medicare GME funds. Nonetheless, they provide valuable venture capital for educational institutions prepared to engage in new and creative education. Over the past three decades, these funds have been instrumental in the development of primary care programs. Their continued presence and potential augmentation will be important. The National Health Service Corps, which funds scholarship and loan repayment for individuals prepared to work as primary care providers in underserved areas, is also significant in this effort. Finally, the training programs of the Department of Veterans' Affairs provide substantial faculty and residency augmentation to academic health centers. These programs have tended to drift with the subspecialty tide of the last decades but, given the aging and needy population of veterans, the potential for substantial upgrading of primary care service and training in these institutions is considerable.

Professional Structure: Primary Care "Architectural" Reform

Primary care has (at a minimum) five different manifestations: family medicine, pediatrics, internal medicine, nurse practice, and physician assistants. While this structure is understandable historically, it creates confusion with the public and uncertainty among payers and providers themselves. Although some degree of ferment within primary care is healthy, five different patterns of schooling, three different professions, and multiple interpretations create an "architecture" of primary care that is unwieldy and a business plan that is almost unmanageable.

Proposals for the merger or realignment of the primary care disciplines, however, have gone nowhere. Collaboration between pediatricians and internists has led to a double residency—a training route that produces an internist-pediatrician with two board certifications. Talks between the board-certifying organizations in internal medicine and family medicine failed to produce a new alliance. The gulf between nursing and medicine remains large and contentious as nurse practitioners increase their training and skill level while insisting that they remain "nurses" and not "doctors." Physician assistants and nurse practitioners are both adamant about their origins and the nuances in their training programs and modes of practice. The possibility of collaboration, let alone codification, within the primary care community seems remote. Nonetheless, new thinking and cooperation are badly needed.

The presence of large numbers of residency-trained family physicians in primary care suggests a starting point for discussions of realignment. Family physicians are more numerous in smaller and rural communities, where their broad capabilities offer an efficient means of primary care delivery. In cities, general internists and pediatricians provide a higher proportion of generalist services, though family practice residencies and practitioners are becoming more common. The doubly trained med-peds physicians, likewise, offer a kind of family-doctor-less-obstetrics model for urban and rural areas. The advent of the hospitalist offers further grounds for reconsidering the arrangement of primary care, with the possibility of dividing the terrain between the ambulatory generalist and the inpatient generalist.

If empirical evidence bears out the promise of nonphysician clinicians (nurse practitioners and physician assistants) providing primary care at the level of physicians, it would make sense to formalize their training at the doctoral level. Such a strategy would unify and upgrade the education of primary care clinicians. Credit would be given for previous clinical experience (as a nurse, for example), training programs for the two disciplines would be standardized, and an internship year would be added to intensify clinical training. Graduating with a doctoral degree, practitioners would join the workforce with didactic and practical training in the full scope of primary care.

Simplification and standardization of the architecture of primary care would help immeasurably in the delivery of service as well as in policy proposals and political debates. Many difficult current issues, such as licensure, scope of practice, referral patterns, hospital privileges, quality assurance, and oversight would be clarified. Patients, payers, and insurers would have a direct and reliable relationship with the primary care sector. Relationships between specialists and generalists would be better understood. And the primary care sector could speak for itself in a far more uniform and articulate fashion than is currently the case.

Communication: A Better Message

While health care professionals may have a clear understanding of primary care, many members of the public do not. The idea is not as simple as general practice once was and not as intuitively obvious as, say, the specialty of cardiology. The mission of primary care is complicated because it is, quite literally, so big. Primary care is complex because it entails caring for people through all stages of life, treating multiple interrelated conditions, dealing with physical and mental health, and keeping an eye on family and community issues as well as public policy as it relates to health. It is difficult to capture this mission neatly with simple labels or phrases, resulting in a considerable lack of understanding about the nature, potential, and persona of primary care.

How, then, is primary care to be packaged, explained, popularized, and publicized? Is there a television series to be made that could feature the work of a family physician and nurse practitioner? Are there profiles for *Parade* magazine or the Sunday supplement to be written about primary care "heroes"? How do we explain the issues of compensation policy or graduate medical education reform on the op-ed pages of the nation's newspapers? These challenges and a dozen more are the domain of communications policy and must be a part of the overall primary care strategy.

Leadership: Who's in Charge Here, Anyway?

For primary care to thrive in the United States, smart strategic leadership will be critical. This premise immediately raises the question of who speaks for primary care? Primary care has many manifestations, each of which has its own educational continuum, certifying authorities, professional organizations, journals, and turf. Family physicians speak with one voice and nurse practitioners with another. Some pediatricians see themselves defined entirely by child health and some internists by geriatrics. The common ground of primary care is not part of their view of the world. There is no alliance that can speak for primary care as a sector, and, as a result, individual organizations tend to develop policy positions or lobby for legislation from the perspective of specific disciplines. Primary care easily falls between the planks of the many organizations active in the field. Many speak *about* primary care, but no one speaks *for* primary care. It has no dedicated publications, meetings, or primary membership. This reality stands in marked contrast to most professional groups.

The creation of a national primary care coalition would address the absence of leadership in the field. Such a coalition would move the representation of primary care from an avocational status to a professional one, playing a principal role in primary care policy issues, engaging in analytical and political activities, providing professional and public education, and representing the primary care community to the government and the public. It would sponsor publications and convene professional meetings. It would give muscle and voice to the primary care movement.

Participation in such an alliance could extend well beyond the medical and nursing groups involved in the delivery of primary care. Citizen organizations, managed care organizations, employers, and payers might all take part. The business community, with a large stake in the future costs of health care, should be heavily involved, as should trade unions, consumer groups, and the public health community. The coalition itself would be a training ground for the leaders who will develop and articulate the policy positions for primary care in the future. Such an organization could radically redefine the mission and effectiveness of primary care.

OUR CHOICE

Our success in these areas of public policy will determine to a great extent the nature of the health care delivery system in the United States in the years to come. The obvious forces at play are political and economic, but the outcome will reflect our values and philosophy as a country. Will we work to give all of our citizens affordable, humanistic care? Will we commit ourselves to principles of equity and effectiveness in health care, a course that will inevitably lead to a primary care–based system? Or, to the contrary, will we promote individualized, technological solutions to medical problems regardless of the consequences for the society as a whole—a direction certain to maintain the irregularities in quality and access in our current system?

I am optimistic. I believe big doctoring will prevail. It will prevail because generalism is a powerful organizing concept itself and has a long history in medical care. It will also prosper because new technologies themselves will create a growing demand for interpretation, coordination, and the human touch to provide entrée to the system, continuity of care, and succor in times of sickness and death. Under whatever name, this will be primary care in America.

Acknowledgments

The idea for *Big Doctoring in America* first took shape more than ten years ago. Since then many people have contributed oral histories, editorial commentary, and helpful advice to the project. Although I will surely fail to mention some, I want to acknowledge as many of those as possible.

First, I thank individuals whose support made the entire enterprise possible. Steve Schroeder, Lew Sandy, and Susan Hassmiller of the Robert Wood Johnson Foundation provided funding and encouragement from early in the project. The Pew Charitable Trusts have also provided generous core support. Special thanks go to Rebecca Rimel and Carolyn Asbury.

Dan Fox, president of the Milbank Memorial Fund, has been an important friend and colleague. In addition to providing financial support, he has been a commentator, critic, and editor of my writings (*Big Doctoring in America* and others) and selected *Big Doctoring in America* for publication in the series California/Milbank Books on Health and the Public. My special thanks go to Dan for his vision, advice, and support.

Seventy-five physicians, nurse practitioners, and physician assistants gave generously of their time and life stories in providing me with oral histories for the project. Fifteen of their stories appear in the book, and the oral histories of the other sixty have been deposited in the Primary Care Oral History Collection at the National Library of Medicine in Bethesda, Maryland. Those individuals deserve special thanks from me and others who will study the history of primary care at the end of the twentieth century. They are Tom Almy, Joel Alpert, John Anderson, Cathy Anderton, Manuel Archuleta, Jeffrey Belden, Elizabeth Berry, Thomas Bodenheimer, Linnea Capps, Arthur Chen, Robert Cohen, William Cole, John Coombs, Terry Crowson, Amos Deinard, Diane Drew, Paul Eneboe, Genia English, Alan Mark Firestone, Virginia Fowkes, Carol Garvey, John Geyman, Catherine Gilliss, Elsie Giorgi, Walter Henze, Bella Hermosa-Villacorta, John Horder, Frank Hubbell, Tim Hughes, William Jacott, Barbara Janeway, Stanley Kardatzke, Jack Kirk, Coleen Kivlahan, Ellen Silverberg Levine, Aliza Lifshitz, David Loxterkamp, John Lucas, Marshall Marinker, Alexander McPhedran, Robert Monroe, Susana Morales, Thomas Nichswander, Stanley Padilla, Richard Perry, Sridevi Pinnamaneni, James Reinertsen, William Robertson, Joseph Scherger, Nancy Schupp, Frederic Schwartz, Terrance Sheehan, Robert Smithing, John Stoeckle, Reed Tuckson, Julian Tudor-Hart, Rodman Wilson, John Winklmann, John Yindra, and Quentin Young.

Numbers of people helped along the way by providing suggestions for good candidates for oral histories. Thanks in this category go to Oli Fein, Steve Cohen, Jack Colwill, Jim Schneid, Dan Onion, Steve Kairys, John Wasson, Gil Welsh, and Elliott Fisher.

Two important figures in American letters and leading practitioners of their particular forms of biography, Studs Terkel and John McPhee, generously coached me on the techniques of personal journalism, the interview, and the recording of oral history.

When the final manuscript was completed, the Milbank Fund assembled a group of experts in primary care, medical history, and health policy to review the draft. As a result of their comments, I undertook major and beneficial rewriting. I thank them for the time and interest they took. They were Ruth Ballweg, Michael Carter, Carolyn Clancy, Jack Colwill, Ann Davis, Nancy Dickey, Mary Anne Dumas, Bob Graham, Gordon Moore, Ed O'Neil, Joyce Pulcini, Richard Roberts, Lawrence Ronan, Lewis Sandy, Barbara Starfield, Rosemary Stevens, and John Stoeckle. Additionally, a number of other primary care physicians reviewed the manuscript and gave me feedback: Joshua Sharfstein, Malathi Srinivasan, Adam Gordon, Scott Gottlieb, Paul Jung, Beaulette Hooks, and Greg Randolph.

During the five years that I spent collecting oral histories and working on the text of *Big Doctoring in America*, I was based at the health policy journal *Health Affairs* published by Project HOPE in Bethesda, Maryland. I thank John Iglehart, *Health Affairs*' founding editor, who provided friendship, advice, and a wonderful place to work during this period. Additionally, the secretarial and editorial support of Nancy Trosky, Meredith Zimmerman, Linda Simmerson, and Judie Tucker was been very helpful to me and the project. Kyna Rubin and Madelyn Ross provided valuable additional editorial assistance. Finally, I thank Lynne Withey and Erika Bűky, my editors at the University of California Press, for editorial help and general good counsel.

Notes

INTRODUCTION

1. Gerard F. Anderson, Jeremy Hurst, Peter Sotir Hussey, and Melissa Jee-Hughes, "Health Spending and Outcomes: Trends in OECD Countries, 1960–1998," *Health Affairs,* 2000; 19(3):150–157.

2. World Health Report 2000. Available at: http://www.who.int/whr, accessed February 26, 2001. See also Barbara Starfield, "Is US Health Really the Best in the World?" *Journal of the American Medical Association,* 2000; 284:483–485.

CHAPTER ONE

1. Fitzhugh Mullan. "The Mona Lisa of Health Policy: Primary Care at Home and Abroad," *Health Affairs,* 1998; 17(2):118–26.

2. *Primary Care: America's Health in a New Era,* ed. Molla S. Donaldson, Karl D. Yordy, Kathleen N. Lohr, and Neil A. Vanselow (Washington, D.C.: National Academy Press, 1996), p. 1.

3. Institute of Medicine, *A Manpower Policy for Primary Health Care* (Washington, D.C.: National Academy of Sciences, 1978), pp. 16–20.

4. There is a considerable body of literature on the cost, quality, and patient satisfaction related to primary care. Particularly useful in this regard is chapter 3 entitled "The Value of Primary Care" in *Primary Care: America's Health in a New Era,* ed. Donaldson et al.; Barbara Starfield, *Primary Care: Balancing Health Needs, Services, and Technology* (New York: Oxford University Press, 1998); and chapter 1 entitled "What Is Primary Care?" in Eric J. Cassell, *Doctoring: The Nature of Primary Care Medicine* (New York: Oxford University Press/Milbank Memorial Fund, 1997).

5. Barbara Starfield, "Primary Care and Health: A Cross-National Comparison," *Journal of the American Medical Association,* 1992; 268:2032–2033.

6. Avedis Donabedian as quoted by Fitzhugh Mullan in "A Founder of Quality Assessment Encounters a Troubled System Firsthand," *Health Affairs,* 2001; 20(1):138.

7. Peter M. Senge, *The Fifth Discipline: The Art and Practice of the Learning Organization* (New York: Doubleday Currency, 1990) p. 3.

8. Important sources on the history of primary care in the context of the medical system in general are Rosemary Stevens, *American Medicine and the Public Interest* (Berkeley and Los Angeles: University of California Press, 1971; 1998), and Paul Starr, *The Social Transformation of American Medicine* (New York: Basic Books, 1982). The later chapters of John Duffy, *The Healers: A History of American Medicine* (Urbana: University of Illinois Press, 1976), are also helpful. The essays in John D. Stoeckle and George Abbott White, *Plain Pictures of Plain Doctoring: Vernacular Expression in New Deal Medicine and Photography* (Cambridge: MIT Press, 1985), tell a great deal about rural medicine in the pre–World War II period—particularly the chapter entitled "Primary Care in the 1930s" (pp. 52–80).

9. Committee on the Cost of Medical Care, *Medical Care for the American People: The Final Report of the Committee on the Cost of Medical Care,* Publication No. 28 (Chicago: University of Chicago Press, 1932), p. 63.

10. American Medical Association, Directory of Approved Internships and Residencies, selected years as cited by Stevens, American Medicine, and the Public Interest, p. 393.

11. Kerr White, T. Franklin Williams, and B. G. Greenberg. "The Ecology of Medical Care," *New England Journal of Medicine,* 1961; 265:885–893.

12. This discussion of the history of family medicine is drawn from *Family Practice: Creation of a Specialty: A Narrative of Events Leading to the Establishment of the American Board of Family Practice in 1969 and Reminiscences of Men Who Were on the Scene* (Kansas City, Mo.: The American Academy of Family Physicians, 1980); Stanley R. Truman, M.D., *The History of the Founding of the American Academy of General Practice* (Kansas City, Mo.: Warren H. Green, Inc., and the American Academy of General Practice, 1969); R. Neil Chisholm, "The History of Family Practice" in *Family Medicine: Principles and Practice,* ed. Robert B. Taylor (Kansas City, Mo.: Springer-Verlag, 1978) pp. 7–12; and David P. Adams, "Evolution of the Specialty of Family Practice," *Journal of the Florida Medical Association,* 1989; 76:325–329.

13. For a more complete discussion of the history of the nurse practitioner and physician assistant professions please see chapter 3 of this volume, "The New Clinicians."

14. Association of American Medical Colleges, *AAMC Data Book: Statistical Information Related to Medical Schools and Teaching Hospitals,* January, 1999. Table B-13, p. 31.

15. *The Registered Nurse Population, March 2000: Findings from the National Sample Survey of Registered Nurses—March 2000* (Washington, D.C.: Department of Health and Human Services, Health Resources and Services

Administration, Bureau of Health Professions, Division of Nursing), p. 50. This survey indicates that as of the year 2000, 102,829 individuals had received formal preparation as nurse practitioners; 91,591 of them were employed in nursing; and 58,512 were working in positions with the title of nurse practitioner. I have chosen to cite this latter figure in the text since it most nearly corresponds to the number of nurse practitioners working in that capacity.

16. American Academy of Physician Assistants, *Information Update*, October 8, 1999, Alexandria, Va., p. 3.

17. Sarah Brotherton, Frank Simon, Sandra Tomany, "U.S. Graduate Medical Education, 1999–2000," *Journal of the American Medical Association*, 2000; 248:1121–1126.

18. Robert M. Wachter and Lee Goldman, "The Emerging Role of 'Hospitalists' in the American Health Care System," *New England Journal of Medicine*, 1996; 335(7):514–517.

19. A. Fernandez, K. Grumbach, L. Goitein, K. Vranizan, D. H. Osmond, A. B. Bindman, "Friend or Foe?: How Primary Care Physicians Perceive Hospitalists," *Archives of Internal Medicine*, 2000; 160(19):2902–2908.

20. Mary O. Mundinger et al., "Primary Care Outcomes in Patients Treated by Nurse Practitioners or Physicians: A Randomized Trial," *Journal of the American Medical Association*, 2000; 283:59–68.

CHAPTER THREE

1. Joel Alpert, "The Ambulatory Pediatric Association," *Pediatrics*, 1995; 95 (3): 422–426.

2. John Noble, Lee Goldman, Sandra Marvinney, and David Dale, "The Society for General Internal Medicine from Conception to Maturity: 1970s to 1994," *Journal of General Internal Medicine*, 1994; 9(8) (Supplement):S1–S44.

CHAPTER FOUR

1. Henry K. Silver, Loretta C. Ford, and S. G. Stearly, "A Program to Increase Health Care for Children: The Pediatric Nurse Practitioner Program," *Pediatrics*, 1967; 39:756–760; Henry K. Silver, Loretta C. Ford, and L. R. Day, "Pediatric Nurse Practitioner Program," *Journal of American Medical Association*, 1968; 204:298–303; and Loretta C. Ford, "Nurse Practitioners: History of a New Idea and Predictions for the Future," *Nursing in the 1980s*, ed. Linda Aiken (Philadelphia: J. B. Lippincott Co., 1982).

2. U.S. Congress, Office of Technology Assessment, *Nurse Practitioners, Physician Assistants, and Certified Nurse Midwives: A Policy Analysis* (Washington, D.C.: U.S. Government Printing Office, 1986), and P. C. Myers, D. Lenci, and M. G. Sheldon, "A Nurse Practitioner as First Point of Contact for Urgent Medical Problems in a General Practice Setting," *Family Practice*, 1997; 6: 412–417.

3. *The Registered Nurse Population, March 2000: Findings from the National Sample Survey of Registered Nurses* (Washington, D.C.: Department of

Health and Human Services, Health Resources and Services Administration, Bureau of Health Professions, Division of Nursing), p. 50. For further information on this figure, see chapter 1, n. 15.

4. Edward Sekscenski, Stephanie Sansom, Carol Bazell, Marla Salmon, and Fitzhugh Mullan, "State Practice Environments and the Supply of Physician Assistants, Nurse Practitioners, and Certified Nurse Midwives," *New England Journal of Medicine,* 1994; 231:1266–1271; and L. J. Pearson, "Annual Update of How Each State Stands on Legislative Issues Affecting Advanced Nursing Practice," *Nurse Practitioner,* 1999; 24:16–19, 23–24, 27–30.

5. C. L. Hudson, "Expansion of Medical Professional Services with Non-Professional Personnel," *Journal of American Medical Association,* 1961; 176: 839–841.

6. Useful reflections on the history of the physician assistant profession include Ronald Berg, "More Than a Nurse, Less Than a Doctor ," *Look,* September 6, 1966; Reginald D. Carter, "Socio-Cultural Origins of the P.A. Profession," *Journal of the American Academy of Physician Assistants,* 1992; 9:655–662; C. E. Fasser, "Historical Perspectives on P.A. Education," *Journal of the American Academy of Physician Assistants,* 1992; 5:663–670; Steven Cornell "Once Upon a Time: Longtime P.A.s Talk about the History of the Profession," *Advance for Physician Assistants,* July 2000, pp. 48–50; and Marianne Mellon, "P.A. Profile: Looking Backward," *P.A. Today,* September 28, 1998, pp. 20–30.

7. American Academy of Physician Assistants, *Information Update,* October 8, 1999, Alexandria, Va., p. 3.

CHAPTER FIVE

1. The earliest history of the HMO movement is captured by Paul de Kruif's *Kaiser Wakes the Doctors* (London: Jonathan Cape, 1944). Paul Starr, *The Social Transformation of American Medicine* (New York: Basic Books, 1982), gives a good description of the early modern HMO movement (pp. 393 ff.), and R. Adams Dudley and Harold S. Luft, "Managed Care in Transition," *New England Journal of Medicine* (2001; 344:1087–1092), provides a review of the evolution of managed care through the late 1990s. The primary-care gatekeeper phenomenon is well explored in two articles: Kevin Grumbach et al., "Resolving the Gatekeeper Conundrum: What Patients Value in Primary Care and Referrals to Specialists," *Journal of the American Medical Association,* 1999; 282: 261–266; and Thomas Bodenheimer, Bernard Lo, and Lawrence Casalino, "Primary Care Physicians Should Be Coordinators, Not Gatekeepers," *Journal of the American Medical Association,* 1999; 281: 2045–2049.

CHAPTER SEVEN

1. I am indebted to Clayton Christensen, Richard Bohmer, and John Kenagy who present this thesis in an article entitled "Will Disruptive Innovations Cure Health Care?" *Harvard Business Review,* September–October, 2000, pp. 102–112.

Index

Index:	Ruth Elwell
Compositor:	Integrated Composition Systems
Text:	10/13 Sabon
Display:	Sabon
Printer and Binder:	Sheridan Books, Inc.

DEMCO

FAITH OF OUR FATHERS

VOLUME EIGHT

Change and Challenge

Jonathan A. Lindsey

A Consortium Book

Copyright © 1977 by McGrath Publishing Company
Manufactured in the United States of America

Library of Congress Card Catalog Number: 77-9551
ISBN: 0-8434-0627-5
ISBN: 0-8434-0640-2 paper

To Joel W. and Ethel S. Lindsey
whose love, wisdom and patience are appreciated.

Table of Contents

Sects and Cults
Women

Chapter Six: Changing Relationships   113

Ecumenism
Mobility and Denominations
Common Concerns
American Judaism

Epilogue: From Adolescence to Middlescence   137

Suggested Reading   141

Introduction

One of the favorite toys of childhood was the kaliedescope. Hours could be spent, or so it seemed, holding the tube to the eye, slowly turning it to see the shapes and designs. Even a slight touch could change the configuration! Something constantly new was being experienced, yet there was some sense of constancy or stability because one felt that he was manipulating the kaliedescope.

America during the past two decades has experienced a new level of crisis response living. Moving from one crisis to another, domestically, politically, internationally, personally has been a sort of roller coaster experience.

Imagine yourself riding a roller coaster trying to look at a kaliedescope.

That is the feeling I have had in attempting to bring some sense of structure to a view of religious experiences in America 1955-1975. Ever changing, the moods and movements during these two decades are not easy to describe or analyze.

Statistics have been used sparingly. Where they have been cited, for consistency only, the Gallup figures have been used unless otherwise noted. Knowing the difficulties inherent in the use of statistical data about things religious, the lack of credibility of many statistical reports, and the necessary caution with which one approaches statistical information about things religious, the reader is forewarned. The use of the Gallup source,

1

however provides a foundation from the view that this organization has established some continuity of information which is of value.

The reader will, no doubt, challenge some of the interpretations, will wonder why some areas of religious experience have been omitted or have received scant treatment. One man's judgment is another's bias. The pages which follow, however, make no claim to a comprehensive review of religious events or religious issues between 1955-1975. Their only claim is the attempt to present one approach to an interpretation of these years.

1

Changing Times

1955 and 1975 stand as parentheses around two decades of change for the American people. Change has entered every phase of American life during these decades. Understanding the changes is made more difficult because the times are so close to us, and we are still living with the implications of some of the events which have affected our lives. Out of the changes which have occurred have come new challenges for Americans to find new ways of living in the world which has been created.

Dwight David Eisenhower, war hero and son of middle America, was President of the United States in 1955. He had been the chief executive who had delivered on his promise of ending the Korean conflict, an undeclared war fought for the preservation of American democratic ideas against the encroachments of Russian communism. He represented the value systems of the nation which still felt that it was the leader of the Western world, with a responsibility to preserve the modes of democracy for the whole world. Regularly he was pictured on the steps of the National Presbyterian Church, being greeted by the pastor following morning worship. Early in his first administration he and the Congress had added a significant phrase to the pledge of allegiance, naming the United States as "one nation under God."

Looking back on the beginning of these decades of change one can be caught by a sense of nostalgia. It was a time in which heroes were still alive in the minds of many. There may be a

3

sense of quiescence about the beginning of this period of our history. But, already the seeds of change were beginning to rise to the surface of American culture.

The most significant change which was being felt in the first year of this era had been enacted only a few months previously in the decision of the United States Supreme Court in the case of Brown vs. Board of Education. Even then, the change had not yet begun, only the anticipation of what the decision meant loomed on the horizon. Now, twenty years later, most Americans have experienced the dynamics of this momentous social decision. Some still resist it.

The cloud of nuclear destruction hovered over the American mind, but was blotted out by a strong sense of progress and a developing affluence. Industry which had been geared for war production during the preceeding decade had been turned to producing items for consumption for a public which once again had a sense of prosperity. Urban sprawl was beginning in a different manner through the development of middle class housing.

In the decade of the fifties a new sense within the middle class was beginning to form. The industries of the war effort had converted the country into an industrialized nation, and the continuing cold war maintained levels of production. Education became available to a larger body within the country than had previously had access to higher education. Through the benefits to veterans, colleges and universities found themselves crowded with a new kind of student, generally upwardly mobile.

In surburbia, as it developed, churches sprang up among the new houses. Construction of churches almost doubled during the six year period 1954-1960, measured in the amount spent for construction. In 1954, $593,000,000 was spent for church construction, and in 1960 the figure reached $1,016,000,000. In 1960 the percentage of the total population of the United States which claimed affiliation with a church reached a figure of 69%, the highest in the history of the country.

Positive thinking was a phenomenon which blossomed during the decade of the fifties. Three individuals, each representing a distinct group of the Judao-Christian tradition, have been identified with this movement. Rabbi Joshua Loth Liebman, a Reform rabbi in Boston, published his *Peace of Mind* in 1946. It was an adaptation of Freudian insights into problems of personal composure. The success of Leibman's thought heralded a rising interest in depth psychology.

Norman Vincent Peale, minister of the Marble Collegiate Church, New York, took a more superficial and individualistic approach. Two books, *Guide to Confident Living* (1948) and *The Power of Positive Thinking* (1952) were immensely popular and influential among the middle class. Peale was even more significant in his understanding of the uses to be made of popular media, especially the budding influence of television.

The Roman Catholic version of both of these approaches to popular religion in the fifties was Bishop Fulton J. Sheen. Bishop Sheen used a low key approach of positive attitudes, which spread through the culture and influenced numbers of individuals as they watched him weekly. In his quiet manner, he spoke directly to the minds of middle class America as he was filmed in a comfortable setting, always with a chalk board on which he could make notes for those who watched each week's performance of reassurance.

Not as generally accepted, but well known among a large following, was Anne Morrow Lindberg, whose *Gift From the Sea* (1955) was a precursor for a rising interest in mysticism, which was later to be influential in the American religious consciousness. Mrs. Lindbergh spoke to American women, many of whom were housewives not yet ready for the explorations of womens' psyche which was to come in the sixties and seventies.

Revival was a phenomenon which received a boost in the middle of the fifties, too. This boost came through the personality and organization of Billy Graham, who had become for many Prostestants the spokesman for their brand of religious thought and experience. Graham, out of a fundamentalist background, established himself as preacher and evangelist through his association with several conservative evangelical groups. By 1956 his organization was using almost all of the mass media then available—advertising, television, radio, paperback books, and movies—with an annual expenditure of two million dollars! This was evangelism as big business never dreamed of by Dwight L. Moody, who served as Graham's model in management and proclamation.

With Graham's successes came an interesting relationship between politics and religion. National prayer breakfasts were begun, held in Washington, and attended by major personalities in government, both elected and appointed. Graham was to become the "friend of the President," a position which he held until the seventies. This friendship was regularly pictured from the clipped greens of golf courses as he and the chief executive would be shown teeing off.

On the youth side of life in the fifties, bobby sox, sweaters, full skirts, crew cuts, duck tails, and leather jackets over pegged trousers were the uniforms of the young. In 1955 James Dean died. He was a young man who had catapulted to stardom through "Rebel Without a Cause." American youth who were reaching maturity in the relative peace of the cold war years were looking to a future which had a sense of security about it. They were learning the routes of success through their entrance into colleges and universities, well paying jobs in industry, and some were finding themselves drawn to a growing professionalism in social services.

In the latter part of the fifties two events occurred which anticipated the development of change within these two decades. The first was the shocking development in the USSR of "Sputnik," a rocket which could orbit the earth. American industry, government, and military strength regrouped itself in an attempt to regain a place of primacy in what was to become the "race for space." 1957 saw the changes in emphasis in American education being geared to assist in the development of minds and skills which would produce for the country a first place among the nations of the world. Science and technology assumed new leadership roles with a goal of making the nation and the world safe.

A year later, Pius XII, pope since 1937, died. In his place was elected an interim pope, Guiseppi Roncalli, who had earned his way in the church through the diplomatic service of the Vatican. Roncalli took the papal name John XXIII, and in his own way sought to refocus the emphases of the church. Through the power of his personality, and through the power he held as pope, he led the church through the opening days of Vatican II, a council which he called as a means of opening the church to the world of which it was a part. His own sense of his humanity influenced the direction which began to evolve toward a greater sense of humanity in all of Christendom.

The decade of the fifties ended with a sense of hope. Americans were striving to maintain their increasing levels of affluence. A sense of unlimited resources, mobility in newer and more powerful automobiles on new highways, opened the continent. Air travel became more accessible, and trains and buses as means of transport began a steady decline. Television replaced movies as a dominant form of entertainment as well as information. Unmanned space exploration anticipated the day when man would orbit the earth. New frontiers beckoned.

John Fitzgerald Kennedy, elected President of the United States in 1960, the first Roman Catholic in American history to hold this office, caught the feeling of the time and became the living symbol of the new day which was dawning. The thousand days of his presidency opened many avenues of experience, hope, and accomplishment for Americans. So many analyses of those first years of the sixties have been attempted that it seems impossible to grasp all that these years meant then, or even now. Kennedy was young, attractive, articulate. He appealed to the growing body of younger Americans, communicating a sense of global responsibility based in altrusim, expressed in a new wave of social consciousness.

Two programs of the Kennedy years were aimed at and captured the participation of youthful Americans. The Peace Corps, which had as its purpose the amelioration of poverty and illiteracy among the less developed nations of the world became a way for middle and upper middle class youth to act out constructively their social concerns. On the domestic side, the development of VISTA provided avenues of social action in cities, rural and geographically isolated regions. The impact of these programs can be seen from the view that some of the denominations in America adopted programs of their own aimed at the same age group of participants, and the same groups to be serviced. The Southern Baptist Convention's Home and Foreign Mission Boards developed explicit programs for Baptist youth. These programs were integrated into the mission ministries of Baptist churches.

In these same early years of the decade of the sixties the seeds of social upheaval were beginning to sprout in other areas of American life. Significantly blacks came to the forefront as the primary minority group. The years of acknowledged second class citizenship, lower standards of income, education, and living were brought to the direct consciousness of the nation through the development of sit-ins, boycotts, and other demonstrable means of calling attention to the quality of life for these people. This movement was not an overnight development, but appeared so from the treatment of it through the media.

The move to obtain equal rights for blacks had begun in the forties, grown in the fifties, but reached a certain maturity in the sixties. At the helm of the movement was the person and personality of Martin Luther King, Jr., who reached prominence in the American mind as the leader of a bus boycott in Montgomery, Alabama. King, influenced by the non-violent concept of Ghandi, recognized and used the dynamics of aggressive quietude as a means of achieving a goal, which he held to be beneficial to all citizens of the land. This movement, too, captured the social conscience of many youth, and provided a means of acting out their altruistic and/or religious concerns.

Future generations may look back at this short period of American life and note that life in the churches of America was taking an introspective turn. Buildings which had been built during the boom times of the fifties were still heavily mortgaged. In some circles talks of merger among denominations took fresh impetus. Vatican II focused attention on the monolith of the Roman Catholic Church, and the world became privy to the fissures revealed in the council debates.

Violence, an occasional undercurrent in American culture, seemed to erupt volcanically during the sixties. The rifle shot from the Dallas School Board Building which killed John Fitzgerald Kennedy, November 23, 1963, seemed to open a volley which still marks the American conscience. The stunned nation was even more stunned when it viewed on live television the action of Jack Ruby, who stepped out of a group of people in a police station corridor and gunned down Lee Harvey Oswald, the President's assassin. To this point in American experience violence was experienced nationally in a second hand fashion. But, this was to change.

Two other assassinations, that of Martin Luther King, Jr., and Robert F. Kennedy, within two months of each other in 1968, increased the awareness of Americans of a strain of behavior among us that was inexplicable. Again direct acts of personal violence were conveyed into American homes through the media—television and print.

Added to these deaths of national figures was the violence experienced in the cities. Watts, 1964, stands as a symbol of the eruption of the conflagration among cities. But, Washington and other cities were to experience the same kind of onslaught during the middle years of the decade. With the impact of urban violence came a sense of fear, but it was a generalized, undefined fear.

On the international scene the United States became more deeply embroiled in another military action. Viet Nam, which had been claiming funds and lives from this country for more than a decade, by 1965 became an undeclared war. The escalation of Viet Nam during the mid-sixties raised the levels of awareness of American youth to a different perspective of their ability to accomplish good in the world. Rather than the hope which had prevailed during the first part of the decade, a sense of despair became general.

College campuses became scenes of reaction. The system—that slow bureaucratic process of effecting change—became the enemy. Delayed goals seemed irrelevant, particularly to a portion of the culture which was disillusioned and disenchanted with the wisdom of its elders. Direct action which achieved solutions immediately seemed to be the goal of a new breed of politicized, activist youth. To achieve change one had to achieve power. The best means of achieving power was the seizure of it from those who held it. Hence, administration buildings were captured, institutional officials were held hostage in their offices, and demands were made which raised the level of awareness of the involvement of higher education in activities basically non-educational. At Duke students demonstrated for the benefit of minimum wages for maintenance employees. At Columbia students raised questions concerning the commitment of the institution to its geographical relationships.

Violence begat violence in the response to students. Police were called in. In some instances campuses reflected an image of armed camps. Kent State stands as the climax of violence meeting violence on American campuses.

At the same time that students on one front were acting out their political ideation, youth of the same age were taking other forms of behavior which caused a large amount of concern among the "straight" adult population. The impact of the drug culture which began developing during the latter part of the sixties had the aspects of nightmare for both the youth and their parents. Experimentation with a variety of drugs, from marijuana to heroin to LSD became a part of the ordinary experience of many students. For some interpreters, drugs had replaced alcohol as the major external stimulant for students.

The general culture and the churches as part of the general culture, were unprepared to deal with this new phenomenon in American life. From some quarters the use of drugs as a means of achieving a heightened religious awareness was suggested. From other quarters the use of drugs as a means of increasing sensitivity to the creative dimensions of the individual was suggested. From other quarters, the sheer thrill of experiencing something new was suggested as a rationale for drug experimentation.

The impact of the drug culture among youth pointed to problems which had been smoldering in American homes for some time. Questions began to be raised concerning the quality of life, the relationships of parents and children, the relationships among siblings. On many occasions it appeared that the time-honored traditions of American middle class life, which had been centered in the domestic tranquility of American households, had been shattered. Increased divorce rates mounted steadily.

On the heels of the drug culture among youth came a religious phenomenon which was identified as the Jesus Movement which acknowledged participants in the drug culture of the West Coast. In dress, demeanor, thought, and expression of the sacraments those in the Jesus Movement seemed somewhat bizarre to main line, middle class, middle aged church attendants. Intensely personal in their commitment to their understanding of the Christian message, appearing in the dress of the former drug culture but wearing the cross as a sort of amulet, questioning the viability of the instituional churches, and expressing themselves openly with the gift of tongues, participants in the Jesus Movement caused more than a mere ripple on the lake of American Christian experience. In some respects it was more like a tidal wave.

Somehow, and we are not really sure how, all the factors came together, music became a focus of the expression of religious experience among American youth. Rock, dependent on the infinite amplification of electronic equipment, had become a dominant form of musical expression. Religious rock followed, gaining slow acceptance because it brought guitars, drums, and other instruments seldom associated with church music into the churches. Through the music expressly written for performance on the commercial stage, religious experience and youth coalesced. "Jesus Christ, Superstar" and "Godspell" were two successful commercial ventures. Out of these two "secular" products there came a view of Jesus of Nazareth which was more human than had been traditionally presented by the churches. Through these experiences, however, some of the joy, celebration, and commitment of youth began to be transmitted to the non-youth audience.

The years from 1968-1970 have been called the "Age of Aquarius." In living through these years both the secular culture of America and the religious culture of America interacted in unique ways. We are not yet able to evaluate all the outcomes of these years because of our closeness to them. The strongest emphasis that we can see immediately from them lies in the increased emphasis of the power of youth to communicate with the world in which they live.

Other significant events in the world of theology and Biblical thought must also be looked at as we attempt to gain a grasp on the nature of change and challenge in the two decades between 1955 and 1975. At the beginning of this era the world of Biblical scholarship was still struggling to find ways of communicating the benefits of historical critical approaches to the study of Scripture. This effort was impeded by the close attachment of Americans to the traditional translation of the King James Version. In the South there had actually been book burnings when the Revised Standard Version of the Old Testament was published in 1952! Slowly, ever so slowly, inroads were made and gradually acceptance came to the Revised Standard Version. Near the end of this twenty year period, however, we find that numerous modern English translations were available, being purchased, and being read by diverse groups of Christians. Probably the leader in the group, at least it was widely accepted first, was the American Bible Society's publication of *Good News for Modern Man* (1966). This New Testament translation, prepared for non-English speaking persons using a limited vocabulary, attempted to communicate the text of the New Testament in a simple, straightforward prose style. Helpful to the communication process were the line drawings which were interspersed in the text.

Shortly following the publication of Good News came the New English Bible. The New Testament had appeared in 1961, but had received little popular acceptance. With the publication of both the Old and New Testaments in a prose form, greater acceptance came for this particular translation which followed the traditional committee structure to assure the best possible translation. A best seller among prose versions of Scripture, however, came when Tyndale Publishing House produced *The Living Bible*. This translation, sometimes using a level of communication which approached slang, achieved a high degree of acceptance among some of the more conservative branches of American Christendom.

The achievements represented in the Ecumenical Bible, 1973, however, demonstrated an unusual milestone in American Biblical acceptance. This translation accepted by both Protestants and Roman Catholics, provided a base for understanding that had not been achieved before. Since Vatican II interest among Roman Catholics in the Scripture had seen some increase. With the acceptance by Roman Catholics of the Ecumenical Bible ways may be further opened for interchange among all levels of American Christian communions for Biblically based conversation.

Neo-orthodoxy reigned as the dominant Protestant theological expression during the middle of the 1950's. The movement which had begun thirty years before was reaching a mature level of scholarship. The "greats" of Protestant theological thought were still publishing. As the sixties dawned seminarians had been introduced to existential thought in their collegiate training. By 1975, however, a seminary professor stated that he was not concerned with his students being too liberal, he found himself trying to open them up!

In these two decades the theological thought of the churches had gone through situation ethics, espoused by Joseph Fletcher.

On the heels of the misinterpretations of Fletcher, which heard him saying "anything goes," came the "Death of God" movement. Time magazine covered the death of God with a black cover bearing red letters announcing "Is God Dead?" Controversy and consternation greeted this announcement and for a while replies were made to those who became the focus of the ideas: Thomas Altizer, William Hamilton, and Gabriel Vahanian.

In the midst of all the discussion some individuals sensed that what was really being brought to the attention of the American public was the almost eternal questions of the immanence and transcendence of God. The rhetoric of the discussion often tended to obscure this question through positions held by those who took opposing sides to defend themselves and their heritages.

Concern with life and death shifted from an emphasis on war and civil strife to an awareness of the quality of life. Early in the decade of the seventies ecology and the quality of life were common themes which faced Americans. The Arab oil boycott made a direct impact on our citizens when their mobility was impaired by increased costs and unavailability of petroleum products. The bubble of infinite resources for energy was pricked as increased prices for gas, oil, and plastics were passed on to consumers. Emphasis on the ecological responsibility of individuals was also expressed through concern for population growth and the means to provide for an exponentially increasing world population. In some churches the theme for Rogation Sunday took the form of a proclamation of ecological responsibility.

Concern for the beginning and ending of life also received emphasis during the early seventies. Abortion laws were overturned by the decision of the Supreme Court, thereby making abortion legal and available on request, through standard medical channels. Death received an increasing emphasis and interest from the point of view of increased publication dealing with this subject, and attempts to understand the dynamics of death.

Euthanasia, often discussed in abstract terms, became a timely topic, and the right to die was raised as an option for the individual. During the latter part of 1975 the question of the right to die was brought directly to the attention of the public in the legal questions raised in the Sharon Quinlan case. At the end of the year the case was under appeal to the New Jersey Supreme Court.

Attempts to measure American religious experience through church attendance has been one way of gauging the religious pulse of the nation. From a Gallup Poll published in 1974 indications were that attendance at church among Protestants or synagogue among Jews had shown virtually no change. The significant difference came among Roman Catholics, with a nine per cent drop in attendance between 1964 and 1973. The nineteen year national average was 45% attendance with a projected figure of 55 million adults. Other indications from the Gallup statistics indicated that more Roman Catholics attended weekly than Protestants or Jews (55%, 38% and 19% respectively); that more women than men attended (43% and 35%); and, that those with less education were more likely to attend church than those with college training (43% vs. 40%). From these same statistics, the South was shown to be the section of the country with the highest record of attendance (44%), and the West with the less probability of attendance (19%). Even with a less than 50% average of church attendance, Americans could still claim to be the "church-goingest" people in the world.

1975 stands as the closure to the parentheses of our two decade period under examination. On the social and political planes of national life we were still dealing with finding effective means of stabilizing the educational opportunities for minorities. Busing as a means of desegregating school systems claimed many headlines during this year. Blacks still sought equal opportunities in education and in the employment market. Enfranshisment of blacks through voter registration drives, particularly in the South, had provided a political clout not heretofore held by this significant minority of American citizens.

Politically the nation also experienced the traumatic change in government leadership during 1973-1974 when "Watergate" became a new word in American vocabulary. Not only was Spiro Agnew unseated as Vice-president, but Richard M. Nixon resigned the office of the President. Questions of the extent of moral decline were raised in both religious and secular fronts. Gerald Ford, a son of middle America, representing middle American values, came to the Presidency. Early in his administration he attempted to regain credibility for the office on the strength of his forthright and direct manner.

In the chapters which follow we shall attempt with some greater detail to examine the areas of changing accents of belief, changing celebration, changing conscience, changing identities, and changing relationships. Even in these looks at American religious experience during these two eventful decades, the metaphor of the kaleidescope is one which is most apropos. The slightest modification of the angle of vision presents the viewer with a new constellation of events and personalities from which to observe the era. Understanding some of the dynamics of change is part of the challenge before us.

2

Changing Theological Accents

Several factors seem to provide an emphasis and interest for theological thought during the third quarter of the twentieth century. Following the war publication was resumed, and this provided a new means for a forum. The development of the paperback book, especially the "academic" paperback, also provided another means for creating a forum. Reprints of classical works, as well as original works, began to be readily available in this form. Also concurrent with readily available materials, theologians who had begun productivity in the earlier decades of the century achieved maturity and recognition. At the same time younger theologians were beginning to achieve early career recognition. Rapid communication of ideas was a phenomenon which had been accelerating during the entire century, but the commercial developments for dissemination of information, especially television, seemed to increase the impact exponentially.

Theological awareness was a mark of the two decades 1955-1975. Although significant change in basic tenets of theology may not have occurred, many people came to the recognition that theology was not static. In these two decades it was seen to be dynamic, open to dialog, and not exclusively the property of academicians.

The Great B's

Four European theologians provided a major impact on the academic side of American religious thought during the 1950s through the early portion of the 1970s. American religious traditions have tended to have roots in European soil, even after the nineteenth century development of strong American denominations. The emphases of the four whose influence is discussed below centered American thought on the nature of Scripture, the nature of man, the role of the church in the world, and the historicity of the New Testament's account of Jesus.

Karl Barth (1886-1968) reformed theological thought early in the twentieth century. His *Commentary on Romans*, 1919, reopened the questions of Biblical interpretation in the modern age. Barth was one who sought to express the ageless messages of Scripture in ways which called for commitment from the individual.

Few theologically trained individuals made their pilgrimage through American seminaries without some contact with the masterful thinking of Karl Barth. His *Church Dogmatics*, fourteen volume repositories of his systematic theology, were basic background or collateral texts in many theological classrooms. This was probably the most definitive work in Protestant theology since John Calvin's *Institutes of the Christian Religion*. Through these, as well as through his preaching, Barth sought to remind men of the authority of Scripture. From his perspective as a Swiss parish minister, as well as from his emphases as a seminal theological thinker of unusual perceptive skill, the Biblical bases of the Christian word were clearly set out.

Barth sought to expound the *sensus literalis* of the Scripture, true to the Reformation principles. In so doing he brought to the revealed word an understanding of the historical-critical methods which had been well developed in Europe. He insisted that the Bible was God's word to man, and was God's word about man. God stood in constant judgment of man, and any who sought to create him in man's image. Barth saw his task as that of rethinking and rearticulating the age-old truths of revelation.

Out of the crucible of Germany's experience in World War I, and the disillusionment which Europe experienced in its wake, Barth sought to clarify the church's understanding of God's word to man, not man's word to himself about God. Thus, revelation, that God revealed himself totally in his Son, was the central theme of Barth's writing. To grasp his thought was like holding a diamond in bright sunlight. From one angle it blinds the viewer to anything else, and from another angle one becomes aware that he is only viewing the single beam reflected by a masterly carved facet.

Emil Brunner (1889-1966) in this same period stood as a major influence, too, in the development of American thought. As a theologian his works also formed a core for theological education. Through his sermons, however, one can see his emphasis on an understanding of the nature of man.

I Believe in the Living God (1959), a small collection of sermons on the Apostles' Creed, presented dialectical theology in it's homiletical form. Brunner emphasized in these sermons problems which face all men—anxiety, guilt, doubt, suffering, and death. Brunner reminded those who approached this collection that true Christian faith was not a matter of belief or intellectual assent to either the creed or the Scriptures. He saw the foundation of faith in trust and obedience to the One who spoke through creed and Scripture.

Through this collection the life situation facing those who heard Brunner's exposition constantly rose to the surface. Brunner as preacher had the skill to speak simply, but never simplistically. In a Europe still ravaged by the impacts of World War II and the Cold War of the fifties, he spoke words of hope as well as responsibility. Man stands always in need of redemption and reconciliation. Only as man submitted himself to the revelation of God could he begin to gain a sense of wholeness in his fragmented world. Only as man recognized Jesus as the redeemer of the world, and as his personal redeemer, could he belong to the community of Jesus Christ.

Dietrich Bonhoeffer (1906-1945), whose martyr's death became the means of placing him higher in the theological world, had a marked influence on theological thought, especially during the 1960s. His *Letters and Papers from Prison* reflected a strong awareness and struggle with evil in the world. Bonhoeffer opposed the Nazi regime in Germany, but returned to Germany to fight through the church. He was tried and found guilty of complicity in plots on the life of Adolf Hitler. During his imprisonment he spent time thinking of the role of the church in the world, the growing secularization of modern man, and the necessity of speaking in a new (secular) way about God. His thoughts were not complete—and from some perspectives there are severe limitations to any attempt to deal with him fully. The most complete attempt at understanding Bonhoeffer and articulating an appreciation of his thought came from the pen of Eberhard Bethge, friend, protege, critic.

In terms of impact, however, his work received an emphasis which was still being examined in 1975. Bonhoeffer's phrase, "religionless Christianity," captured the minds of disillusioned youth who, in the sixties, were acutely aware of the failure of the church to act as a redemptive agent in the world. This phrase focused the polarities of institutional forms of Christianity and the personal affirmations and faith actions of the individual Christian. Bonhoeffer provided a type of rationale for several movements in the sixties, some of whose proponents were not reading his work accurately against the historical background in which it was created. Bonhoeffer sought a form of Christianity which could accept a Biblical faith without requiring its expression in traditional religious forms.

The effect of Rudolf Bultmann's (1884-) thought on American Christianity was an anticipation of the development of popular theology. In the classroom Bultmann was presented as one who raised legitimate questions concerning the historical accuracy of the New Testament records of the life of Jesus. His was not a new search, but a new emphasis in a more than century old search for historical evidences which would verify the gospels. When his work, called "demythologizing," came to the attention of the popular mind, however, the reaction was sometimes harsh.

Bultmann's writings which were translated for American audiences raised the question of how accurately the gospels presented the events, as well as the teachings of Jesus. He was building on what for nearly one hundred years had been the search of both form and source criticism. These two forms of Biblical study sought to examine the language, internal historical references, and external information such as that provided by archaeological discoveries, in an attempt to provide an authenticated picture of the real events surrounding the life of Jesus. This was not an attempt to deemphasize the role of faith in the lives of men, but an attempt to provide a better understanding of the realities on which faith was based.

Through the Gospels to Jesus, or a continuing search for the Jesus of history, was an apt description of what he was attempting. His attempts, however, were interpreted negatively, rather than positively. He was accused of stripping mystery away from the Christ event to such an extent that nothing was left to the believer.

Bultmann's earlier interpretations of Jesus emphasized the radical commitment Jesus demanded of those whom he called out and whom he summoned to decision. In his later works he emphasized a concept and program of demythologizing, calling for the interpretation of the narratives of the gospels in light of historical and literary evidences. He insisted that these narratives would require reinterpretation to modern man so that the kerygmatic word could be communicated.

These four individuals had a powerful influence in twentieth century theological thought. Their thinking was filtered through theological classrooms to the pulpits of the nation. In some instances they were read by those without theological training. Some of their phrases became catchwords for movements as superficially diverse as social reform and Biblical criticism. They contributed to the changing accents of theology both directly and indirectly.

Dialog Theology

One of the products of the impact of theological thought between 1955 and 1975 was the development of what can now be called dialogic theology. To a mind-set which received theological thought with a sense of absoluteness the development of a new dialog with a popular base was a significant opportunity. It was not easy to achieve dialog outside the realms of theological education. Several writers, among many, can be used to illustrate this movement. They are chosen as illustration because their writing to some extent entered the level of popular theological thought. The extent to which their work penetrated the popular mind cannot be known fully. In years to come it may be seen that their penetration was only superficial. However, to fail to note this popularization of theological thought would fail to shed some light on the mixed picture of these decades.

John A. T. Robinson, churchman, educator, bishop, and pastor, was among the first to achieve a popular hearing. *Honest to God*, 1963, was offered as a writing which could provoke dialog among the theological world. In this small volume Robinson challenged the traditional concepts of the universe and the relationship of God to the universe. One of the words to which he gave emphasis was depth. Through challenging the traditional cosmology—heaven, earth, hell—he was pointing to the need for a language which would communicate with a world then entering the space age.

His book became a best seller, with a large readership on American college campuses. Part of the popularity of the writing was out of Robinson's conviction that truth is more likely to lie in a tension than in a choice of opposites. This struck a cord among collegians and theologians who were learning to live in a world of tension. Another feature of Robinson's dialog was the attempt to bring together some of the thought of Paul Tillich, Dietrich Bonhoeffer, and Rudolf Bultmann. That success was seen in the development of this triad as the central figures for mid-century theological thought. For some, Robinson heralded the beginning of radical theology in the twentieth century, for others he was not radical enough.

Following closely on the heels of Robinson was the work of a young Harvard bred theologian, Harvey Cox. In *The Secular City* Cox focused thought on the role of the city and the opportunities and limits which the city offered. The work pointed to the new life styles forming in American culture in the early sixties. The city had been the stronghold of one form of American evangelicalism since the mid-nineteenth century. In the city, Dwight L. Moody, Billy Sunday, and other evangelists in the evangelical tradition had developed their crusade mode of witness. But in the sixties Cox saw the city in a different light.

He focused on the urban inapplicability of a religious experience which had been developed and nourished from small town and agrarian models. The city provided anonymity to those who sought to lose themselves in it—and even for those who lived their whole lives bounded by the concrete and steel megaloposes of the continent. The simplicity of the "I-Thou" popularized in Christian interpretations of Martin Buber's Jewish-fed humanism, had added to it a third dimension of the "it." "I-it-thou," as a category of understanding relationships, recognized the function of providing services without entering into a personal relationship.

Like Robinson's work, when the popular mind was confronted by the dialog, there were limits to the extent in which dialog could be engaged. Cox was analyzing the states of life in our culture in an era when the popular mind was not yet prepared to receive the analysis. The reaction was loud, but short-lived.

Two other themes of the sixties eclipsed discussion about the work of Robinson and Cox. One confronted American consciousness with the relative nature of its ethical decisions, and the other challenged the traditional categories of thought about God. Joseph Fletcher, a respected ethicist, raised the hackles of complacency when he offered an agape-based method for making ethical decisions. Three young theologians challenged the ways men think about God with their assertion, "God is Dead."

Fletcher proposed in *Situation Ethics* (1966) a way of making ethical decisions which would involve the decision maker in a determination of what could be the most loving action, given an understanding of the circumstances affecting the decision. The differences between ethical decision making and moral behavior were not clearly articulated in the debates which ensued. Sometimes the behavior which resulted from the ethical decision cut at the base of middle class morality. Fletcher was intepreted as advocating immorality, when in fact, he consistently placed before his audience an understanding of the principles by which men make decisions which determine morality.

His three categories—the legal, the antinomian, and the situational—were a summary of the historical means used for making decisions. He openly recognized the basically relative nature of the decision process and the behavior which resulted from those decisions. The popular response to Fletcher's thought may have caused him to overstate the behavioral forms in which the decisions were actualized. He was consistent, however, in his demand that one seek the agape-base in decision making.

Thomas J. J. Altizer, William Hamilton, and Gabriel Vahanian, aided by the popular press provided the real "shaker" of the decade of the sixties. *Time* magazine's cover, April 8, 1966, proclaimed in bold red letters on a black background "Is God Dead?" It had taken six months, October 1965 to April 1966, for the opinions of Altizer, Hamilton, and Vahanian to reach the popular mind.

Altizer, the chief spokesman for the position, was a young professor of Bible and religion at Emory University, a Methodist affiliated school in Atlanta. He articulated in 1965 the thought of Friedrich Nietzsche, who in the nineteenth century had proposed ideas about the death of God. The church had faced this question early in its existence, since as theology developed questions arose concerning the relationship of Christ to God, particularly in the death-resurrection mystery. One branch of the church, later declared heretic, said that Jesus only seemed to die, thus protecting the eternality of God. Another group, also declared heretic, said that God died in the crucifixion of Jesus. The orthodox position has been to hold the mystery of the death-resurrection as central, affirming both as actual, but not resolving the questions of identity between God and his son. Altizer held that the best understanding of his view could be described as the death of God in Christ in which God no longer exists, but is embodied in the humanistic teachings of Jesus.

Hamilton and Altizer were interviewed on the tenth anniversary of the popularization of their views. Both were no longer identified professionally with religiously related institutions. Hamilton was dean of a state university, and Altizer was professor of English at a state university. Each affirmed his belief in the value of the death of God controversy, a decade previously. They said the major benefit was an opening in the theological world for other forms of theological understanding which have evolved during the decade, namely what is known as black theology and feminist theology. Each lamented the loss of a sense of dialog in the theological world.

Politicized Theology

The dialogic nature of theology became evident during the sixties. As the dialog developed, it was seen in some circles to be a new experience, and others viewed it as the continuation of the role theology should play in the lives of men. For once, at least in the twentieth century, it became popular to talk about religious ideas. The two most difficult areas of social conversation came into vogue at the same time. Politics and religion ceased being odd bedfellows, and for a while there appeared to be the development of a relationship between the two.

Some of the development of the relationship between theology and political matters probably came as a result of the skillfull use of religious thought and experience in the civil rights movement. For the blacks, the power of the movement was centered in the mobilizing efforts of black churchmen. For some the center was the galvanic personality of Martin Luther King, Jr. For others the center was their participation in civil rights activity as a direct response to their sense of discipleship. Regardless of the motivations, however, religious motivation to political action was a phenomenon of the sixties. Another look at this dimension of

American religious experience will be assayed in the chapter dealing with changing conscience. In this instance we must focus our thought toward the theological dimensions of the political behavior of some people. For instance, the term "politicized theology" must strike some readers as a discordant term. How can you politicize theology, even with the penchant in recent American English to create verbal forms? The thought of three men, whose influence on this era varies, helps one grapple with the means of politicizing theology. Reinhold Niebuhr, Jurgen Moltmann, and Helder Camara have each contributed to our understanding of how politics and religious experience interact.

Niebuhr's influence developed over a long period of time. The experiences of his early parish where he faced the reality of the basic sinfulness of man marked his thought throughout his life. *Leaves from the Notebook of a Tamed Cynic*, diary entries of a young parish minister, had a remarkable sense of social relevancy during the sixties, even though the experiences which were recorded were thirty years old. To be convinced of the sinfulness of man, however, led Niebuhr to seek means of communicating reconciliation to man.

By the mid-fifties, with the popularity of neoorthodoxy, Niebuhr was one of the most read American theologians. He has been compared with Jonathan Edwards, in being the only two theologians indigenous to America to achieve international reputations. His influence was felt directly by those who preached weekly, as well as those who worshipped regularly. Man is sinner was the theme. But God had provided the means for man's redemption. When man accepted God's grace, and chose to live in grace, change was the result. The impact of change, however, had to be felt in all areas of man's life, including the political sphere.

The Nature and Destiny of Man, Niebuhr's Gifford Lectures, 1940, was the systematic treatment of sin, and man as sinner. He argued convincingly for the idea of original sin (not, however, for the old doctrine!). He led the forces in the theological world against an optimistic view of the nature of man. But even more important to an understanding of the political sphere was Niebuhr's concept of power and the meaning of power. In 1940 in an essay, "Politics and the Christian Ethic," Niebuhr began with the statement, "All life is an expression of power." When he retired from Union Theological Seminary in 1960, after thirty-two years of teaching, he was still reiterating this theme.

Both *The Nature and Destiny of Man* and the 1940 essay on "Politics and the Christian Ethic" were aimed at an understanding of the dynamics of power. No special "spiritual power" accrued to the Christ follower. He was still a man in need of redemption living in a world of sin.

Helder Camara and Jurgen Moltmann, both non-Americans, raised issues for politicized theology which influenced American thought. Camara was not well known by many Americans because he represented an area we call the third world. He was a leader in Latin America for nonviolent social change. Moltmann, professor of systematic theology, Tubingen, heralded a new era when his work made its way to America. Moltmann spoke about hope, to a world that had given up hoping.

Camara as the Archbishop of Olinda and Recife, Northeastern Brazil, represented the thrust of social action in the developing nations. He has been influential in the work with urban poverty, land reform movements, and as a formulator of Vatican II's statements on social justice. He was a Nobel Peace prize nominee.

Camara spoke incisively about the problems of developing nations. The issues were not between East and West, but between the Northern and Southern parts of the world, between developed and underdeveloped countries. He denied the Western panacea of birth control, not with a traditional Roman Catholic argument, but pointed directly to economic imbalances as a basic problem for developing nations. He saw the participation of the forces of religious institutions committed to the alleviation of social problems as the most hopeful sign of vitality in the church during the late sixties.

Camara was one who lived his convictions. He refused to live in the Archbishop's palace. Instead he lived among the people in two rooms behind a delapidated church in one of Recife's slums.

Moltmann's word of hope came at a time when hope appeared absent among theologians. Moltmann returned the attention of the theological world to eschatology, but not the negative eschatology of many American revival preachers. The eschatology pointed to by Moltmann was to remind churchmen that Christianity is a world-transforming and world-overcoming hope. He saw this dimension of Christianity acted out in the ecumenical, church renewal, and student movements of the sixties. At the same time he protested the development of an attitude characterized by the view that pious students do not protest, and protesting students had nothing to do with Christianity.

In the *Theology of Hope* Moltmann provided a statement of the nature of twentieth century Christian action politically, and generated through it a sense of the eschatology in which true Christian hope is based. He failed, however, to describe the practice of hope. He later corrected that oversight by suggesting that Christian hope is not a naievely blind optimism, but a discerning sensitivity which sees suffering and at the same time believes in freedom. But, even more, he declared hope is the art of perseverance. The perseverance is acted out in the lives of Christians who engage themselves in the decision making processes of the world.

Deaths of the Greats

One of the great fears among religious systems is the silence of the gods. To assure the continued support of the faithful, the oracle at Delphi always had a word. Even among the ancient Hebrews the silence of God was to be feared. This is true, even in our enlightened times. We fear the time when the prophets pass on, afraid that there will be no new word from the Lord. The fears may be realities, because between 1955 and 1975 the greats of the twentieth century theological world passed to their eternal rewards, and some strained to hear the cry of a new prophet in the land.

Reinhold Niebuhr died in 1971. His brother, H. Richard Niebuhr, equal scholar in interpreting the American scene, died in 1962. Karl Barth died in 1968, and Emil Brunner in 1966, both of whom we have noted whose influence molded the century. Albert Schweitzer died in 1965, having influenced the thought of the entire century. John XXIII (d. 1963), the only pope many people can identify by name, followed the pontificate of Pius XII (1937-1958) and opened the windows and doors of the church. Several, however, should be noted at greater length for their impact on different segments of the American experience.

Paul Tillich, 1886-1965, German bred and educated, came to the United States in 1933 to avoid the persecutions of prewar Germany. Forty-seven, already a recognized theologian, he was to have an unusual influence on American theological thought in the post-war years. Like other European thinkers, he was an able preacher, and many people are familiar with three collections of his sermons: *The Shaking of the Foundations, The New Being,* and *The Eternal Now.*

Tillich's popular and some academic writing retained the same themes consistently: man's estrangement from God and his anxiety, man's attempts to find his salvation in what Tillich called "idolatries" identified as status, sex, nationalism, or at times the church! Against these idolatries and man's anxiety, Tillich proposed God. Not the God of easy understanding or quick conversion, but who was beyond man's ability to concieve. His thought was difficult for many people to grasp. He understood religious experience in terms of symbols, charging always that the symbols should never be mistaken for the unknowable thing they represented. Thus, God, Christ, resurrection were the symbols for an unknowable mystery, unknowable in the pedagogical ways of man. God was the "ground of man's being" in Tillichian thought.

Tillich described faith as ultimate concern. As such it demanded an act of man's total personality, which involved man's spirit, body, and soul. Even while dealing with the concepts of ultimate concern and the essential mystery of the Christian faith, Paul Tillich always seemed to be grounded in the human situations in which faith lives.

By the time of his death in 1965 Tillich had made an ineradicable mark on American and international theological thought. He described his life as one lived "on the boundary," a title given to a posthumously published "spiritual autobiography."

Reinhold Niebuhr, 1892-1971, was responsible for bringing Paul Tillich to America. His experience for thirteen years as pastor of a Reformed Church in Detroit had introduced him to the suffering of man and the faltering skill of the church to minister to men. He rejected the optimism of social and religious thinkers in the early part of the twentieth century, those who insisted that man was good and would respond to goodness.

Niebuhr was a hard-headed realist who insisted that the church take its stand in the political and social spheres of man's life. He did not mouth words asking others to take action, but involved himself in the political arena, at one time running for Congress on a Socialist ticket. He demanded personal responsibility for actions, even interpreting the Biblical story of Adam, Eve, and the apple in terms of personal responsibility. Men tend to take the easy way out to excuse themselves, to pass the buck as Adam did when he blamed Eve because she gave him the apple! In this act Niebuhr saw the central focus of man's greatest evidence of sin, pride.

Twenty books and about a thousand articles in a fifty year span provided those who followed Niebuhr and his thought with a clear articulation which judged events in American life. As an American, son of a mid-western pastor, Niebuhr was the greatest American-born theologian since Jonathan Edwards. He died at his home in Stockbridge, Mass., where Edwards spent the years of his exile before he became President of Princeton, 1758. Niebuhr's funeral was at the church in Stockbridge where Edwards preached. His insight into the human events of his time, and the role the church must play in those events caused him to speak continually on political issues. Socialism, pacifism, cold war political maneuvers, civil rights, and Viet Nam were issues which he faced and on which he demanded responsible action. As early as the Depression years he suggested a

Gandhian-like passive resistance move as more productive for civil rights than dependence on benevolence. This was a form of the lesson he had learned in Detroit in his opposition to Henry Ford's public generosity in view of the dehumanizing conditions of the developing automotive industrialism.

The Nature and Destiny of Man, Niebuhr's major theological treatise, delivered as the Gifford Lectures, University of Edinburgh, as the world was facing the inevitability of World War II, profoundly spoke then, and continued to speak to man's role in God's world. He insisted that only the Bible provided a proper image of man, whom he described as a self transcending being whose freedom contains possibilites for good and evil. He found man intrinsically evil, but capable of good as he understood God's mercy active in history through the cross of Christ. In this way, only, could man become fully conscious of both his guilt and his redemption. Guilt and redemption describe the nature and destiny of man.

Paul Tillich and Reinhold Niebuhr provided the intellectual foundations for Christian theology in America between 1955 and 1975. They worked in the same spheres, and influenced American thought and action. One started with the human situation, but pointed to a concept of God which often seemed outside of the human realm of awareness. The other remained grounded in the human situation and sought to provide a view of God active in the lives of men. Both men provided the foundation for political activism in the 1960s, some of the details we will explore in the chapter on changing social conscience.

Three other theologians, however, whose deaths occurred during these two decades, must be considered. Their impact on the broad picture of American religious experience may not have been as central as Tillich and Niebuhr, but to ignore their contributions would leave a gap unfilled. Thomas Merton, a Trappist monk, raised the issues of contemplation and mystery which foreshadowed popular interest in these dimensions of Christian thought and experience. On the side of Jewish thinkers who had a profound impact on American religious experience we must also consider Martin Buber and Abraham Joshua Heschel.

Thomas Merton entered the abbey of Our Lady of Gethsemane, Bardstown, Kentucky, at the age of twenty-six after a peripatetic youth. He was ordained in 1949, and the abbot assigned him to continue writing. His first major book appeared in 1948, *The Seven Storey Mountain*, a spiritual autobiography which detailed his search for personal and religious meaning. It attracted wide attention to Merton as well as to the monastic and priestly vocations. Merton's influence with the pen was expressed on a variety of causes, many of them social concerns. He was an absolute pacifist, and gave support to any anti-war cause.

Merton's strengths as a man, as a Trappist, and as a writer were unusual. He was a poet whose sensitivity to the world was expressed as poignantly in prose as in verse. He was a contemplative whose understanding of the interchange between the world of ordinary life and the necessary withdrawal for a life of silence and prayer for this world was constantly in tension. In the last years of his life he was allowed to withdraw from the community life of the abbey and pursue an anchoritic existence in a small cabin about a mile from the monastery. His life ended tragically, by an accidental electrocution from a fan in his quarters at Bangkok. He was on a special leave from the abbey to attend an ecumenical conference of Christian and Buddhist monks.

To be able to feel the pain of men, to pray for their salvation, and to live a life apart from the world were some of the things Merton represented. But, to be able to feel the pain of men was his finest gift; because, in feeling the pain he communicated to others their common responsibility to alleviate that pain. That this occurred in a life devoted to silence, in a remote mid-Kentucky monastery was even more remarkable in the pain-filled world of the sixties. Merton was an atypical Trappist, who fulfilled the goals for which Trappists stand.

The import of Merton internationally was seen in the following of his available writings among young Roman Catholic intellectuals in Poland in 1974. Invariably when the writer raised questions concerning who was read by this group of Polish society, Merton was named among the first three. Usually he was first.

Martin Buber's death June 14, 1965, ended the life but not the influence of one of Judaism's most interesting spokesmen. He was born in Vienna, 1878. Buber's grandfather was a distinguished Talmudic scholar, in whose house Buber spent his boyhood. He did not take Talmudic studies, however, but moved toward philosophy and art history at Vienna, and at the University of Berlin he earned a doctorate in philosophy.

One of the earliest avenues pursued by Buber was Hasidic lore, exploring the writings of the Hasidic rabbis, as well as the legends of the tradition. Five years were devoted to the collection of these tales and stories, which began the publication of a dozen volumes of Hasidic stories and teachings, plus one novel, *For the Sake of Heaven*. Buber also made a remarkable translation of Scripture from Hebrew to German.

Buber's achievements lay in many fields. He was a theologian, philosopher, philosophical anthropologist, literary artist, teacher, sociologist, and existential humanist. These fit him like a Joseph's coat. He was a leader of German Judaism until 1938 when he immigrated to Israel. In Israel he was a Zionist, but one about whom some of the Orthodox complained. Although he held a chaired professorship in social philosophy at Hebrew University, the Orthodox rabbinate refused to allow him to teach religion until after his 1951 retirement.

Martin Buber was not bound by many limitations. He understood the mysteries and the practicalities of life in the twentieth century. In 1937 he published *I and Thou* which recieved large public attention in the fifties and sixties. The acceptance was so widely spread among Christians that some did not know Buber was a Jew. He understood and articulated, as few men have been capable, the polarities and mutualities of Judaism and Christianity. *Two Types of Faith* was not an attempt to reconcile the incompatibles but to examine openly the complementary natures of the two traditions. Buber once said, "To the Christian the Jew is a stubborn fellow, who in an unredeemed world is still waiting for the Messiah. To the Jew, the Christian is a heedless fellow, who in an unredeemed world, affirms that salvation has, somehow or other, taken place." His study of Hebrew prophets provided the basis for his criticism of Christian idealism, which he said was too individualistic and sentimental. For him the Hebrew prophets were germaine for their calls to radical justice.

Buber influenced most of the theologians of the twentieth century. His emphasis on dialog, that theology is essentially a dialog, helped move theologians away from the older forms of propositional theology.

"When I marched with Martin Luther King in Selma, I felt my legs were praying." This was the statement of Abraham Joshua Heschel, 1907-1972, whose central motif was the belief that life should be full of sacred moments that taste of eternity. Heschel was a modern mystic who believed God was active, and his theology was never passive. Not only was Heschel with King at Selma, he went to Rome in 1964 to appeal directly to Paul VI for a statement from Vatican II which would absolve Jews of corporate guilt in the crucifixion of Jesus. He was also founder with Daniel Berrigan of Clergy Concerned about Viet Nam, and was the first Jew appointed to a faculty role at the prestigious Union Theologican Seminary, New York. Heschel was a Jewish ecumenicist, whose morality included an open concept of brotherhood.

Raised in the Orthodox ghetto of Warsaw, Heschel was a teenager when he purchased his first book. Educated in Germany, his study for his doctorate produced the first of more than twenty volumes. In 1940 he escaped to America, but was unprepared for the unsettled rationalistic Judaism which he found here. Prior to coming to America he served several faculty appointments, one at Frankfurt with Buber, and immediately prior to his American immigration he founded the Institute for Jewish Learning, London.

Heschel's major works, *Man is Not Alone: A Philosophy of Religion* (1951) and *God in Search of Man: A Philosophy of Judaism* (1955) placed him among the major theological voices of the century. In these writings he sought to establish some clearer answers to the problems of religion faced by modern men. The work was poetic (his first publication was poetry), and showed mastery of skill as a writer, thinker and apologete. He revealed the essential mystery of religious experience without violating philosophical canons.

Emphasis on the Activity of the Holy Spirit

The Pentecostal phenomenon in American religious experience has surfaced at least once each century since 1700. The advent of revivalism provided the first general awareness of this dimension of religious experience on the American scene. The twentieth century, however, has seen the development of this facet among American churches to the point that some chronicle of it has been achieved.

In the sixth decade of this century the phenomenon, until then considered a fringe or cult occurrence, began to be noted among middle class church groups. The response to the glossolaliac dimensions of Pentecostalism was mixed, and often rejected by the main-line bodies of American Christians. The movement turned underground, but other groups formed which reflected some of the theological emphases of Pentecostalism, especially with an emphasis on personal salvation.

Among the first groups to be identified, not as Pentecostal, but having an emphasis on personal evangelism was Campus Crusade for Christ. In October 1951, Bill Bright, then a business man who was also attending Fuller Theological Seminary, experienced a vision of personal evangelism which he began on the University of California, Los Angeles campus. The central thrust of the movement begun by Bright was a confrontation of an individual with a perception of his lost and sinful state and to offer him the experience of salvation through conversion and commitment. Bright developed a simplified approach to the conversion experience.

"The Four Spiritual Laws" was developed by Bright in 1957 as a response to a challenge he heard in a conference for Campus

Crusade staff training. Initially an approach to personal evangelism was prepared for staff members, who memorized the full twenty-minute presentation of "God's Plan for your Life." This was later modified by Bright into the "Four Spiritual Laws," emphasizing the love of God rather than man's sinfulness. To achieve this emphasis Bright reversed the original position of the first two laws, immediately before the final draft for the first publication of the laws was prepared.

During the late fifties and through the decade of the sixties Campus Crusade for Christ grew in its impact on the American religious scene. Organization became necessary, along with careful training of staff. All staff of Campus Crusade are volunteers, who provide the foundation for their personal income through gifts solicited for the organization. The early years of the movement retained an emphasis on campus ministries, but during the sixties broader horizons of ministry were incorporated. By 1975 the movement and its staff represented an international dimension, as well as providing a ministry of assistance to churches in the development of personal witnessing skills.

In 1972 Campus Crusade sponsored a youth convocation at Dallas, Explo '72. Eighty thousand youth met in this mass meeting with the purpose of learning to tell others about the love of God revealed through Jesus Christ. In 1974 an international Explo was held in Seoul, drawing more than 300,000 reported attendance. Crusade leadership saw this meeting as the move which would make Korea the first country in the world to be totally evangelized.

Campus Crusade for Christ denies participation in the Pentecostal phenomenon. Like another group, the Full Gospel Business Men's Association, its primary aim is personal evangelism in the form of personal witnessing with a goal of conversion and commitment to discipleship by the one to whom witness is offered. In both groups, the heavy emphasis on dependence on the activity of the Holy Spirit in conversion and the life of the individual places them in the broad category of charismatic Christians.

By the late 1960s other developments in the American religious experience brought to common usage the term "charismatic." Significant in the development of the use of the term was the impact of the Jesus Movement, 1967-1972. Popular treatment in the secular and religious media blurred the differentiation between "charismatic" and "Pentecostal," to the extent that the two became connotatively synonymous. This has been unfortunate for clear communication concerning the goal, mission, and ministries of groups like Campus Crusade as well as other groups with a long history of Christian tradition.

A clearer delineation of charismatic Christians as those who seek to live their discipleship with a sense of awareness of the direct guidance of the Holy Spirit offers all Christians a rationale for claiming this dynamic of faith. Pentecostalism, more clearly defined, is a movement within Christendom which claims the essentiality of glossolalia for the full experience and expression discipleship.

The blurring of this distinction came through the development of the Jesus Movement. It began in California in 1967 as a spin-off from the drug culture among youth in that area. The emotional articulation of religious experience, often accompanied by glossolalia, as well as the anti-institutionalism which the movement directed toward established lines of denominationalism, and the adoption by the youth of the dress and behavior patterns of the drug culture were some factors which drew sharp lines of demarcation for it. As part of the general pattern culturally the Jesus Movement may now be seen as a phenomenon which provided a religious sanction for the radical withdrawal of youth from previously accepted cultural patterns. The intense personalism of the religious experience and the development of models of Bible study which emphasized a literal approach to Scripture interpretation as well as its apocalypticism placed the movement ideologically in the spectrum of religious movements usually identified as fundamentalistic.

Only as the decade of the seventies was reaching mid-point were analyses of the Jesus Movement being developed. These offered more than reporting on the activities of the movement or an emphasis on its more spectacular phenomena.

Biblical Translation and Scholarship

One other dimension of the American experience ought to be noted for its impact on changing accents of belief. Biblical translation and scholarship blossomed between 1955 and 1975, producing an impact analogous to that of the development of moveable type in the fifteenth century. Until the twentieth century American Protestants read, memorized, and swore on the third authorized translation of Scripture into English, commonly called the King James Version. Roman Catholics maintained the authority of the Rheims-Douay Version, and Jews accepted the Masoretic text which dates to the tenth century.

Biblical scholarship in America had been through the throes of the development of the historical-critical method, through reactions to that method by conservative interpreters, and through the renewal of interest in this realm of scholarship by the time of the second world war. Renewal of interest in Biblical scholarship following the war came after the discovery of the Dead Sea Scrolls in 1947. The chronicles of the discovery, first marketing, and later exploration of the content of the scrolls has been clearly recorded. The discovery among the scrolls of a complete text of Isaiah validated the accepted texts. To have a text which is a thousand years older than any extant text, and for the two to be so close represents an achievement in calligraphy which is unusual. The scrolls and their reflection of life in the first and second centuries, as well as the Biblical texts they represent, were a part of the initiation of a new era of Biblical study and emphasis.

The first important translation which should be noted was published between 1946 and 1952. The Revised Standard Version, a product of careful translation by committees, fulfilled the goal of the International Council of Religious Education, which in 1928 had acquired the copyright to the American Standard Version (1901). The Council appointed a committee of scholars to deal with the question of whether a new translation should be attempted, and adopted the 1937 report of the committee favoring a new translation. The revision committee of thirty-two scholars and a fifty member advisory board submitted themselves to the task of providing a version which reflected the advances of twentieth century scholarship, but which retained the stylistic qualities of the King James Version. The New Testament translation was published in 1946 and the publication of both Testaments as the Revised Standard Version of the Bible was voted by the Council in 1951.

Reception of this translation was mixed. Little popular reaction was evident until after the publication of the Old Testament. Reaction came from those groups and individuals whose allegiance was to a literal interpretation of the English of the King James Version. Particular objection was raised to portions of the Old Testament which in the Revised Standard Version seemed to question the legitimacy of the virgin birth. Some book burnings were held, but gradually objection to the new translation receded.

The great thrust of translation activity came after 1965. The American Bible Society led the development of public consciousness of translations with the publication in 1966 of the Today's English Version, commonly called "Good News for Modern Man." Prepared for a non-English speaking audience, this translation/interpretation used a limited vocabulary, a prose style, and line drawings appropriately illustrating sections of the text.

The New English Bible (New Testament, 1966, Old Testament, 1970) was a prose version translated by the committee method. In a few instances English colloquialisms have been noted, and acceptance by the American public has been slow to develop. The total change of style may have been a factor in the popular acceptance of this translation. Among some groups, however, another prose version has received a high level of popularity. *The Living Bible* has been marketed aggressively among select groups of more conservative Protestants, and has in some instances replaced the King James Version.

On the whole, however, a 1971 Gallup survey indicated that 71% of adult Protestants had read the Bible in a home setting within the preceeding year. The South showed the highest percentage of Bible readers (81%), and generally women were dominant (81%, 64% men). The King James Version was the dominant version read, with 62% readership. The poll was conducted prior to the publication of the New English Bible. It does, however, indicate the attachment to the King James Version, even over the Revised Standard Version, which at that time had been published eighteen years.

Although clear evidence is unavailable, it may be conjectured that the Bible reading population would fall among those groups of Christians who would tend toward the more conservative, fundamentalistic, or literal groups. Among the youth who reflected attachments to Bible reading and study during the early seventies, it could be observed that their methods of study did not include the assistance of standard commentaries. They appeared to transfer the literal interpretative approach long associated with the King James Version to their preferred modern English version, thereby developing a new form of English Bible literalism.

The development in Biblical scholarship 1955-1975 has produced a continuous series of publications to provide both laity and religious professionals with more adequate tools for Biblical study and interpretation. *The Interpreter's Bible* and *The Interpreter's Bible Dictionary* both provide extensive critical and historical information generally well grounded in accepted scholarship. Several single volume commentaries were published during the latter portion of this period, aimed particularly at the nonprofessional audience. Two which received wide acclaim were *The Interpreter's One Volume Commentary* and *The New Abingdon Bible Commentary*.

Signal achievement in Biblical publication came in 1973 with the production of the Ecumenical Bible. This was a revised Standard Version text which received the approval of Protestant, Roman Catholic and Eastern Orthodox ecclesiastics.

Changing accents of belief among American Christians can only be gauged by trends which developed during 1955-1975. No sharp changes in basic beliefs were to be noted. The change in accents must be viewed from the perspective of consciousness raising, which occurred. Traditional theological lines remained evident; although there may have been some blurring of the demarcations inherited from prior generations.

Gaps continued to exist between the academic theological world and the world of daily religious practice and experience. The political role of religiously motivated individuals achieved visibility through the media. We have reserved comment on the impact of Vatican II and ecumenical developments for later exploration. Even the power of these movements may not be seen to be significantly altering basic beliefs. Their major contribution appeared in the realm of broadening the bases of conversation and modification of practices among communions.

Touch the kaleidescope and the configurations change.

3

Changing Celebration

The developments of changing emphases in worship seem to crystalize around the early events of Vatican II and its consideration of worship. The promulgation of the Constitution on the Sacred Liturgy, passed by the august body of bishops before they spoke officially on the nature of the Church, opened a window to the world, and the breath of the Spirit was felt by some to be a whirlwind. The most striking products of the changes from Vatican II were the reversal of the bodily position of the priest in celebration of the mass. For centuries his back had been turned to the faithful. With the adoption of the more ancient basilican form, a form datable to the second or third centuries, the priest faced the congregation at an open table near the entrance of the sanctuary. The other readily noted change was the adoption of national languages in the celebration of worship. The use of the vernacular, widely accepted and at the same time opposed, demanded a different level of participation. The change shifted spectators to active roles in worship.

Among Protestants this dramatic change modified the idea of "mumbo-jumbo" which had been associated with the Latin rite. Now they clearly could understand what was being said and what was transpiring in the service. Faithful Roman Catholics had the same experience, although through careful catechetical teaching they had been exposed to the meanings of the Latin. Vatican II did not change the meaning of the mass. All its provisions required was a change in the way the mass was celebrated. Thus we were confronted with a changed form which had in it the potential for clearer communication of what was taking place. Clearer communication among the participants in worship was a remarkable achievement. This achievement crossed denominational lines. The Episcopal Church in America adopted a modern English liturgy, seeking a clearer communication of the dynamics of worship. The introduction of new forms of music into worship among many communions could also be interpreted under the umbrella of clearer communication and reversal of the spectator roles of communicants. Liturgy regained its base meaning, the work of the people.

In the following pages we shall look at the Constitution on the Sacred Liturgy, examine some of its specifics, and then interpret some of its implications. We shall also be concerned with looking at the development of what some writers have called the festival spirit in worship. Liturgical reform, not already treated, will be noted, along with the development of mysticism and other forms of personalized religious experience. Finally we shall attempt an evaluation of the steady witness of evangelicalism. Once again we tackle a large assignment.

Vatican II and Liturgical Change

For centuries part of the mystique of the Roman Catholic Church and its worship through the celebration of the mass was the language used. Latin provided a tangible link with the past, and spoke to the slowly changing (for some unchanging) stances of the church through the centuries. In the middle ages the cup had been removed from the laity, partially at their request. The architectural shape of the churches was modified with the development of thirteenth and fourteenth century Gothic form. In some instances, due to the physical distance as well as the illiteracy of the laity, bells were introduced to signal appropriate movement. The mass was theologically interpreted as a sacrifice, hence the need for genuflection on approach and departure from the physical presence of the body of the Lord. Color, pageantry, incense, music, movement all coalesced in the actions of worship, in which the people retained only a spectator role. Liturgical change was not an innovation with Vatican II. The road to change had been traveled within the church for several decades prior to the papacy of John XXIII. As early as the twenties and thirties pioneers in evaluation of the liturgy began investigations which would be incorporated in the actions of Vatican II. Frs. Virgil Michel, Gerald Ellard, H.A. Reinhold, Martin Hellreigel, and others developed a movement which became the Liturgical Conference. Twenty-five years of development clearly indicated that liturgical change was not merely the work of a few theologians in Europe and America. Fr. Joseph Jungman became a leading spokesman for liturgical reform, laying a groundwork carefully based on a clear understanding of the historical traditions of the church.

When the Council was called, Cardinal Gustav Cicognani was named chairman of the preconciliar commission on the liturgy. The work of the commission was enhanced when leaders from Trier and Paris were added to its force. In four months of intensive study, the commission's subcommittees worked out the details of each chapter of the Constitution, and the whole commission evaluated the entire text three times before it was submitted to the Council.

The focus of the document was thoroughly Biblical. It stressed salvation history, and at times used the words of Pius XII's encyclical *Mediator Dei*. The Council debated the document from October 22 to November 13, 1962, providing 328 oral commentaries on it. On November 14, 1962, 2,162 Council fathers approved the Constitution, with only 46 dissenting. One year later final approval was provided, revisions and modifications from the lengthy debate of 1962 having been examined and incorporated. The document was officially promulgated, pronounced an action of the Council by Paul VI on December 4, 1963, and became the first Constitution published by the Council.

The process and some implications of change had been worked out. The challenge facing the church in 1964 and in following years was the implementation of the document. Two dramatic changes in the experience of worship were immediately instituted. Both of these have been mentioned previously but attention to their import should be reiterated. The language of the mass was Latin for more than seventeen centuries. The Constitution provided for national councils of Bishops to make the determinations on the use of the vernacular. The United States Council of Bishops approved English for the celebration of worship in 1964. This change was instituted specifically to allow more participation by the people in the actions and words of worship.

The second dramatic change was a modification of the physical location of the central action of worship, the sacrificial action of the priest in the celebration of the mass. For centuries the priest had performed the action of consecration of bread and wine with his back to the people, facing an altar far removed from them. The Constitution provided for the location of the altar in a more central position, with the consecratory action of the priest being performed facing them. By this change the church adopted the more ancient basilican form for the celebration of the altar sacrifice. These modifications, while the more immediate to be noted, are not to be considered the full accomplishment of change. Equally exciting for the experience of worship were the foundations within the Constitution on the Sacred Liturgy which provided for more complete sharing by the communicant in all dimensions of the experience of worship and the receipt of grace thereby.

Traditionally the priest was the central human figure in the celebration of the mass. The Constitution on the Sacred Liturgy recognized the officiating role of the priest, and raised to a new level of conciousness the participant role of those worshipping. The liturgy was declared to be an exercise of the priestly office of Jesus Christ, manifesting man's sanctification through signs perceptible to the senses. The priest is the contemporary human agent of the priestly office of the Lord. The Constitution requires the priest, as a fulfillment of his pastoral office, to assure that the faithful participate knowingly, actively, and fruitfully. Only through the interaction of priest and people could the liturgy become the central thrust of the life of the church. One entire section of the Constitution deals with the catechetical responsibility of the church for assuring that priests are prepared to provide adequate leadership for the laity to participate knowingly in the activity of celebration.

In some instances participation without preparation was a liability to the introduction of new levels of involvement for the people. Those who were accustomed to using the time in the mass for personal devotional actions were not easy to convince that they played an important role in worship. Music in the vernacular became a part of the worship experience. In the first years following the publication of the Constitution, new music had to be written. In some instances hymns long familiar to Protestants were used, even "A Mighty Fortress is Our God!" Other hymns used were "All Hail the Power of Jesus' Name," "To God be the Glory," and "Amazing Grace." Gradually new music for worship was written, and the early days of borrowing or using poorly written music with a questionable theological base decreased. In 1966 the folk mass was introduced, with some greater benefit on the levels of communication and theological perception.

Another significant emphasis encouraged by Vatican II was the strengthening of the use of Scripture and preaching in worship. The presence of Christ in the worship experience was affirmed not only in the elements of the sacrifice, but also in the words spoken when the Scripture was read. The Constitution required readings which were more varied and suitable. To accomplish this purpose lectionaries had to be revised and rewritten. The New Roman Missal was published in 1970 in the United States. It provided many optional texts for various parts of the mass. The content of the sermon was to be based in the Scripture, and should be a proclamation of God's work in the history of salvation. Calling men to faith and conversion before they came to the celebration of the liturgy was to be achieved through the emphasis on Scripture reading and the sermon. Faith and repentance must be proclaimed even to believers as the foundation of appropriate grace achieving experiences.

The sense of community which liturgical reform sought to implement via the Constitution was developed in the exchange of the "sign of peace." At the central point of the mass, between the words of institution and the reception of the element, the priest turns to the people and speaks the words, "Let us offer each other the sign of peace." The priest would shake the hands of the lay reader and others while the congregation would extend greetings to each other with the words, "May the peace of Christ be with you." Direct, personal, face-to-face interaction prior to receiving holy communion revitalized the corporate experience of people in worship. It further had the benefit of incorporating meaning into the actions of worship, deemphasizing the singularity of the individual.

Finally a significant development of the implementation of the Constitution has been the modification of the Church year. To accomplish this goal the feasts associated with the saints took a necessary secondary role to the central dimensions of the liturgical calendar which proclaims the history of salvation in the life and work of Christ. The medieval and Tridentine emphases on saints, their special feasts and festivals and statuary were seen as secondary. Appropriate modification of this emphasis was necessary to implement the Christocentric dimensions of the liturgy. Further, the Constitution even provided for the development of a fixed date for the celebration of Easter, an ecumenical overture which could approach a bridging of the fissure between Eastern and Western Christendom which has lasted since the fourth century.

The challenge of implementation of liturgical change has not been accomplished by decree. The development of appropriate forms and rites which reflect local emphases have been continuous since 1964. The New Roman Missal (1970), five years in development, was a testimony to the process of liturgical change. The continued efforts of theologians and priests will be required to provide the necessary catechetical functions for providing a corporate entity which assures that the faithful participate knowingly, actively, and fruitfully.

The Festival Spirit in Worship

Irony? Coincidence?

In the middle of a period in the life of the nation which was facing a volley of problems which ranged from the increasing awareness of the futility of the Viet Nam conflict, revolts among the students on leading campuses, youth dropping out through an increasing drug influenced culture, some areas of thought began to talk about the role of play.

The thought forms which began to be heard in American culture were influenced by Robert Neale who developed an anthropology of play in *In Praise of Play.* He said that man is basically a player, not a worker; and, that man's true nature is distorted when he sees work as the most important facet of his life. Man becomes the slave of his percept of work, thereby causing a loss of the spirit of adventure. Eventually he loses the ability to respond totally to his environment in the same way that a child loses a sense of adventure in the process of reaching adulthood. In the examination of work and play new inquiries into the Puritan background of American culture were explored. Through the approaches to life exemplified by elementary text book levels of understanding American colonial Puritanism, work had become a primary value.

In the world of religious experience and expression, the dynamic understanding of the festival spirit of worship took its incentive from the culture to which the church ministered. In many respects this was a Protestant movement, since the work ethic in American cultural experience had achieved the designation "the Protestant ethic." Robert Neale suggested that full play is what religion really is. This idea rang strongly in the ears of those whose childhood had been underscored with the parental admonition, "Don't play in church!" But the emphasis on play provided the opportunity for a reevaluation of the action of Protestant forms of worship.

On examination Protestants found that worship experiences in the mid-twentieth century had tended to lose some of the elements of spontaniety, participation, and involvement which had been a part of nineteenth century or earlier worship experiences. The heritage of Puritanism had an effect through the long sermon, the long prayer, and the occasional congregational hymn. For the most part, however, Protestant middle class worship forms were oriented on the axis of leader and spectator. Nineteenth century developments of participation had stemmed from the revival emphases which came early in that century. The mourner's bench had been abandoned. Only among Pentecostals and blacks was there to be found the vestiges of this heritage. The impact of the crusade forms of revivalism from Dwight L. Moody to Billy Graham may also contain the seeds of retarding congregational activity in worship.

Contemporary with the emphasis on play, and a raising of the levels of consciousness concerning the actions of the worshipping community, another force entered which had some effect in molding Protestant attitudes. The youth musical or folk mass, depending on the liturgical proclivities of a denomination, began to develop. The folk mass was introduced among Roman Catholics in 1966. The youth musical, complete with electronic sound systems (sometimes with mega-amplification), choreography, and costuming entered the sacred palaces of worship. For older generations the cacaphony was inimical to effective worship, but for youth the emphasis was on relevancy and communication. The sound was contemporary. To be contemporary became the hallmark of relevance. Communication was more than the aural level, although this was dominant. Some attention was given to content, but evaluations of content often judged it as being theologically weak. Two successful commercial productions of this genre, *Jesus Christ, Superstar* and *Godspell* both raised a level of consciousness outside the churchly world.

Basic to an understanding of this new consciousness of movement or action on the part of the worshipping community was an awareness of the role of nonverbal communication. Action was interpreted as the essential ingredient of worship. Verbal communication was seen as the support for the action. James F. White reported in 1971 a service of communion for ministers and seminarians which was totally silent. The individual was fully participant in the action of worship, even creating his own sermon from a form of cue cards. In *New Forms of Worship* he indicated that the activity of the worshipper and the worship leader were integrated, particularly in the celebration of communion.

In some worship settings dance became a form for experiences in experimental worship. Biblical foundation for this phenomenon was established from the temple practices of Judaism, and on the bases of some analogies of the movement of the mass. Thomas Merton made an interpretation of the priest's movement in celebration as a form of stylized dance. Interactive dance forms were observed, particularly among the youth developments, at the same time that it was being recognized that this activity was appropriate for limited experiences in worship. Generally, when dance was used as a portion of worship activity, it was interpretative, performed by an individual or group as a chancel or dias activity as a support for other elements of the worship experience. "Dancing in the aisles" did occur, but this was not a regular phenomenon of worship.

Notably it was among black churches that the tradition of participation of the worshipping community has maintained the greatest degree of vitality. Out of the traditions of congregational support for the preacher, particularly in examinations of the sermon as a form of oral literature, the role of participants was actively observed and commented on. The sermon in this tradition was an extemporaneous oral creation with a degree of the impromptu element in it. It cannot be called wholly impromptu because of the reality of culturally acquired and developed motifs which appear in transcriptions of the sermons. There is a basic level of material, both Biblical and illustrative, with which both preacher and congregation must be familiar in order for the creative dimension to function. Thus as an extempraneous experience, with some degree of antiphonal expression, the sermon was the joint creation of people and proclaimer.

All dimensions of worship, especially among Protestants, converged in the development of an awareness of the festival spirit in all experiences of worship. Festival came out of the boxes of Christmas, Easter, and some national holidays, so that each worship experience was interpreted as a part of the ongoing festival or celebration. Words like joy and celebration entered the vocabulary. Banners hung from balconies or clerestories, on walls, and against reredos. Color, both the traditional liturgical colors and new brilliant combinations, was employed to heighten the festival awareness for the worshipping community. Somber colors were overshadowed in some instances by plaids and stripes. All of these ascribed the elements of celebration. Color was also adopted by the more conservative dimensions of Protestantism, and a noted evangelist's wardrobe approached a peacock's hue from emerald green velvet sports coats to the offical blue pinstripe. Vestments were adopted by traditionally non-vested clergy, and in some instances worshippers wore crepe paper stoles in brilliant hues.

The goal of the festival spirit as it developed was the creation of a new consciousness of participation on the part of the worshipper. As he entered into the dynamic of activity, he became co-celebrant with the leader, thereby approximating from some quarters a truer interpretation of the Reformation doctrine of the priesthood of believers. After 1973 less emphasis was heard about the festival, lending some credence to the view that this was another fad which had run its course. The impact of the movement, however, could still be seen as Protestants were generally more willing to attempt new forms in an effort to find more effective means of communication.

Other Liturgical Reform
Already note has been made of the liturgical reform via Vatican II and as it was a product of the festival spirit among Protestants. Specific reforms of liturgy were active on many fronts, however. The impact of Vatican II was a movement among Protestants causing them to review their own levels of experience in worship.

The Episcopal Church in America was among the first to attempt the challenge of providing a new focus for the worship
experience of all communicants. The development of a trial
liturgy, wherein the language of worship was significantly modified was a continuing project after 1968. As late as 1975 even
with the publication of a new prayer book, pockets of resistance
remained highly vocal. Rubrics were not significantly changed,
but greater emphasis on the role and participation of the laity
was the goal. Modern English failed to provide the familiar
qualities of Elizabethan cadences, and canticles needed new
musical forms appropriate to the rhythms of the language being
used.

The impact of liturgical change has been seen to be a continuing dimension of the life of the church. Modes of worship reflect
the continuing response of the church to changing cultural conditions. Realization of the needs of men as they approach the life
rejuvenating function of worship has been at the base of liturgical change.

Liturgical change in some instances has not been as dramatic
as the examples from Vatican II or in the Episcopal modifications. For some it has come in a recognition of the values of
appropriate recognition of traditional seasons in the Christian
calendar. Advent, Lent, and the Trinity season have been recognized for their basic value to the Christian tradition. Even among
Southern Baptists, long recognized as an anti-liturgical body,
there were evidences that individual congregations were adopting with appreciation Advent and Lenten disciplines in public
and private worship.

Also, one can speculate that the dual factors of higher educational levels as well as more open attitudes among denominations were leading to an adoption of some changes in the
actions of worship. The former may be seen in the growing
acceptance of traditional church music among communions
where a quarter century earlier little appreciation of Bach or
Palestrina would have been noted. The latter may be seen as the
product of community worship at stated seasons of the year,
particularly Passion Week.

Whatever the forces, liturgy by 1970 was not as negative a term as it had been, and the Protestant reactions to it seemed to be less on a "Protestant-Catholic" continuum. Worship showed evidences of being clearly "people centered" and thereby fulfilled the true meaning of liturgy.

Mysticism and Personal Piety

Worship is not only a public activity. For many individuals personal religious devotion is as important as the activity of public worship. In the decades 1955-1975 fresh emphases on personal religious experience ranged from the conversion experience which is basic to some forms of understanding personal religious life to the flowering of a renewed interest in the practice of the traditional forms of Christian mysticism. This gamut of experiential religious life has been augmented by a consciousness of the interior life and the role of the Holy Spirit as the energizer of religious life. As we look at this dimension of changing celebration some examination of popular forms of piety will be attempted.

Personal expressions of religious experience have tended to be centered around the traditional crisis occasions of life. Birth, baptism, marriage, and death form the focuses of personal religious experience. The church has ministered at these crises for all the centuries of her existence. These are still the cardinal events when the ministry of the church has represented the means of grace for the faithful. Personal piety continues to anticipate the ministration of the church in these central life events.

In the past two decades attention to the central life crises of individuals received fresh emphasis. One of the ways the church sought to respond was through the development of the pastoral care movement. Through specific training in the disciplines of counseling and crisis intervention, seminaries developed curricula and faculties with the goal of equipping ministers with skills which would aid them in their ministry to individuals. Leaders in the movement came to prominence in theological education during the fifties. Wayne Oates, Seward Hiltner, and Ruel Howe are only three among the many whose skills in relating psychological and theological insights were formative for several decades of ministers. Their emphases on ministering to individuals in crisis called new attention to a perspective of the professional ministry. The blending of skills from two disciplines raised the general level of consciousness of the churches toward this responsibility of their ministry. One of the impacts of the pastoral care movement lay in the heightening of awareness of religious experiences of individuals. Thus, personal piety was the benefactor.

Another dimension of personal piety which achieved emphasis came through the development of cell groups. In this move small groups within a congregation, or among congregations, were formed for study and/or social interaction. The thrust of these groups was to heighten personal identity, to provide an opportunity for depth study, to provide social action teams, and to develop trust relationships in what was seen as an increasingly depersonalized culture. The cell group approach applied to a group obtained some of the same dynamics that pastoral care held for individuals. In some instances the cell group concept took on some of the dynamics of group therapy within a religious context.

Sensitivity Training and Transactional Analysis were also methods which were employed among church groups as these phenomena became widely accepted in the general culture. Shortly after Eric Berne's publication of *Games People Play* another publisher produced *Games Christians Play*. One wonders if the market for the second item was actually aware of the pattern on which this humorous treatment of congregational life was patterned. Sensitivity Training and Transactional Analysis interacted in a religious culture which by the late sixties and early seventies had become accustomed to the joining of insights from the fields of psychology and theology. These, too, were avenues through which one may see further development of an emphasis on personal piety.

Personal piety in this era also received an undergirding from a segment of American religious life which did not fit some of the norms of earlier denominational structures, offering the opportunity of high levels of individual commitment for individuals whose religious goals were more intense. The Church of the Savior, Washington, D.C., under the leadership of Gordon Cosby provided a religious community for a limited group of people. The congregation offered a variety of worship, learning, and service opportunities for some people who responded to discipline and commitment. Elizabeth O'Connor's writings interpreted the ministries of this congregation, and there were many attempts to imitate some of the accomplishments of this group. Church of the Savior was among the first Christian groups to develop the coffee house as a form of ministry. This, too, was often copied with greater success than was achieved by those who attempted to emulate the disciplinary standards of the Washington congregation.

Elton Trueblood, not so much as a Quaker, but as one who understood the strains of twentieth century life, proclaimed a form of religious experience which has some of the marks of personal piety. Trueblood's emphasis on personal commitment and discipline pointed to some of the concerns of personal religious experience. Yokefellow House and the Yokefellow groups became synonymous with a concept of piety which had a center in discipline, prayer, and sharing.

Significant, however, among all of the areas which raised an emphasis on personal piety, was the absence of the traditionally strong emphasis on Bible reading and private prayer. In the fifties and sixties these may have been included in some phases of the various movements, but they were not central. This caused, to some degree, a change in the meaning of piety. In many instances piety and pious were confused, pious having a negative connotation associated with a fundamentalistic and otherworldly form of Christian expression and experience. Some individuals who reacted against their more rigid backgrounds in conservative branches of Christendom found that the newer forms represented a level of sophistication more compatible with their cultural experiences in adulthood.

Prayer and responsiveness to the leadership of the Spirit of God active in the world seemed to take two forms during these decades of change and challenge. One form found a responsive audience mainly among the conservative, conversion oriented sectors of Protestantism. The other found an audience among a more intellectually oriented group. The first had a celebrity base, and the second seemed to eschew the popular celebrity.

Among the first group Dale Evans Rogers stands as an individual who spans the entire two decades. Ms Rogers first came to national attention as a spokesperson for the conservative, conversion oriented groups through the publication of her testimonial *Angel Unaware*. This small volume, describing the experience with a retarded child, captured the hero imagination of a broad segment of the American populace. Her own established reputation contributed to the acceptance of the religious views represented in the writing. Other established celebrities, whose religious experience fit the conversion motifs of conservative groups also published testimonials. These writings provided a base for religious biography and autobiography which became a popular literary form.

In most of the popular writings there appeared a strong emphasis on the conversion experience and the struggles of the biographees to retain a sense of the presence of God active in their lives. Prayer was an important phenomenon of religious expression, and the types of prayer recorded were intensely personalistic. The awareness of the presence and activity of God which was reported was also described in highly personalized terms. Some emphasis was given to the Bible as a guide for daily living, but the writings tended to be weak in their articulation of an understanding of revelation in Scripture.

Another note which sounded from these works was a sense of serenity in surrender. A type of self abengation was voiced which approximated Milton's slough of despond and the leap of faith from Kierkegaard and Schliermacher. Rejection of self dependence and total dependence on the provenance of God was articulated. Not only Dale Evans Rogers, but also Pat Boone, Johnny Cash, Catherine Marshall, and others provided a popular testimony which appealed in terms of personal piety to a segment of the American populace.

Another segment of the American religious consciousness responded to a more contemplative approach to religious experience. Mysticism became a means of achieving a sense of the active presence of God in the lives of men. Classical mysticism was studied for clues to the dynamics of this form of religious experience. Thomas Merton, the Trappist monk at Our Lady of Gethsemane Abbey, near Bardstown, Kentucky, had a large following. Although Merton achieved one level of acclaim for his social awareness, it was through his understanding and articulartion concerning mysticism that his greater contribution came. As a Trappist he specialized in the practice of the traditional mysteries of the church. As novice master of the Abbey he communicated to each group of novices the essential disciplines of the mystic's life of prayer for the world. As a prolific author who was encouraged to publish his work he had a profound effect on the consciousness of the mystically inclined among both Protestant and Roman Catholic Christians.

Merton's was not the only voice heard to proclaim the vitality of the mystic's way. Henri Nouwen, a Dutch priest, provided sensitive insight into the ways of the modern mystic for a limited public. In 1972, this sensitive and aware man had achieved the status of unofficial chaplain to the Divinity School of Yale, where he then taught. His human responsiveness to those in that setting provided them with a living example of the power of the mystic's perception of the activity of God in the lives of men.

Two other phenomena which may illuminate an understanding of personal piety and mysticism require attention for a rounded picture of this aspect of changing patterns. Both of these were more restricted to academic communities and interests. One attempted to analyze some forms of religious consciousness in terms of religious humanism. The other emphasized the strengths of religion as story, particularly in terms of biography and autobiography.

Among the interpreters of the first view were those who sought to explain the anti-institutional expressions, but social consciences, of American youth in the late sixties as a form of religious humanism. Few dispute the rejection of the institutional churches by youth in the sixties. But when the social conscience of these same youth was examined, they were found to be acting on a religious-like motivation. Some have sought to explain the popularity of the Peace Corps and VISTA programs as essentially humanistic concerns which captured the social conscience of many middle class youth. Through these secular agencies they were able to act out the religious behavior which they had been taught, but in rationalistic and humanistic forms.

Intense personalization of religious ideation was made possible in academic settings through the emphasis on story. Religious mythology, carefully examined in mushrooming departments of religious studies, seized on this mode of expressing religious experience in a non-confessional setting. This provided for the development in this approach for the emphasis on biography and autobiography. Spiritual biography and autobiography became a means of approach for the study of religion as a cultural phenomenon without doing violence to the recognized personal features of religious experience. In the academic atmosphere a sense of objectivity and comparison was offered. Personal piety in modern dress lay at the base of these studies.

Although there may be a disparate nature to these suggestions of the impact of personal piety and mysticism, there is a connecting thread among them which relates them to the emphasis on changing celebration. First, in most instances they tended to provide a raised consciousness to individual needs and crises which could be met by religious experience. Second, they provided an interdisciplinary base for approaching an understanding of man as a religious creature. Third, they provided a heightened sense of the presence of God active in the lives of individuals. Fourth, they found expression in a community structure. Fifth, they accented a positive approach to the life experience of the individual. Sixth, their public articulation was in a vocabulary which can be called celebrative. Seventh, they emphasized in some instances the traditional disciplines associated with Scripture and prayer. Eighth, they provided a base for openness toward and interaction with the forms of worship being developed in the same era. Finally, collectively, they sought to maintain some sense of balance between religious experience as a personally based and as a community based phenomenon.

The Steady Witness of Evangelicalism

Evangelism and evangelicalism are not the same thing. For many people, however, the terms became inseparable. The energy associated with evangelism, proselytizing innovations, and the emphasis on personal conversion have long been marks of evangelicals in America. Evangelicals are activists. As activists they carved a clear niche for themselves in the annals of American religious experience.

One of the ways in which evangelicals have gained high visibility on the American religious consciousness was through their awareness of the positive values of the media as an effective communication tool. The dicta of Marshall McLuhan, "the medium is the message," was not lost on the evangelistic efforts of evangelicals. Television, radio, magazines, newspapers were used effectively by these groups for the proclamation of the word. The effective power of a mass audience, the hallmark of the crusade form supported by many evangelicals, was another characteristic trait of these energetic proclaimers.

Billy Graham and Oral Roberts, both symbols of evangelism via the crusade movement, have both understood the power of television. Roberts may have preceded Graham in the adoption of the television as a communication tool. Who was first is not as important as the recognition that both of these men represent a distinctive use of visual media for effectively maintaining a level of consciousness among the populace. Graham's use was mainly through televising the essential elements of crusade meetings—songs, sermon, and call to discipleship. Roberts, however, developed the use of the medium through careful programming and production, particularly in the years after the establishment of the Oral Roberts University.

Each of these men has large personal followings among the

grass roots levels of America. Graham's following has lasted longer, or has been more firmly entrenched. The high levels of acceptance among Presidents Eisenhower through Nixon, though diminished in the latter Nixon years, provided Graham with the aura of being the evangelical spokesman for the country. To see him pictured on the golf course with government dignitaries, greeting the chief executive following worship at the White House, or participating in the annual ritual of the National Prayer Breakfast provided him with a national image separate from the crusading evangelist.

In American experience evangelicalism is a particular manner of interpreting Christianity. It has not been clearly identified as a denomination, nor has it been a total feature of any single denominational group. It has represented cultural movements among diverse religious groups, ranging from the National Holiness Alliance to interdenominational educational institutions like Moody Bible Institute, Bob Jones University, and Wheaton College. It may even be seen as a cultural base for the positive thinking movement of the fifties. Robert Ellwood described it as a religious form of popular culture in *One Way*, but also acknowledged that within it are seeds of a culture denying mood.

At the base of the evangelical spirit in American religious expression is the belief and practice of a personal, deeply felt experience or relationship with Jesus Christ. A single, powerful mystical experience has in some instances been the sine qua non of evangelicals. Some emphasize an awareness of the precise date, time, and place of such an experience. This allowed no room for Bushnellian Christian nurturing, which sought to speak to the nineteenth century emphasis on the demand for precise conversion experiences.

In some instances the emphasis among evangelicals has moved toward the necessity of the Pentecostal glossolalia experiences. When this has been the emphasis, men have been offered the opportunity to live post-conversion sinless lives. Generally, however, except for the Pentecostal experiences, evangelicals have emphasized spiritual rebirth, infallible Scripture, signs and miracles, imminent eschatology, and a sense of exclusivism which cut them off from interaction with other Christians.

With some exceptions the worship practices of evangelicals have centered on music, Scripture, prayers, and sermon. The music was popular, folk, gospel, and in some instances rock. As the youth influences were felt more strongly in the late sixties and early seventies the unique form of "Jesus Rock" became associated with evangelical worship practices. Few visual symbols were used in evangelical places of worship. Flowers, an open Bible, and occasionally a cross may be placed in the worship center.

The sermon was the focal point of evangelical worship forms. It may be supported by direct testimony, and required subsequent testimony. The sermon was based on Biblical truths which emphasize the sinful state of man and his need for salvation. It was a confrontation of man with his natural state and presentation of his potential as a redeemed individual actively living in the grace of God. Grace, however, was a word foreign to the vocabulary of many evangelicals. The ultimate goal of the sermon was to present the hearer with the alternatives of accepting or rejecting the salvation of God provided by the sacrifice of Jesus. Two choices, salvation through Jesus Christ, or the torment of eternal damnation for rejecting him, thereby committing the unpardonable sin, were the options proclaimed.

Evangelicals in America have been activists, but seldom social activists. They promoted rallies, Sunday school attendance, tours, programs, and revivals. Sometimes the militant spirit of their activity overflowed into their language, reflecting a self concept of the army of the Lord which must conquer the world, routing sin and Satan.

Significantly among some Protestant groups the evangelical spirit has prospered in the churches with burgeoning Sunday schools. Of the ten churches in America with the largest Sunday school enrollments during the early seventies, all represented the force of the evangelical spirit. Central to each was a powerful personality at the helm of leadership.

One of the leading publications of the evangelical movement, *Christianity Today*, was founded in the mid-fifties as a conservative voice for American Christians. This publication provides a reactionary interpretation and platform. It does not hesitate to judge. Often its content has a polemical style, or it is at least described as absolutist. Carl F. H. Henry, first editor, was among the leading spokesmen for a literalistic approach to Scripture interpretation during the mid portion of the century.

Finally, to be noted among evangelicals was an apocalyptic tone. Eschatology was a favorite theme. Preparation for the end time, particularly to assure that all men have the opportunity to be confronted by the gospel, was a motivating force. The mass movement—revival or crusade—was the medium most suited to this approach. Evangelicals appear to be the backbone of these continuing movements in American religious experience.

Worship, in this chapter called celebration, received large attention during the decades 1955-1975. In the mid-fifties new buildings were equipped with the accoutrement of an affluent, upwardly mobile middle class. Dignity in public worship was a goal for many churches, especially those in the free church traditions. With the early sixties and the developments in Vatican II new emphases in worship were focused on the participation of the individual, sharing the experience with the leader. American culture tipped the kaleidescope and a new angle of vision brought emphases in personal piety, and even experimental forms. New music, new liturgies, new ways of communicating the truths of the religious experience were developed.

But, amid the new sounds the basics remained unchanged. The mass was still the essential grace imparting sacrifice. From the Protestant right the emphasis was still on the sinful state of man in need of conviction, confession, and commitment to discipleship. All sectors of Christendom, however, sought means of communicating their perceptions of religious truth in language, symbols, and settings which communicated with mid-twentieth century man.

4

Changing Conscience

One of the strong heritages of Western Christendom has been its social awareness and interaction. Service, the earliest function of the diaconate, became a trademark of the church. The exercise of a social conscience was expressed through the development of schools, hospitals, and other charities through the monastic system. Until well into the Renaissance the monastic houses of Europe were the centers of education, care for the poor and dying, as well as providing hospitality for travelers. The foundation of the church's social conscience appeared to be securely set on an understanding of koinonia, that all men are one and need support and care through the fellowship of the Spirit of Christ alive in the world. The Reformation did not alter the social conscience of the church, but contributed to it by emphasizing the responsibility of individuals as well as groups.

The Reformation heritage of individual social conscience became a strong force in American religious experience via the strengths of Calvinism and the impact of what came to be called the Puritan work ethic. In the past several decades there have been new attempts to understand the American psyche via an understanding of Puritanism as it was expressed in New England Congregationalism. This has lead to a clearer understanding of the social awareness of the religious groups in America.

Twentieth Century Social Conscience

From the perspective of 1975 it appears that the social conscience of Americans in the twentieth century was molded by the impact of two concepts. The first, a collective view of responsibility, and the other an individual view of responsibility. Each view had many proponents, but two names seem to represent each view quite clearly. Walter Rauschenbusch, Baptist, immigrant influenced theologian provided a rationale for the social gospel. Charles M. Sheldon, Congregationalist, preacher, and pastor represented the view of individual responsibility, through the question "What would Jesus do?" Sheldon has continued to have a high level of influence as individuals sought to walk *In His Steps*.

Rauschenbusch came to his views of social responsibility out of the crucible of life in Hell's Kitchen, a slum section of New York City, where he was pastor of the Second German Baptist Church. In 1917 he published his major treatise, lectures at Yale under the sponsorship of the Nathaniel W. Taylor Foundation. *The Theology for the Social Gospel* was his attempt in a systematic manner to provide a rational foundation to his views, conceiving Christian doctrine in social terms, and to relate the Christian message to the regeneration of the social order. The thrust of Rauschenbusch's thought was to undercut an oversimplified or simplistic concept of individual sin and personal salvation which fails to consider the nature of sin in man's collective efforts and in the institutions of society. The situations out of which Rauschenbusch developed his feelings as well as his thought were life experiences.

The doctrines of sin and redemption, two central concepts to Rauschenbusch, clearly placed in perspective the necessary tension between man's personal and collective actions. The view of sin as selfishness is more in harmony with Rauschenbusch's views that a view of sin as rebellion against God. For him sin was transmitted by means of social customs, institutions, and traditions which the individual absorbed from his social group. On the view of original sin, a thoroughgoing social gospel theology would have to argue for a view that original sin is partly social. Personal and social salvation is a goal of the social gospel. To achieve this, the Kingdom of God is central. The social dimension of the kingdom was weakened in the teachings of the early church when emphasis was placed on the concept of individual salvation vs. social redemption. In the Medieval and Renaissance eras the church held a high view of social responsibility, but did not exercise this responsibility in a manner which emphasized corporate action. The height of Renaissance piety saw the development of monastic orders which had a social sense, but they were not active in molding the policies of the social order. Savanarola at Florence at the time Columbus sailed to America was the closest the Renaissance came to developing a concept of social responsibility.

Rauschenbusch's emphasis on the kingdom had an eschatological note, but it was one which insisted that the kingdom was present and yet to come. Man could not achieve the kingdom by means of earthly labor, a denigration of popular Calvinism, but present labor was preparation for the kingdom when it would come. The present symbols of the kingdom were identified as worth of personality, freedom, growth, love, solidarity, and service. In some instances these represented the optimism of American thought prior to and during World War I.

The Theology for the Social Gospel was a classic piece of twentieth century religious literature. Close to it was Rauschenbusch's *Prayers of the Social Gospel*. Through the prayers one can see clearly the human situations which motivated the man's thought. Concrete, precise, directed to the events and concerns of ordinary men, the prayers lose little in their late nineteenth and early twentieth century language. Reinhold Niebuhr, like Walter Rauschenbusch, found the plight of ordinary men in the vices of the city a crucible which forged a passionate social compassion.

Charles M. Sheldon, Congregationalist minister in the midwest used Sunday nights as an opportunity to speak in a type of serialized account about the activity of God among men in his world. His most popular, well known, or lasting novel was published in 1896. *In His Steps* was the attempt to communicate the power of the social implications of the gospel. But, the social implications were seen in terms of the salvation experience of an individual who pledged to live one year of his life taking for himself as the guide or rule for living the question, "What would Jesus do?" Each situation or decision of the individual must be determined on the basis of the response to that question. The individual had two basic guides to assist him in achieving an answer to the question: the Bible, and the Spirit of God. *In His Steps* was not unique, because it was one of more than ten novels produced by Sheldon. All had the same basic theme. *His Brother's Keeper*, set in a new mining district of the mid-west, provided the same stock characters in the same stock situations, responding to the call of God and seeking to serve him fully as they subjectively perceived his will. It did, however, contain some lyrics of Salvation Army songs from that era which were probably authentic.

The impact of Sheldon's work was that its continued acceptance maintained a norm of Christian piety into the seventies. The evangelical nature of the writing fed the evangelical emphases of the sixties and seventies. Sometimes those who offered themselves in response to the call of Christian social service had been influenced by reading Sheldon and becoming convinced that only through changed individuals could there eventually be a changed social order. Although no concrete evidence is available, it could be suggested that this was the level at which evangelical piety remained for the most part during the twentieth century.

During the last half decade of the fifties the last days of colonialism began to dawn on the world. In 1945 war ravaged countries needed help. In 1955 the United States was beginning to see the development of some ideas of global responsibility, and by 1975 global responsibility was hotly debated between hawks and doves. By 1975 the stress on individual experience, of man being confronted by the claims of the gospel, was one of the distinguishing marks of large groups of Christians.

Both men, Rauschenbusch and Sheldon, were important in shaping the social conscience during the fifties, sixties, and seventies. Their works, then, are a part of the unique background of American religious experience. They were theoretical and practical, representing that which applies to group norm and that which is an adequate individual norm.

One final dimension of interpretive background for the social conscience of America is the reminder that the social legislation of the sixties was a product of the far reaching influence of mid-twentieth century pietists whose influence lay within the system of the law. Sometimes it is difficult to recall that much of the legislation of the sixties was a means of providing a sense of the corporate nature of man as creature, as sinful creature, whose life was to be lived as a testimony to the love of God in the world.

Another way of describing the impact of the developing social conscience of the churches of America is to see their actions as described by the phrase "souls vs. systems." Religious dominoes was the game for one group in the souls vs. systems game. Only in the game the object was to "save" as many individuals as you could. Some of the more conservative student groups would identify quite well with this emphasis.

In the megalithic society of the twentieth century the systems needed to be reworked. Reworking the systems of institutions could make them operate more efficiently, as well as retaining more clearly the central purposes of the institutions. Some hoped that as men interact with each other in a changed environment, they will be responding to each other on a higher level of the redemptive experience of mankind. The theme was to change the system in order to change the people in it. Another theme was that changed individuals can effectively modify the system so that it is effectively changed for the greatest mutual benefit. These are still the polarizations of the social consciences of most Americans.

In the late sixties and early seventies several issues arose in American life which challenged both sides of the social conscience of the country. One way the church responded was by developing social agencies. Earlier models of the institutional church, staffed by social workers, and recreation leaders was one response. Thus, we shall look at some of these issues and reflect on their meaning.

Theological education broadened between 1955 and 1975. Both Protestant and Roman Catholic seminaries increased their curricula to include specific training for students to meet the social problems of these decades. Some institutions included specific training for social workers. In a few instances fears were expressed that the traditional disciplines of theological education would be undermined by the social training. From another perspective, however, the schools insisted that they were responding to the needs of the culture and preparing men and women to minister effectively in the culture. The question posed by this change in educational emphasis cannot be provided with a definitive answer. The effect, however, was one in which the church saw itself as part of a broader cultural experience to which it attempted to minister.

Three areas of emphasis became important near the end of the sixties. Each emphasis raised a new set of questions for the individual and the institutions in which he was a participant. The questions revolved around the nature of man in the world. The first question came on the axis of life control. Its poles were birth control and euthanasia. The second question centered on poverty. The third centered on the convenient word, ecology. In each instance the social conscience of the church was increased particularly as it sought to be an agent seeking solutions to the problems.

Life control, raised in the questions of birth control, was an issue which began to surface in the late fifties. With the development of effective and easily accessible oral contraceptives, by the early sixties the social conscience of many individuals was sharpened. For the first time in the history of mankind a viable choice concerning parenthood became possible. One could effectively and conveniently make a positive decision not to become a parent. True, some individuals had made this choice in prior years, but the effectiveness of the choice lay in the exercise of continence. Through the development and public acceptance of oral contraceptives the choice could be made in positive terms. By the end of the decade the effect of decision making on birth control was demographically evident. The birth rate had declined.

The Roman Catholic Church refused to recognize any artificial contraceptive. In 1968 Paul VI spoke in *Humanae Vitae* even denying abortion for therapeutic reasons. He spoke against the advice of a broad group within the church. In reaching his decision he voiced the traditional teachings of the church against violation of the sacredness of human life, the potential threat to accepted moral behavior, and the danger of a view of man that was based in materialism or rationalism. As late as 1973 studies among Roman Catholics showed the lack of effect of the papal view. In 1955 30% of Catholic women between the ages of 18 and 30 practiced contraception. By 1965 the figure had reached 51%, and by 1970 it had risen to 68%. It was estimated that the figure reached 75% for women under thirty. This figure was significant because it was also correlated for women whose piety included monthly communion.

Abortion is another mode of birth control. In 1973 the United States Supreme Court set the individual privilege of abortion on the mutual consent of a woman and her physician. Much reaction developed over this decision, and the lines of support were still being drawn in 1975. Right to Life groups were still being established in many states in the effort to obtain reversal of the decision. Also, during this same period, but without the emotional fanfare attached to the contraceptive and abortion questions, increasing numbers of men submitted to voluntary vasectomy as an effective means of birth control.

The other side of life control is decisions about death. The question came in two forms: euthanasia and death by decision. Both of these questions have long been a part of ethical discussions, but their popular consideration was a phenomenon of the early seventies. In 1975 the question focused on the case of Karen Quinlan, a twenty-one year old woman who was comatose for nine months. Her parents requested court permission to have the life maintaining technology of the hospital removed, and that she be allowed to die. The case achieved national attention. The appeal of the parents was denied, and at year's end the case was in an appeal status to the state supreme court of New Jersey. In March 1976 the New Jersey supreme court granted the parents the right to seek physicians who would execute their decision on the basis of the probability that the patient could not regain a viable, self sustaining life system.

Euthanasia is legally a criminal offense. Medical personnel are placed in a precarious position when they consciously or even indirectly remove life maintaining technology from a patient. Leroy Augenstein cogently raised the question and pointed to decisions to be made in *Come, Let us Play God.* His unfortunate accidental death ended his dialog on the question. By 1975, however, the publication industry was responding with a steady flow of volumes to discuss the questions. As well, medical schools were developing seminars, faculty, and courses to deal with the questions of bioethics.

Poverty was another major problem which sharpened the social conscience of religious America during the decades of the fifties through the mid-seventies. In one approach to the problem the United States government sought means of relieving poverty within the continent. The establishment of a minimum wage, an official poverty level income, and assistance programs in the areas of housing, food, and medical care were developed during the late sixties. The impact of an inflationary economy negated some of the benefits of these programs, and the cost to tax payers mounted. Poverty, like civil rights, gradually gained less racial emphasis, although the critical dimensions of both problems were ethically centered.

Poverty in the United States was not the only concern of religious groups. World poverty gained great attention. Massive programs of assistance were developed. Bangladesh became a word synonymous with acute poverty. Third world nations, whose ability to produce adequate food for starving populations was impeded by severe drought and poor technology received considerable attention and donations from the more affluent Americans. For one of the few times in modern history food products became issues in international diplomacy.

A third problem which sharpened the social conscience of American churches was grouped under the designation ecology. This emphasis was related to the preceding discussions of life control and poverty. Sensitivity to the idea that man is the steward of the planet on which he lives was raised in the late sixties with the articulation of the concept "spaceship earth." As the nation reached the peak of its space exploration of the atmosphere, climaxed in one great leap for mankind in the first moon walk, July 19, 1969, awareness was raised to the reality that the planet can support a maximum number of people in a viable life style. Natural resources, rather than being limitless, were forcefully recognized to be limited by the oil embargo in the winter of 1973. Conservation of energy resources became a requirement which altered life styles in an affluent culture, at least temporarily.

In some instances the social conscience of American ecclesiastical bodies sought to make men aware of their responsibilities to conserve and replenish the resources of the planet. Rogation Sunday became an emphasis on ecology, even among some religious groups who were not normally followers of the traditional liturgical calendar.

As American religious bodies, and individual practitioners of American religious groups, faced the impact of the variety of problems associated with life control, poverty, and ecology, the polarities of the old social gospel versus redeemed individuals came to renewed evaluation. The thrust of the dilemma was a raised consciousness level to the view that man is not a creature in isolation. The concept of man has been under continual reevaluation. As individuals have been able to particularize the problems of the culture, and from that particularization to extrapolate to a world view, the inevitable complexity of the situation has been awesome. Sharpened social awareness has not been an easy experience in these two decades. Many more problems than the three isolated above have cried for solution. The power of individuals to effect global, national, or regional change has been ineffective. Thus, institutions have been sought which collectively could work toward change beneficiently.

The conclusions being reached at the end of 1975 were in the same camps with which the century began. Both the social order and individual men were considered in need of redemption and grace. The effect of a sharpened social conscience was best seen in the closing of the gap between the two alternatives. No longer was this being interpreted as an either/or but as a both/and phenomenon.

Civil Religion

Since 1967 interpreters of American religious experience have often grouped their dialog around the catch phrase "civil religion." This phrase was used by Robert N. Bellah in his essay, "Civil Religion in America." He acknowledged that the term was one used by Rosseau, and indicated his amazement that it had not earlier been taken up as a means of identifying and describing the American experience. Prior to looking at the impact of Bellah's arguments and developments related to it, attention should be directed to earlier works or ideas which were important in molding some of the ideas related to what is now called civil religion.

Basic to an approach to the civil religion of America is a concept of the mixed motives of the colonizers, as well as of the founders of the republic. Profits and proselytizing were the conflicting motives of colonizers. The founding fathers used a set of symbols which relied on Biblical imagery to describe their experience. God and American destiny have been related in the conscious and subconscious lives of the citizenry. With this relationship, nationalism and patriotism obtained a religious identity. That this occurred in the development of American history and culture is not considered unusual. It is part of the European heritage. Awareness of the civil dimensions of American religious experience was, however, a product of the more recent decades.

In 1955 Will Herberg published *Protestant-Catholic-Jew; An Essay in Religious Sociology*. By 1960 he had completely reviewed and revised the work on the basis of written and oral evaluations. The impact of *Protestant-Catholic-Jew* was that it signaled an approach to interpreting American religious experience from a synthesis of critical disciplines. Herberg's reputation as a scholar in areas of overlap among religion, philosophy, and the social sciences provided him with a platform for his evaluation of the American experience. Herberg's central point was to present an acknowledged interpretation.

"The American Way of Life," a system which has seldom been defined, was described by Herberg as the common religion for the functioning society of America. It provided American society with a necessary sense of unity. The American way of life was described as an "organic structure of ideas, values, and beliefs that constitutes a faith common to Americans and genuinely operative in their lives" (p. 77). The impact of the concept of the American way of life was described as the integrating factor for the official religious bodies of the country. It judged them. Their validity, so to speak, was dependent on their relationship to the American way of life.

To be a Protestant, a Roman Catholic, or a Jew was seen by Herberg to be a type of ethnic identity. To be an American who was involved in the American way of life, whether Protestant, Catholic, or Jew was the major evaluative criteria. The three dominant religious groups in this country had been Americanized to the extent that non-Americans observed that American religious bodies often appeared to have more in common with each other than with their European counterparts. This was a process of secularization which was not achieved along traditional theological lines, but was achieved out of the unique ethos of the American development socially, politically, and culturally.

The American way of life was described as a system which

believes in the efficacy of religion. Religion is good. To be without it is to be judged evil. Poll takers continually reaffirm this
basic tenet of the American ethos. In 1971 the Gallup polls reflected that 98% of Americans expressed a belief in God. Women
outranked men by only one per cent. Non-college graduates
outranked college graduates only by four per cent (99 and 95%,
respectively). Age, political identity, income, region, and size of
community all represented percentages above 96, with a devia-
tion of not more than three per cent. In contrast, a survey of
Europeans reported in April 1971 showed Greece to be closest to
the American figure, 96%. The European countries from which
the backbone of American religious heritage was developed—
England, Germany, France—showed significant deviations from
the American figure. Germany reported 81%, England 77%, and
France 73%.

Herberg used the term civic religion as a means of describing
the celebration of the "values and convictions of the American
people as a corporate entity" (p. 89). But civic religion was not a
description of the American way of life. For him the American
way of life developed "through a devitalization of the historic
faiths, and inner, personal religion that promises salvation to the
disoriented, tormented souls of a society in crisis" (Ibid.). This is
a faith in faith, a belief in the basic necessity of religious experience and its affirmation described above. The American way is
congruent with the culture. It celebrated noble civic virtues functioning in much the same way as the civil religion of Greece,
Rome, and ancient China.

In 1967 when Robert Bellah chose to use Rosseau's term to
describe what he meant by civil religion, he pointed to some of
the same characteristics and dynamics to which Herberg had
directed attention. The difference in the two approaches was one
of degree and emphasis. Herberg saw the denominations interacting with the American way of life, sometimes so sufficiently acculturated that they lost their independent identity. Bellah
articulated civil religion as a phenomenon which existed parallel
to the denominations. In this emphasis he made the same point

about faith in faith which had been made earlier by Herberg.

Bellah analyzed the 1961 inaugural address of John F. Kennedy, and noted the three references therein to God, a concept which most Americans accept but on which there is no concensus. His analysis indicated the American political allegiance to the sovereignty of God, noted specifically in the motto on coins, "In God we Trust," and the inclusion in the pledge of allegiance of the phrase "under God." He suggested that the entire address was a call to Americans to implement God's will on the earth. Even in his analysis of the Declaration of Independence, Bellah asserted the same themes. The significant point which Bellah raised via his examination of presidential addresses and actions of the Congress 1789 to the time of his writing, emphasized that the American way was a collection of beliefs, rituals, and symbols which were neither sectarian nor Christian, nor was it antithetical to the basic positions of Western Christianity. In fact, the average citizen has difficulty separating civil religion and the denominationally centered religious affirmations of the populace.

In academic circles, and it must be recognized that questions about civil religion have been largely limited to academic circles, writing about the American religious experience demonstrated a change in form from 1955-1975. The earliest writings of religious history in this century were defenses of the missionary motives of the settlers. Rereading these documents, one is faced with a sense of the apologetic quality in them. In the nineteenth century, with the rise of denominationalism, history writing took on a polemical flavor, defending the growth and development of each denominational body in the face of pluralism. In the twentieth century William Warren Sweet concentrated on the development of the relationship of the frontier as the normative avenue of American religious experience. Only near the end of his career did he begin to view the task of writing about American religious experience from an interpretative point of view. Students trained by Sweet, or others who began to publish during these latter decades, developed a mode of church historiography which was basically interpretative. Cultural and intellectual history became an area of concern for these individuals. They sought to bring other disciplines into a critique of the American religious scene.

The two major disciplines which came to be a part of the interpretative tools were sociology and anthropology. In some instances psychology was also a discipline. Sociology, however, came to a certain maturity academically after 1955, and its methods were applied to studies of religious phenomena. Sociology moved from an axis of institutional study of religion to the more personal orientation of Max Weber and Emile Durkheim. Within that discipline, however, there continued to be an active dialog about the appropriate emphases and methodologies for the study of religion. This led to the development of criteria for the scientific study of religion, phenomenologically, both in its institutional and individual manifestations. At the end of our two decades of observation civil religion had emerged as one way of describing a cultural phenomenon with unique bases in the American experience.

One final means of describing the interaction of civil religion and its impact on American life is through a look at the activity of prayer. Prayer is a basic ritual in the denominational expressions of religious experience. It has two primary manifestations, private and public. The public dimension of prayer was exercised in the worship experiences of the people. But public prayer also had a civil feature. Until recently, prayer, specifically the recitation of the Lord's Prayer, was a daily feature in the classroom experience in many of the nation's schools. After the Supreme Court ruled against prayer and Bible reading in public schools, the practice was curtailed, but not terminated. The South was the area with the greatest resistance to accepting the dicta of the court. Prayers at inaugurations of government officials, openings of shopping centers, and other clearly civil functions have been a part of the acting out of the interrelationships of the American way. Civic prayers are a ritual which continue to point to American civil religion as an ongoing phenomenon.

The study of the phenomenon was not entered as a means of judging, but as a means of describing and articulating experience. As such it has continued value academically, politically, and emotionally. The religious value of this study can assist in defining the religious response of people, providing them with some sense of demarcation between healthy affirmation of religious experience and clear awareness of nationalistic or patriotic expressions which have acculturated religious overtones. This is not a secularization of religious experience, nor a sacralization of civic experience, but an attempt to articulate the dynamics of interactions of the two experiences. Civil religion adopted the motifs of the Exodus, chosen people, promised land, new Jerusalem, sacrifical death, and rebirth from the symbols of the Judao-Christian traditions. In their civic expressions these Biblical archetypes have a distinctively nationalistic tone. Acceptance of these symbols does not negate their religious significance except where their religious origin and meaning has been abandoned.

In 1975 when America was preparing for the celebration of the Bicentennial the nation had passed through a wrenching emotional experience. The devastation of Viet Nam and the termination of the Nixon presidency left the nation in a sense of moral disillusionment. The American way had been violated. Many voices were raised in the anticipation that the two hundredth anniversary of the republic would provide the opportunity to refocus on basic values. The Bicentennial had the potential for being a religious event reunifying the fibers of civil religion as the ethos of the American way may be recaptured. Even so, this awareness is part of the social conscience in the American religious experience.

Missions ... Evangelism

At first it may seem strange to include missions and evangelism in a discussion of changing social conscience. On reflection, however, it seemed an appropriate inclusion because through these ministries of American churches, mission has been the avenue of awareness, change, and new accomplishment. The combination of mission and evangelism, actually the two are almost the same thing, was the force of American activism. Between 1955 and 1975 significant world changes faced American churches which brought to the forefront of much thought an emphasis on mission, changing one basic set of concepts. Missions was a program generally outside the continent, although sometimes continental programs were called missions. Evangelism was more often accepted as actions within the local geography of a denomination. Another way of saying this is in the terms that missions was a program of the denomination collectively supported by the congregations, but evangelism was the active ministry of the congregation.

To take a long view of the development of this dimension of the life of Christianity in America one needs to recall that in the first two centuries of American experience, the country was the mission field for European based bodies of Christendom. After the Revolution national church bodies had to be formed. This formation did take place, not without some wrenching of relationships, however. By the end of the first quarter of the nineteenth century, however, the present national bodies of Christians had established basic organizations.

American aspects of mission initially were directed toward the Indians. During the colonial era this was the primary focus of American mission experience. If the pagan Indian could be converted, this would provide a safer country for all inhabitants. The goal of converting the Indians to Christianity was noble, worked at with some energy, but the expanding nature of the settlement of the continent continually interfered with the accomplishment of this goal. Land became more important than souls, specifically the souls of red men.

During the nineteenth century new areas of mission activity opened for all of Christendom. Asia, Africa, and some parts of South America became the focuses for concern. The Roman Catholic Church had been active in South America since the sixteenth and seventeenth centuries. Protestant missions focused on Asia and Africa. Each denomination developed independent programs once the system of independent mission societies was seen to be less effective. The twentieth century saw the development of the International Missionary Movement, 1910, in Edinburgh, a century after its initial suggestion. This provided some bases for cooperative enterprise on foreign fields, but the basic thrust remained denominationally sponsored and financed.

After 1955 American missions overseas experienced several crises. The impact of political situations in some instances forced the removal of American missionaries. India was one of the countries which refused to provide entrance and residence visas for persons who would spend their time proselytizing. Skilled technical and professional personnel were accepted, however. This forced a change in the thinking concerning appropriate training for missionaries. Agriculturalists were recruited, as well as medical and educational personnel. When this occurred Americans became more aware of the social problems which their missions could share in moving toward solutions. Social consciousness on an international scale began to be developed.

As more countries of Asia and Africa achieved national status the nineteenth century concepts of paternalism were challenged. National Christian bodies began to be formed, receiving support from American personnel and from American finances. The shift from paternalism to brotherhood did not occur overnight, nor without frustration for both groups. Paternalistic forms were slow to disentigrate. Gradually, however, both nationals and Americans tended to recognize that interdependence was a more viable means of achieving goals. In some instances paternalism was seen as imperialism. In developing countries the political rejection of any form of imperialism was applied to all foreign relationships, including the church.

American affluence contributed to an awareness of the needs of other parts of the world. With the convenience of jet travel and American wanderlust, all parts of the globe became open. As Americans traveled over the world some sense of human need impinged on their consciences. Missions was one way of providing for some means of ameliorating the living conditions of poorer nations. For those Americans who did not travel, the experiences of other travelers became a vicarious insight into the life styles and living conditions around the globe. For some, this vicarious experience raised their levels of perception of needs and they contributed through regular denominational channels for missions.

In the sixties the development of the Peace Corps provided another window on the lives of individuals in all parts of the world. When the federal government sought to use the motivation and energy of youth as a force in assisting developing nations and the people of those nations, the altruistic response of youth touched the basic altruism of the nation. Through the eyes of young people older generations gained a different perspective on suffering humanity. Assistance and aid were the means toward the goals of self sufficiency. Self sufficiency was the American self-image as well as the goal for individuals in foreign lands. Hard work, bootstrap economics, and American initiative were too simplistic an approach for the complexities of indigenous poverty, illiteracy, and pre-technological cultures caught in fast paced political and social change. But, the impact of the Peace Corps was in the unmeasurable avenue of increased social awareness.

The Peace Corps and VISTA had three effects on the religious organizations in America. From one perspective the altruism which was at the base of the response to these two movements had the form of fulfilling from a secular perspective some of the latent religious motivation of youth. Many of the youth who responded to the humanistic goals of these organizations had backgrounds in the main line bodies of American religious institutions, but they had rejected their religious heritage because they perceived its ineffectiveness. To offset this some denominations developed domestic and overseas short term programs which would provide within established institutional structures mission experiences for qualified youth. The effectiveness of these programs may be illustrated through their continuation, presently. A third effect may be seen to be more general, but it provided a rise in the consciousness level of both the churched and the non-churched areas of American culture. Here, again, the American way and its influence came into play.

During the sixties, concurrent with Vatican II, there developed a sense among the denominations when the word "mission" began to be heard as much as "missions." Missions was a phenomenon external to a local congregation or parish. Mission, however, was integral to the function of the parish. This came in the wake of a general self awareness which permeated American Christendom as the Roman Catholic Church opened itself to scrutiny internally and externally. Mission became one of the "in-words" for a time, even evidenced by the American Baptist Convention renaming its journal, *Mission*. Central to the renewed thrust of interest in mission was the raison d'etre for the parish. This introspective period came at a good time to anticipate the development of social action directions for the churches at a time just prior to the cataclysmic need for human involvement in social programs in all areas of American culture. The increased awareness of local social needs provided an opportunity for the development of local action which sought to meet problems and provide depth solutions, or at least encourage individuals to be a part of the solution process. Once again a slight shift of the kaleidescope provides a slight shift in the development of a changing social conscience.

Regardless of the local interpretations of the words "missions," "evangelism," or the newer emphasis on "mission," all are related to the function of Christianity of testifying to the redemption which God has provided. Saving souls, providing schools and hospitals, or providing after school supervised recreation and tutoring for children of working parents, and numerous other local applications of the meaning of ministry to the social needs of men has had a beneficial effect on the social conscience of Americans. Almost with certainty by 1975 a prediction could be made that where parishes had no sense of personal mission acted out in some form of social ministry, there was a concurrent diminution in the vitality of the congregation. The impact of these two decades was to see the acceptance of missions and evangelism in social terms, interpreted as meeting the life situation needs of men, women, and children.

Black Religious Experience and Civil Rights

The most dramatic change to occur in the social conscience of America between 1955 and 1975 was centered on movements among blacks and minorities. The civil rights movement spans the century, but in two decades more concrete change occurred than had transpired in the preceding hundred years. The civil rights movement, especially among blacks, brought to center stage the role and function of the church for this significant minority. Caucasian awareness and changing attitudes did not come easily. In the long view of these two significant decades, however, much change has taken place. As a creative force in effecting changing social attitudes Caucasian awareness of black religious experience has been an added benefit of the civil rights movement. Once again we need to be reminded that the culture wrenching forces of the civil rights movement was greater than a racial issue, even though the focus at times seemed aimed only at that experience of American life. The foundation of the civil rights thrust, subsequent legislation implementing some of the goals of the movement, and reflective approaches to interpretations of the movement point to a concept of man. At its foundation was an anthropology.

The Supreme Court's 1954 decision in Brown vs. Board of Education declared unconstitutional the separate but equal forms of education which had been legislated or allowed to develop. The early reaction to the court's decision seemed to be rejection and a certain heel setting to see that the implementation was impeded. One by one schools were challenged, boards of education faced the responsibility of providing facilities, and colleges and universities opened their classrooms. Little Rock, New Orleans, Tuscaloosa, and many other cities stand poignantly as symbols of bravery and resistance in the memories of a generation of Americans.

In the late fifties another phase of the civil rights struggle began to surface. Lunch counter sit-ins became a means of focusing attention on another dimension of discrimination. Again the struggle was intense. Local and state law enforcement was necessary to maintain civil peace, or to restore civil order between citizenry and local officials. The lunch counter movement adopted an operative of passive resistance.

The leader in American civil rights movements who encouraged and lived by the dicta of passive resistance was Martin Luther King, Jr. King achieved national prominence as the leader of the Montgomery, Alabama, bus boycott. This developed when Rosa Parks, a member of the Dexter Avenue Baptist Church where King was pastor, refused to move to the back of the bus. From the reaction which her arrest caused, the black community organized itself to effect a transportation boycott within the city. Because the church was the only place they could meet, no civic meeting places were open to them, and because clergy provided leadership, the civil rights movement found its identity closely allied to churches among blacks.

As the civil rights movement gained momentum and direction it achieved some of the external trappings of a crusade or pilgrimage. To be a part of the movement was a means by which some individuals acted out their religious convictions about the brotherhood of man. Progressive college chaplains and socially conscious students saw a sense of hope in the aims of the movement. The church centered leadership also provided some of the pilgrimage or crusade aura. Unfortunately, while the movement declared itself non-violent, and tried to live by that goal, response to the movement was often violent. The violence provided several martyrs, again adding to the pilgrimage and crusade images. The murder of Martin Luther King, Jr., provided the ultimate martyr to the movement.

Some observers of the black church during the activity of the civil rights protests suggested that the movement was the focus of black religious experience. This implication was that the means and ends had been reversed. Even in 1975 it is difficult to recapture the images and experiences of the preceding decade. Five years, especially 1965-1970, were the most complex years for the civil rights movement, the churches which provided support for the movement, and the entire fabric of American culture. Not only were Americans struggling with civil rights, Viet Nam had been escalated into a full scale undeclared war, cities were erupting (Watts, Washington), campuses were erupting (Berkeley, Columbia, Kent State), and there were other forces which impinged on the attitudes of the American public. The social conscience of the nation was stirred.

Still the question persisted, to what extent was the civil rights movement a religious quest? Observation showed the movement centered among religious institutions, that the language of the leaders was filled with religious imagery, some of the symbols of the movement were religious symbols, and the goals of the movement were based in religious ideas. Civil rights became a focus of a large portion of the black religious experience in America, but it did not engulf and vitiate the vitality of the black religious experience. There were deeper factors in the religious culture of blacks which were more stable than the temporary focus on civil rights issues. In looking at some of these factors a view of the significance of religious experience among blacks may be gained.

Concurrent with the civil rights emphases, awareness of the American Negro and his church became more apparent. The black Christian groups in America were dominantly composed of seven separate denominations, numbering between eleven and twelve million members in 1974. Four of these groups were Baptists, and three were Methodists. These twelve million black Christians constituted a separate division of the general church. Among dominantly Caucasian churches black membership was less than one percent of the one hundred twenty three million members. The Roman Catholic Church tripled its black membership during the third quarter of this century, claiming 722,609 members, outnumbering three of the all black denominations. Methodists also included a large black membership, claiming 225,000, and the American Baptist Convention claimed a black membership of 200,000 in 1966. In view of these figures and the pragmatic dimension of church life, Liston Pope, late dean of Yale Divinity School, called the church the most segregated institution in American society.

Awareness of the black religious experiences must be more than statistical, however, This significant minority was ignored as a viable subject for sociological study until the mid-sixties except for the classical work of W. E. B. DuBois. Early in the sixties, however, awareness of the social dynamics of black religious institutions began to surface among some academic circles. Joseph Washington initiated some phases of the study with his 1964 publication of *Black Religion*. The previous year, but to less notice, E. Franklin Frazier published *The Negro Church in America*. Frazier, a distinguished social thinker and diplomat, provided a commentary on the historical development of the religious experience of blacks in America. He pointed to the total reculturation of the slave with the exception of rhythmic dance. Significant in his analysis, however, was the evaluation of the church as a social institution which spawned other cooperative endeavors like death insurance societies and education. He called the black church an invisible institution, pointed to the beginning of urbanization of blacks during World War I, and the subsequent development of a clearly recognizable black middle class. His evaluation included an awareness of the restricted role of minority groups in the general American society.

Washington, however, published at a time when greater recognition was accorded his work. His initial evaluation of the black religious experience among Christians was that it lacked a sense of historicity, a theological framework, and a sense of ecumenical inclusiveness. He called black religion a folk religion in the sense that he found it ethics oriented, stressing socialization and social protest. Socialization was a strong emphasis in the black experience, with social protest being relatively recent.

He also asserted that black religion had no theology, and was roundly attacked for such a claim. Some verification of his observation came, however, when shortly the theological world was offered several claimants for unique black theology. James Cone received the greatest attention for his combinations of traditional theological language with the language of black power leaders of the mid-sixties. Washington further concluded that the only viable theological base for the black church lay in mergers with Caucasian churches, thereby claiming the total history and theology of the church for blacks.

The groups of black Protestants who comprise the "Black Church of America" have the same problems of any sect group. Caucasian churches which are exclusive, history denying, and otherworldly oriented, can be viewed from the same perspectives as black churches. Black churches imitated the structure and thought forms of the Caucasian churches out of which they originated.

Black religious experience, however, has a positive contribution to the total understanding of American religious experience. Attention needs, therefore, to be directed toward its positive contributions. Three areas of black experience seem to be important to understanding its vitality and as providing some contributions to American experience: an emphasis on the word, a unique musical heritage, and a sense of celebration.

Oral tradition is a dimension of black religious experience which makes it distinctive. The role of the sermon and the preacher was a central focus of the worship experience. In eras when blacks were dominantly nonliterate the preacher was among a small group whose literacy was demonstrated in his reading of Scripture and his communication of its truths to the people. Among blacks was developed a sense of the mythopoetic aspects of religious language of Scripture and religious experience. The sermon was a mutual creation of preacher and people in the setting of worship. The antiphonal nature of the creation process for the sermon demonstrated the shared dialog between preacher and people. Monologic sermons, the patterns of Caucasian preaching, was foreign to the black worship experience.

The preacher and people responded to each other in the development of the sermon, depending on the spontaneous creation of the mood for worship. But the mythopoetic dimension of the black religious consciousness goes beyond the sermonic experience. It is transferred to an attitude toward Scripture which allowed an internalization of the language and symbols of Biblical truths. One of the clearest examples of this spirit may be found in James Weldon Johnson's *God's Trombone*. In this literary medium he captured the essential dimension of the transfer. Vitality and personal identity speak eloquently to the tradition which found expression in the lives of the people.

Henry H. Mitchell in *Black Religous Experience* characterized black religious attitudes toward Scripture as non-literalistic in contrast to many non-black attitudes. Nor has the black experience faced the curtailing experiences of the arguments about science and reason versus faith. Experience is the base and goal of black preaching, and experience embraces all of life, even politics. The style of the black preacher was described in terms of language and mannerisms, both colorful. The style of preaching connotes freedom, a freedom in which the people share vicariously and in actuality in the mutual creation of the sermon. He pointed to the aural images which are imperative in the communication experience between people and preacher. Finally, he pointed to imagination as an integral component of black preaching.

Dependence on oral communication, a heritage in which the story is a valid part of experience, and a recognition of the experiential nature of religion in the lives of people are essential factors in understanding the mythopoetic framework of black preaching. This stands in sharp contrast to the levels of Caucasian religious experience.

Music is a second factor in black religious experience which makes it distinctive. The vitality of religious music has been greatest when it has arisen from the life experience of the people and captured for them symbols of their world view. The contribution of black religion to music was the spiritual. Born in the slave experience of the blacks, the spiritual was a synthesis of African rhythms, life situations, and new world perceptions of religious symbols. Again the mythopoetic dimension of black heritage and culture may be noted. The songs were built around Biblical themes of creation, deliverance, miracle, the prophetic word, and the life and ministry of Jesus. Almost unanimously they contained a testimony of hope, in concrete terms. Initially the musical form was simple, as was the thought form. When spirituals were arranged for concert presentation, brilliant syncopated accompaniments were composed for them. Yet, in the complexities of syncopation the basic simplicity of the musical form was retained.

Caucasians stand in awe of performances of the religious music of blacks. They fail to achieve involvement and articulation of this medium. Blacks claim that "soul" is the essential to the spiritual and its role in their religious experience. But as spectators Caucasians in many instances have a keen appreciation for black contributions through music.

Third, a black contribution to American religious experience can be viewed under the word "celebration." Earlier I described the development of celebration in worship. For blacks the worship experience is celebration with the elements of freedom and spontaneity. *Homo ludens*, playing man, was an emphasis among Caucasians in the early seventies. They needed the emphasis, having been constricted by their cultural development. Blacks brought to the celebrative event of worship the primitive festival concepts found in Biblical and non biblically oriented religions. Again, attention may be directed to *God's Trombone* as a classical example of celebration. To picture the interaction of God and people in the setting of a fish-fry, and to gain an image of the strength of this picture as celebration is to see the essence of the mystery and poetry integral to the foundations of the Hebraic underpinnings of Christian tradition.

The civil rights movement provided the opportunity for raising the level of perception of American culture to the black church. In the early sixties it may have been well described as an invisible institution. Through it social consciousness was focused, leadership was provided, and marked social change was accomplished. When the cultural situations in America changed, however, a greater legacy was opened to view a previously unexamined phenomenon of American religious experience. The troubled era of 1955-1975 afforded this opportunity. The social conscience of American religious experience was broadened beyond the parameters of black-white civil rights to a new appreciation of the vitality of the church among this important minority group.

We cannot say that the social conscience of the American public has changed en masse during these two decades. But we can look back and see the progress which has been made both inside and outside the churches of the land. The slow process of attitudinal changes has been seen to be developing. In some instances the churches participated in actions which were culture forming rather than culture reflecting. Even the acceptance of selective conscientious objection, although it was limited, is another reflection of changes in the social conscience of the American people.

5

Changing Movements

Within the decades 1955-1975 American culture generally and religious bodies within America experienced, with what appeared to be greater intensity than was previously observed, the introduction of new groups and phenomena into the life of the nation. Some of the groups which developed challenged the traditional religious establishments of the country. In some instances the challenge came in the form of indifference, especially among students. In other instances the challenge came in the form of adoption of bizarre religious practices. This, too, was a phenomenon most noted among the youth culture. In some instances, however, movements from within the church developed, seeking recognition, status, and participation in the decision making process. Women, long the silent partners, began by the seventies to seek admission to overt leadership.

These movements do not lend themselves to common trends, except that they represent responses within and outside organized religious bodies to events and movements within the general culture. Each of the movements has at its base a sense of youthfulness, and that may be a common denominator. But, there is little common ground between movements as diverse as Transcendental Meditation and young women seeking ordination and full functioning within the life of the organized church.

Therefore, while we choose to discuss students, sects and cults, and the role of women within the broad heading of "changing movements" we shall not struggle to find for them a common set of characteristics.

Students

The role of students in the American religious scene has been important since the seventeenth century. Harvard College was established in 1636 in order to avoid leaving the churches with an illiterate leadership. The early history of higher education in America was a story of the actions of religiously motivated individuals. The real push for public higher education came after the Civil War with the development of land grant colleges. Until the twentieth century students in state supported institutions and those in private institutions were basically from the same strata of the culture. They reflected basically the same sets of values and religious concerns. They reflected a homogeneous culture.

The twentieth century has provided the opportunity of education for the largest and most significant group of Americans in the history of the country. Collegiate education has moved from the status of privilege toward the status of a right of citizenship. In the 1967-68 school year 6,963,687 students were enrolled in 2,252 institutions of higher education. Between 1900 and 1965 more than 800 junior and community colleges were established. By 1985 some estimates pointed to a student population of 17 million, thereby almost doubling the 1975-76 student population. The American college student, then, was a phenomenon whose attitude toward religious institutions was important.

In 1950 a Gallup poll asked on a college questionnaire for the respondent to name the four Gospels. Thirty-five per cent of the respondents named all four, 47% named at least one correctly, but 53% failed to name either Matthew, Mark, Luke, or John. In 1971 Gallup polls indicated that college age youth showed a decreasing acceptance of the view that organized religion was a relevant part of their lives. Eighteen year olds responded 51% yes, 49% no; by age 21-23 the responses were 38% yes, 62% no.

The same poll reflected that collegians over 24 years old responded 41% yes, 59% no.

Changing attitudes among students during the twentieth century help to place the above figures in some perspective. In the early part of the twentieth century, especially prior to World War I, students were concerned mainly with the social and extracurricular aspects of college life. Fraternity membership, athletics, school pride, and campus rules seemed to be the major issues. Victorian restrictions on social interaction were strong. With the exception of suffrage, which became an issue in women's colleges in the East, some political awareness was evidenced in the formation of Socialist political action groups. Neither doctrinal questions nor personal spiritual nurture concerned the pre-war student. Some religious feeling or social concern was evidenced in broad humanitarianism, tolerance, and social concern. The strongest religious movement among students during the era was the Student Christian Volunteer Movement, a coalition of various Protestant groups of evangelical mein, including the YMCA and YWCA.

After the first world war the image of the typical college student changed. During the twenties, a decade of relative prosperity and optimism, old values were challenged. The Victorian and Puritan moral codes were challenged. Women raised their hemlines from above the ankle to above the knee, were known to attend movies without escorts, began smoking cigarettes in public, and would even admit to necking and petting. Male students were characterized by raccoon coats, hip flasks, roadsters, and some articulation of ideas of free love. Sex, drinking, and new and exciting "things to do" were the most discussed topics of campus conversation. Prosperity allowed students to have a good time in college, and the collegiate mood was pictured as light, sophisticated, and optimistic. Student concerns about religion seem to be unclear for this decade. Some indications showed interest in personal religious experience, but little interest in organized religion. By the end of the decade several observers of the religious attitudes and activities of students noted what they considered to be decided diminution of interest.

The thirties brought another dimension to collegiate life in America. Economic depression cut into the "frill and play" image of universities and colleges. Enrollment in courses in economics, history, and social sciences showed steady increase. Student concerns centered around economic, political, and social issues. In 1933 the *New York Times* described the typical student as a skeptic, one who had been disillusioned by political corruption. Political activism among students rose during this decade, with students affiliated with regular adult social and political organizations. Marxism-Leninism occupied the economic consciences of students for the first half of the decade and then was replaced by growing concern over the approaching European war, with many students adopting an anti-war stance. In 1934 a student strike for peace occurred in April, with one of its focuses being an anti-ROTC movement. The April strike occurred annually until 1939.

The second world war came and interrupted the education of many American youth. After 1945 the veteran returned to American campuses. In his wake education was serious business. He brought a wife, and sometimes he brought children. The married student was a new phenomenon which demanded adjustments in many areas of American educational concern. Veterans were interested in degrees that would provide jobs. Extracurricular activities were of little or no concern.

The fifties entered on a somber note for the collegians. Another military action demanded the attention of American youth. Domestically liberal ideas were feared, particularly in the wake of the "Red Scare" of McCarthyism. In 1955 the Ford Foundation created a program to encourage political discussion groups on campuses. Marxism, political criticism, race, and even religion were undiscussed topics on college campuses. In the wake of a quiescent student generation, however, religion did gain some visibility on two scores. Some schools reported increased attendance at voluntary worship or other religious activities. Religion also began to be accepted as an academic discipline. Late in the decade some evidence of change began to surface as the external dimensions of Western political relationships of the Cold War began to thaw. The last years of the decade were a transitional period.

The decade of the sixties can be described generally as the great era of crises and involvement among students. If the preceding decade was accurately described as one of fear engendered quiescence, the sixties may be described as an era of freedom. Students began to be involved in the social and political movements which swept the decade. Civil rights captured the participation of many, and reached its zenith in the August 23, 1963, march on Washington. The Berkeley revolt of 1964 was interpreted as an extension of the freedom and involvement experienced via participation in the civil rights movement. Students learned that they had political power.

1965-1970 was the great period of student reaction, political activity, and use of power. The issues were the Viet Nam war, escalated in 1965. In 1967-68 student opposition to the war was at its height. Secondary concerns among students during these years were university reform, black power, and action against injustice and poverty. Radical student groups like the Students for a Democratic Society attained national attention for campuses through strikes, campus take-overs, confrontations with deans and presidents, and a revolutionary rhetoric new to the collegiate scene. The media cooperated by providing national coverage of student activism. Kent State, May 1970, stands as the end of radical activism among students. Two students had been killed by National Guard weapons at Jackson, Mississippi, and then four students were killed at Kent State.

1970 began as a decade of changed concerns. The Viet Nam War was reduced to a nonentity, deescalation of the war reduced the draft and eventually terminated it, university reforms were taking place, and civil rights were being achieved. The energy of students was channeled toward some counterculture objectives, but students almost suddenly began to thrive on academic pursuits. One faculty member noted, however, that the student of the seventies had no sense of humor.

Religion became a viable topic again. The Jesus movement became a symbol of one phase of religious concern and participation. Objective study of religion as a social science or as a literary phenomenon began to be noted. Involvement in organized religious institutions in some instances showed slight increase. For the most part, however, students reflected a high interest in personal religious experience, but low levels of commitment to the established religious structures of American culture. During the seventies a clearly evident religious counter culture manifested itself.

It should be noted, however, that while the radical behavior of students gained a large amount of attention during the 1960s, and the counterculture achieved attention in the seventies, students involved in these activities represented only one side of the academic scene. These years were also the prime years of federal assistance to education during which funds were made available for student loans and scholarships, many institutions upgraded or developed research centers and graduate programs, and there was a phenomenal growth on most campuses across the nation. The seventies were also characterized as a period of developing personalism or privatism in students' religious ideation. With the demise of issues and the action of campus radicals, it may that this silent majority came into greater visibility.

Surveys of values of collegiate youth have offered some indices about attitudes which provide some indications for a picture of youth. Daniel Yankelovich has examined youth values since 1967. Some of his information from *The New Morality: A Profile of American Youth in the 70s* offers an interesting picture of change.

	%1973	%1971	%1970	%1969	%1968
I. Very Important Personal Values					
a. privacy	71	64		61	
b. changing society	24	34		33	
c. patriotism	19	27		35	
II. Welcome Value Changes					
a. more acceptance of sexual freedom	61	56		43	
b. more respect for authority	48	45		59	58

III. Moral Issues (activity thought wrong)

a. violence to achieve worthwhile end   66   56
b. having an abortion   32   27   36
c. relations between
   consenting homosexuals   25   26   42
d. casual premarital sex   22   25   34

IV. Marriage and Family

feel institution of marriage
becoming obsolete   32   34   28   24

V. Belief in Traditional American Values

a. people should save money regularly   71   67   76   59
b. hard work pays off   44   39   56   59

VI. Criticism of American Society (Agree strongly or partially)

Police should not hesitate to
use force to maintain order   55   53   32

Yankelovich also provided data on non college youth as a comparison. One section of his study concerned activities thought to be morally wrong. Its findings were interesting.

	%Total non-college	%Total college
Destroying private property	88	78
Taking things without paying for them	88	84
Collecting welfare when you could work	83	77
Paying for college by selling dope	80	64
Interchanging partners between couples	72	57
Using violence to achieve worthwhile ends	72	66
Cheating big companies	66	50
Extra marital sexual relations	65	60
Having children without formal marriage	58	40
Living with a spouse you do not love	52	41
Having an abortion	48	32
Relations between consenting homosexuals	47	25
Casual premarital sexual relations	34	22

While the Yankelovich study, and others similar to it, does not deal with a precise picture of religious experience or ideation among youth, values are related to the realm of religion in American culture. In the light of other surveys of the general culture there was some evidence that religion was thought to be decreasing in its influence on American life. The result of these Gallup surveys provide an interesting picture of trends. To the question, "At the present time do you think religion as a whole is increasing its influence on American life, or losing its influence?" the following responses were made:

	%1970	%1969	%1967	%1962
Losing	75	70	57	45
Increasing	14	14	23	31
No difference	7	11	14	17
No opinion	4	5	6	7

In the 1969 survey there were indications that a greater number of younger adults considered religion to be losing influence (85%) than older adults (67%).

From these data clear trends or conclusions would be difficult to use as a projection. They do, however, provide some indications of attitudes of youth during the turbulence of the sixties and early seventies. They reflect changing movement among youth. Religious movements which attracted some youth during this era gained a relatively high level of visibility through the media. Youth generally, attained a high level of visibility in all sectors of the culture.

Sects and Cults

One of the new phenomena on the American religious scene during the sixties and seventies was the development of sects and cults, both Christian and non-Christian in orientation. In earlier years American youth tended to follow patterns of mainstream religious groups, or if they became disillusioned with organized forms of religious experience, they dropped out. A normative curve was at one time used to indicate that during the collegiate years youth may drop out of organized religious institutions, but with marriage and children they rejoined the churches. This approach was most used during the fifties, the period called the fourth revival of religion in America. Following the student reactions of the sixties, the impact of the drug culture which developed, and a massive record of youth expressing a sense of alienation from the norms of the adult culture, a group of sects and cults developed.

A common characteristic among the sects and cults of the sixties and seventies was the role of ecstasy. The groups which surfaced in all sections of the country had a strong ecstatic or personal experience dynamic. Lacking among many of them was a clearly articulated base of doctrine or governing principles. Also, noted among these groups was their dependence on a central personality or small group of personalities for leadership. Few of the groups have reached second generation status in terms of longevity, hence little can be said for their stability in the absence of their initial or founding leadership.

Robert S. Ellwood, Jr., in a 1974 study of *Religions and Spiritual Groups in Modern America* (pp. 28-30) provided a list of characteristics which may be found among the cults and sects of this period. His list was instructive as a preface to an examination of specific groups.

1. a founder who has had or knows the secret of ecstatic experience
2. an interpretation of the experience as possession or marvelous insight
3. a band of supernormal helpers
4. a desire to be "modern" and to use scientific language
5. a reaction against orthodoxy
6. eclecticism and syncretism
7. a monistic and impersonal ontology
8. optimism, success orientation
9. emphasis on healing
10. use of magic techniques
11. a simple, definite process of entry and initiation
12. establishment of a sacred center or headquarters
13. emphasis on psychic powers
14. tendency to attract isolated individuals rather than families

15. increasing emphasis on participation by all members in the ecstatic experience.

All characteristics will not fit each group discussed below, because of each group's distinctive emphases. The list does, however, provide a succinct means of identifying a body of common characteristics. The groups arbitrarily may be classifed as the Jesus Movement, Oriental movements, the occult movements, and fundamentalistic Christian movements. The latter seem less likely to fit characteristics of sects and cults because of their identity with established ecclesiastical bodies in America.

The Jesus Movement is difficult to date with precision prior to 1967. At that time the youth drug culture had centered itself on the West Coast in the Haight-Asbury district of San Francisco, or on Los Angeles' Sunset Strip. Documentation of the development of the movement is scarce if one would depend on sources from within the groups. The media provided some documentation, and some critics charged that the media must bear some responsibility for the development of the movement. "Jesus People," "Jesus Freaks," and other terms were used to describe almost any long-haired, blue jean and tee shirt wearing, sandal footed youth who gave evidence of a Christian testimony. In some instances the commercialization of the movement was evidenced with the sale of Jesus Christ jockey shorts and bikinis! Two major musicals were created at this time using rock music format. *Jesus Christ, Superstar,* and *Godspell* became part of the marketing of a pop culture.

The hippy culture in California was the first locale in which the Jesus Movement attracted attention. Hippies were a body of youth who had drifted to this locale, many seeking sustenance in the drug culture which had developed there. A unique characteristic of the hippy movement was the solid middle class base from which it came. This separated them from the genuinely poor or downtrodden of American culture. As a group they achieved visibility, interest, and concern. This concern was expressed by individuals who chose to develop a ministry among them—a unique kind of missionary. Generally those who ministered among the hippies were of a more conservative or fundamentalistic strain of American Protestantism, with a strong apocalyptic emphasis.

The Jesus Movement was presented having success in turning youth off drugs and turning them on to Jesus. They reported intensive conversion experiences; held mass baptisms in swimming pools, rivers, and the ocean; adopted a literalistic approach to Biblical interpretation; disdained organized or "straight" Christianity; and, were soundly apocalyptic in their thinking. In many instances they reported experiences of glossolalia.

"Success" among this amorphous group was not measured in traditional terms. Those who tried to provide organization or to relate them to established churches tended to find their following diminishing. Arthur Blessitt's experience on Sunset Strip was an example of this phenomenon. Blessitt declared himself the minister to Sunset Strip and attained recognition, if not notoriety, for some of his tactics. By the early seventies, however, he had difficulty pointing to the thousands of converts he claimed. He later made an attempt to convert the Times Square area of New York City, but with limited impact.

One group among the large designation of the Jesus Movement established and maintained an organizational identity. The Christian Foundation was founded by Tony and Susan Alamo in Hollywood. Alamo, born Bernard Hoffman in Montana, changed his name when he entered show business because of his perception of the popularity of singers with Italian sounding names. He switched from performance to promotion on the basis of a reported vision from God of threatened death if he did not give up show business and begin to preach the gospel. He eventually began working among the youth of the strip, preaching and providing a domicle, receiving support from a business men's group. Eventually the Alamos obtained a former restaurant in Sagasus, which formed the headquarters for the communal life of the group. Alamo declined the use of the term "commune" because of the negative connotations held over from the drug culture.

Most of the Alamo converts were former drug users, but in

Christian Foundation they lived drug free lives. Relations between the sexes were carefully controlled. Handholding was forbidden, as was dancing, and conversation was limited to meal times. Smoking, however, was allowed. Marriage was permitted, if approved by the Alamos, but only after the couple had submitted to a ninety day period of fasting and prayer.

A distinction of the Alamo directed Christian Foundation was its emphasis on a harsh message, "Repent or be damned." Most Jesus Movements emphasized love. The King James Version of Scripture was the only translation approved by Alamo, although many Jesus groups used more modern translations. The Alamos insisted that the numerous modern translations were a sign of the apocalypse.

The Children of God was another group which achieved major recognition. They were seen in demonstrations at the funeral of Everett Dirksen, proclaiming that he was the last public official in America who cared about the Bible. They were highly apocalyptic, predicting the end of the world within two decades. They were exclusive in the sense that the rest of the world was evil and damned.

The Children of God was founded by David Berg, son of a rather traditional traveling evangelist. Berg had been associated with a radio evangelist, Fred Jordan. In 1967-78 Berg became director of "Teen Challenge," a coffee house in Huntingdon Beach. By that time some mainline churches were adopting coffee house and youth night clubs as a form of ministry. Berg, however, developed a following from whom he demanded and received absolute loyalty. Youth who attached themselves to Berg's movement cut all ties with home, family, and friends, and submitted themselves to communal living under the direction of Berg or his designates. In 1968 Berg and his followers began a period of wandering because of fears of earthquake then rampant in California. By 1970 the group had settled on a four hundred acre ranch in Texas owned by Fred Jordan. This began a brief period of mutual aid between Jordan and the Children of God, whom he used on his television programs.

By 1972 the Children of God claimed some three thousand

members in sixty colonies spread throughout the country. Berg was reported to be living in England in the early seventies, and there were later reports of a developing relationship with Colonel Mu'amman Gaddafi, the military revolutionary leader of Libya. The radical political orientation of the Children of God was obscured because they presented themselves well scrubbed, clean shaven, neatly clothed, demonstrating courtesy, pleasantness, and friendliness. With this image an NBC program in 1971 grouped them among the Jesus groups.

The Children of God were charged with brainwashing converts to the movement. Parents claimed that their children in the movement appeard "drugged," in trances, or in hypnotic states, and that they quoted Bible verses in a parrotlike state. For a time in 1973-74 Ted Patrick a former lower echelon California state government official, obtained recognition for "deprogramming" youth he removed from the quarters of the Children of God. A Denver court conviction was the result of one of Patrick's deprogramming episodes.

Former Children of God members have reported life experiences which tended to substantiate the charges of parents. They said that on joining the group they were never alone, for long perods of time they were forced to memorize Scripture passages, and that they had given to the Children of God all personal possessions. Anonymity was a feature of the Children of God. All members adopted Biblical names, and former identities could be unknown. In the communes was a high spirit of community and acceptance, a sense of joy and sharing.

Berg's leadership of the movement during the early seventies was provided by letters, tracts, and memoranda which he sometimes signed "Moses." These directives could be vitriolic in their attacks on life outside the communes.

Another leader of a group with some affinities to the Jesus Movement was Sun Myung Moon, a Korean who had led his movement internationally for more than ten years, but who moved on the American scene after 1972 when he had a speaking tour. In September 1974 he staged a rally at Madison Square

Garden. Moon, too, preached an apocalyptic message, declaring that these were the last days, that the end was near, and a new messiah was about to come. Some observers imputed that Moon claimed to be the messiah. Moon's movement was called the Unification Church.

Converts to Moon's movement were described as being from middle class families, in their late teens and early twenties. Campaigns on or near college and university campuses provided recruits to the movement. Moon obtained property in Tarrytown, New York, and a former Christian Brothers monastery reportedly valued at 1½ million dollars. No clear indications of the source of this income have been available. Devotees of Moon operate small businesses or sell street-corner style commodities such as flowers, peanuts, candles, and dried flower arrangements. The followers live communally, often in near poverty conditions. The extent of the movement in numbers was uncertain, but during 1975 it was functioning primarily in urban areas of the Northeast and mid-west.

In 1972 attention was directed among the American churches to a group of theologically conservative, activist churches. Dean M. Kelly, a staff executive of the National Council of Churches, in *Why Conservative Churches are Growing* pointed to Southern Baptists, Assemblies of God, Pentecostal and Holiness sects, Mormons, Jehovah's Witnesses, Seventh-Day Adventists, and Black Muslims as examples of vitality among the religious groups of America. He suggested that the sources of their vitality were doctrinal strictness, uniformity of life style, and enforced standards of discipline. Kelly prescribed concentrating on the main function of providing the meaning that makes life whole, guarding the entrance and membership requirements, accepting the basic conservatism of religious institutions, and developing a core which will perpetuate and provide the norms of participation.

Kelly caught the malaise of some of the mainline bodies of Protestantism at a time when declining income and increased costs were taking their tolls from a declining membership. Also the interdenominational influence of clearly defined, goal directed groups like Full Gospel Business Men's Association, Gideon International, and Campus Crusade for Christ were shown to be having growth and income increases.

One other phenomenon which attracted youth during the late sixties and early seventies was the glossolalia phenomenon associated with Pentecostalism. The movement was called the charismatic movement, and had a broader base than the Jesus Movement. As noted earlier, tongues speaking was a common occurrence among the Jesus movements. One feature of this broader glossolalia centered movement, however, was its impact on Roman Catholics in America. It began about 1966, initially under the leadership of Kevin and Dorothy Ranaghan, who said the first to become involved were faculty at Duquesne University, near Pittsburgh. At first the movement was called the Catholic Pentecostal Movement, but later became known as the Catholic Charismatic Movement. Meetings were held at Notre Dame and Michigan State universities which attracted attention via press reports. This group managed to remain in the bounds of the church, but by late 1974 some indications of a sectarian separation were being noted.

Religious movements with an Oriental base also came to public view during the late 1960s. Three of these were the Divine Light Mission, the Hare Krishna Movement, and Transcendental Meditation. Each of these had an appeal to youth. These have also had appeal to young adults, as TM required some degree of affluence for initiation.

The Divine Light Mission was a movement at whose helm was Guru Maharaj Ji who came to leadership at the age of thirteen. He first came to America in 1971. By 1973 his followers arranged to rent the Houston Astrodome for a three day festival for which they were still paying in 1975. Guru Maharaj Ji was the son of Shri Hans Ji Maharaj, an acknowledged Indian guru who spent his life among the poor. At his death in 1966 leadership passed to his youngest son. Maharaj Ji, his mother, and three older brothers were known as the holy family. His followers responded to him as God.

The Divine Light Mission was begun by Maharaj Ji's father in 1960, and by 1973 it had grown to more than four hundred fifty centers in thirty-eight countries. The mission had film, record, newspaper, and magazine production and marketing subsidiaries. These, and proceeds from followers provided the guru with prince-like living accomodations. Followers of the guru lived in communal settings called ashrams. Some worked for the organization, others in organization directed business concerns, and some had outside jobs.

The movement had no elaborate theology or philosophy. Sacred texts of all religions were acceptable, although the Bhavagad Gita, as the oldest, received the greatest attention. The major appeal of Divine Light was experience, not articulation of a creed or doctrine. The experience, called Knowledge, came to the initiate only through the ministration of a mahatma. One Westerner, an Englishman, has achieved the status of mahatma.

Followers of Guru Maharaj Ji described the experience in general terms. Defectors have described the experience as pressing on the eyelids until light was experienced, pressing on the ears until music was heard, movement of the head and neck to achieve nectar, and then the provision of a secret word for meditation. Each of these portions of the experience was designated by a descriptive term: Divine Light, Divine Harmony, Nectar, and Word. Satsang was a type of devotional or cultic experience in which teaching took place, preferably from the guru or one of the holy family, although mahatmas could provide satsang.

The Hare Krishna movement was the most Eastern looking of the Oriental groups operative in America. Devotees shaved their heads except for a ferule or pony tail, and wore dhatis and saffron colored robes among the men. Women wore brightly colored saris, and their long hair hung freely. All members were required to wear a tilaka, a streak of white clay or paint down the forehead to a point between the eyes. This was a mark of Krishna. Followers of the movement hesitated to call it a religion, but preferred to describe it as a cultural movement with a distinctive life style.

In 1965, A. C. Bhaktivedenta Swami Prabhupada brought the movement to the United States. Prabhupada arrived via merchant ship with a suitcase full of Vedic scriptures, seven dollars (because of currency restrictions), and the goal of fulfilling an instruction received when he was forty years old. He was seventy when he arrived in the United States with a letter of introduction to an Indian family in Pennsylvania. Advised to adopt Western dress, he refused, and Indian dress became a cardinal requirement for those who entered the movement.

Members lived an ascetic life in their ashrams. Bedtime was 10 p.m., with a 3:30 a.m. arisal for meditation prior to breakfast at 7:15. Meals were vegetarian, with drugs, alcohol, tea, and coffee prohibited. Sex among the married was forbidden except for procreation. Even a kiss was illicit if given or received at a time other than the most fecund. One of the rules of the movement was reconciliation with parents, thus negating some parental anxiety over adoption of the movement by their children. Hare Krishna followers were aggressive in their proselytization.

Transcendental Meditation was the latest Oriental based movement to attract a following among Americans. More a technique for meditation than a religion per se, TM was the creation of Maharishi Mahesh Yogi. As early as 1950 he began efforts to spread his message. Early adherents were from the entertainment world, notably George Harrison of the Beatles, and Mia Farrow. The Maharishi purchased the assets of Parsons College, Fairview, Iowa, in 1975, and from that vantage point began to direct a large organization. He established the Maharishi International University, and made the appropriate moves to become an accredited, degree granting institution, with a clearly set purpose, curriculum, and faculty. From this location trainers were prepared to provide lectures, teachers, and others who spent their time spreading the word about Transcendental Meditation.

In 1970 TM received a boost from sectors of the scientific world. Research reports were published which indicated certain psychomotor modifications for subjects experiencing meditation. Heart rate and oxygen consumption decreased, and electroencephalograms showed changes in certain frequencies.

These findings indicated verification for the claims of TM that meditation provided tranquility and relaxation. TM claimed to assist increases in productivity, to provide better concentration for study, and to aid in interpersonal relationships. By 1975 these claims attracted wide attention of students, and some educational administrators. The pragmatic technological dimensions of meditation were functioning with less relationship to the metaphysical foundations of the movement. TM had gone commercial, and was one of the spiritual toys of an affluent middle class. In late 1975 the course fee was $125.00 with initiation at which time the mantra was given.

Another side of cultism which was recognized in the late sixties and early seventies was an interest in the occult and satanism. Earlier popularizations of occult phenomena had captured the public mind with extrasensory perception, fascination with ghosts and poltergiests, and other phases of parapsychology. The reality of a spirit world began to be almost a daily topic of conversation. The film and literary world provided grist for the mills of conversation, the most spectacular being Warren Blatty's *The Exorcist*. After the emotional orgy of *The Exorcist* earlier Hitchcokian interludes had the aura of childishness. Interest in the occult, particularly witchcraft, reached proportions that in 1974 the Daughters of the American Revolution passed resolutions condemning public school teaching of material related to this movement.

Both witchcraft and satanism were attempts to provide some explanations for the nature of evil. Though they have some cultic trappings of religions, they tend to be attractive only to a small portion of the population.

Women

For some readers a section on women in the religious world of America should have been treated in the chapter on changing social conscience. Other readers will wonder why it has taken so long to get to such a vital group in the total history of American religious experience. Still others would be appropriate in expecting a full chapter dealing with this significant body of individuals, who in 1971 were reported to comprise 52% of all church membership in the United States. This represented a majority which had probably been constant for the twentieth century.

The women's movement was in the past two decades an effective force in changing consciousness and consciences. But it is a forceful movement which has a history reaching directly into the nineteenth century. The nineteenth century movement, like the current one, called to question the full spectrum of institutions which tended to discriminate against or subjugate women: political, economic, social, and religious. The nineteenth century movement was initially related to the abolition movement. They were, however, barred from speaking in public and refused membership in some anti-slavery organizations. Women formed their own organizations, to the consternation of some male leaders. At the World Anti-Slavery Convention, London, 1840, women delegates from the United States were not allowed on the main floor of the convention hall, but were relegated to the balconies as observers. In 1848 at Seneca Falls, New York, women held their own meeting. This marked the official beginning of the woman's suffrage movement.

During the Civil War women worked mainly on the anti-slavery issues of the conflict. In 1865 they made efforts to have the word "male" deleted from the fourteenth amendment. They tried again on the fifteenth amendment to gain rights by having the word "sex" added, thereby assuring suffrage regardless of race or sex. They failed.

In 1869 the movement split into two factions over the central issue of suffrage. The more conservative group limited themselves to specific issues on suffrage. The other had a broader base of concerns, but to which suffrage was thought to be the key. The first group was led by Elizabeth Cady Stanton and Susan B. Anthony, and the second was led by Lucy Stone and Julia Ward Howe. They rejoined forces in 1890 in an organization which bore the name National American Woman Suffrage Association. This organization lasted until 1920 when suffrage was achieved.

Elizabeth Cady Stanton (1816-1902) denounced the church for being the main obstacle to the equality of women.

Prior to the general development of the women's movement which appeared to gain momentum after 1963 with Betty Freidan's *The Feminine Mystique*, the Methodist and Presbyterian churches officially removed all barriers to the ordination of women. The Methodist action in 1956 came after four years of intensive activity following the 1952 General Conference when the issue was laughed off the floor. In the four year interval the Women's Division of Christian Service obtained 2,000 petitions to the General Conference. But 1963 is the touchstone date for the development of a movement which has had direct effect on the whole fabric of American life.

Women throughout the history of the church reached isolated roles of leadership. But they tradionally were overlooked when it came to questions of active visible roles in the decision making processes of ecclesiastical organizations. Women did not sit on the official boards of church organizations, or if they did, their representation in no way reflected the fact that women comprised more than half of the church's membership. Employment by denominational agencies also reflected the lack of women in executive leadership.

In 1969 the National Council of Churches surveyed 156 denominational boards and agencies. Responses were received from 65 boards and agencies representing 17 denominations. At that time three fifths of the respondents indicated that women held administrative positions, and one-third indicated they had no women executives. While eighty per cent of the respondents indicated an opinion that women were as capable as men in performance, only 25% of the 1,558 positions reported were held by women. Significantly on the basis of salary only 9.2% of the women earned $15,000 minimum, while 24.4% of the men were reported at this salary or above. Salaries under $10,000 were reported for 43.2% of women in administrative work, but only 16.1% of the men were in the lower salary bracket. Only two of the responding agencies reported specific programs aimed at recruiting women for top level executive positions. The evidence of salary discrimination has been an issue among women inside and outside the church during the past decade.

Ordination, the full acceptance of women to perform all roles of the ministry of the church has been another area of concern. In 1965 this question was raised at Grace Cathedral, San Francisco, with the ordination to the diaconate of a woman. During the nineteenth century Quakers, Universalists, and the Congregational Church were among the first to provide ordination for women. The United Methodist Church claimed a century of ordaining women, and in the early seventies reported some 300 women ordained. American Baptist Churches recognized the ordination of women prior to the turn of the century, but in most recent years reported only between 20 and 35. In the decade 1964-1974 the Southern Baptist Convention, the largest body of Protestants in America, reported possibly thirteen ordinations of women, with the majority of those functioning in institutional chaplaincies. The one woman serving as a pastor of a congregation served a church dually alligned with the Southern and American Baptist national bodies.

In 1970 the Episcopal Church's General Convention approved ordination of women to lower orders of the clergy, specifically the diaconate. During the first five years of this decade attention was focused on ordination among Episcopalians when eleven women were ordained without authorization. This will be a major issue at the church's General Convention in 1976. Roman Catholic women have also been active in their pursuit of full clerical status. At Detroit in October 1975, 12,000 conferees met to discuss the issue of women priests and to develop strategies, contacts, and tactics. Both the Episcopal and Roman Catholic churches are bound by canon laws and traditional authoritarian structures which will require change before ordination for women ecclesiastically can be declared legitimate. Each of these bodies of Christendom has throughout history provided for active service roles for women through vocational orders.

During the early seventies the rabbinate was also opened to

women. In 1975 four women had been ordained, and one of them was married to a rabbi.

Church leadership in America has been a bastion of male dominance. Women created separate organizations in most denominations, devoting their energy to local or foreign missions support. Even among denominations which claim a strong allegiance to the decision making roles of the laity, decision making boards and committees tended to be composed of clergymen. The experience of women in the American Baptist Convention has pointed to some of the issues and problems.

In 1955 the Women's American Baptist Home Mission Society and the Women's American Baptist Foreign Mission Society were merged with the American Baptist societies for these two areas of mission. Initially personnel were merged, but in the ensuing decade executive leadership by women suffered attrition. They were replaced with men, or not replaced in the organizational structure.

In 1969 the Women's Division of the Board of Missions of the United Methodist Church affirmed a position that separation was a viable role for women. Their affirmation was based on the conclusion that separatism provided a visible power base for women, and to lose visibility by merger would require separate organization at a later date.

Tactics for women in the church to alleviate discrimination may fall into three categories. They should

1. challenge traditional theological positions which place women in a secondary role to men;
2. question tradition or ecclesiastical law which forbids the function of women as ordinands; and,
3. pressure to assure that women at all levels of employment receive salaries and benefits on an equilateral basis with men.

Movements may not be adequate barometers for measuring change in a culture. They lack definition in some instances, especially when the fluctuations of the student mentality in America is considered. In the case of cultic or sectarian movements, illustrated by the Jesus Movements or the Oriental based movements, one may look at the fad sense in which these groups developed. Transience is a phenomenon which mitigates evaluation of their impact on the culture of the nation as a whole.

The women's movement appears at the middle of the seventies to be the one group which has achieved measurable change in the culture. The ordination of women has opened the issue of the ongoing role of women in the church from one end, and the growing acceptance of women in decision making roles provides opening within the church at another end. Central to the question of the effective acceptance of women in leadership roles in the church will be the modification of prejudices of the culture.

6

Changing Relationships

In some instances American religious experience in the nineteenth century has been interpreted as the time when denominationalism was a major issue. The development of national bodies for most of the branches of American Christianity, and even for American Judaism, developed before 1900. During the first half of the twentieth century the lines of denominationalism were sharply drawn and lived by. Following the second world war, however, small breaks in denominational lines began to be evident.

The first half of the century provided several cooperative organizations among national and international Christian bodies. The Federal Council of Churches, founded in 1907, eventually became the National Council of Churches, 1950. The National Council claimed membership from thirty Protestant groups with collective memberships of twenty three million. Absent from the National Council were the Roman Catholic Church, the Southern Baptist Convention, and several Lutheran groups. In 1972 Roman Catholic membership was recommended.

Missions was an area in which cooperative endeavors were a nineteenth century phenomenon. The World Missionary Conference met in Edinburgh, 1910, to discuss the state of disunity of world mission enterprises. Between 1928 and 1948 several international meetings laid the groundwork for the formation of the World Council of Churches. In 1938 the Faith and Order and Life and Work movements proposed a World Council. In 1948 at Amsterdam the first World Council meeting was held with delegates from 147 denominations. Conspicuously absent were delegates from the Roman Catholic Church. At its second meeting, 1954, Evanston, Cardinal Stritch of Chicago forbade Catholic attendance. In 1968 at the fourth meeting, Roman Catholics were elected to membership in the Faith and Order Commission of the Council.

Between 1955 and 1975 unusual changes in relationships among the religious groups of America took place at both the parish level and at the organizational level. To approach some understanding of theses changing relationships we will look at ecumenism, mobility and denominationalism, and some common concerns. Finally in this section a brief interpretation of American Judaism will be offered as a means of rounding out some of the dynamics of American religious experience.

Ecumenism

In December 1960 Eugene Carson Blake, Stated Clerk of the Presbyterian General Assembly since 1951, preaching at Grace Cathedral, San Francisco, to the opening of the annual meeting of the National Council of Churches, proposed a relationship among four American Protestant groups. He suggested that the Episcopal, Northern Presbyterian, Methodist, and United Church of Christ combine into one large denomination of American Christians. Blake indicated that the idea had developed in his mind about six weeks prior to the sermon in which it was proposed, but it had been nascent in his thought for some time. Precedent for the choice of the four denominations he named to begin the move to an organic American Protestant church lay in the 1947 merger of Anglican, Methodist, Presbyterian, and Congregationalist churches into the Church of South India.

Blake presented no organizational blue print or plan for the merger he suggested. Instead he voiced some principles, drawn from the traditions represented by each of the four churches. In the proposal he attempted to point to the values of the traditionalist catholic churches with their emphasis on liturgy and sacrament. For the Bible-centered, Reformation oriented churches he pointed to their emphasis on preaching and the priesthood of all believers. These emphases he felt would strengthen and complement each other in what he interpreted as the growing dynamism of Protestantism. Greater unity would provide the appropriate crucible for the expression of that dynamism.

More specifically, Blake suggested that from the catholic tradition could be drawn a sense of historic continuity within the church, both preceding and following the Reformation. This would be essential for the Episcopal Church, which has held to a strong position of apostolic authority, even though the first American bishop was consecrated by non-juring bishops. Also from the catholic tradition the new church would be trinitarian and provide an emphasis on the sacraments, particularly the two central ones of baptism and holy communion. From the other pole, the churches of the Reformation tradition, Blake suggested their contributions would be an emphasis on democratic governance, a sense of brotherhood and fellowship. The combinations from all traditions would provide variety in the intellectual formulations of faith and in the expressions of worship.

The thorne in Blake's proposal was admittedly the question of ordination. In the Church of South India all orders were initially accepted, but susequent ordinations came under the umbrella of apostolic authority through the Anglican tradition. Closely connected to the question of ordination in the new structure would be the opposition from the free church tradition to the role and authority of the bishop, and the fears of some churchmen of loss of congregational autonomy in an episcopal system. Among Methodists and Episcopalians some talks of merger had been held as early as 1948, but the size of the Methodist contingent deterred Episcopalians who feared the consequences of being outnumbered three to one.

Blake's proposal provided for a great deal of discussion among the Protestant bodies of America, who in 1960 numbered more than 250 separate denominations. Blake's proposal was not submitted into a vacuum. Mergers of different bodies of Protestants had been in the making or were being accomplished during the preceding decade. The United Church of Christ in Blake's proposal was a group which had been created in 1957 from a 1947 proposal that the Congregational Christian Churches and the Evangelical and Reformed Church unite. Other mergers prior to and following the Blake proposal are shown on the next page.

In 1962 the Consultation on Church Union was organized with representatives from nine Protestant denominations:
Protestant Episcopal
United Presbyterian Church
Methodist
United Church of Christ
African Methodist Episcopal
African Methodist Episcopal Zion
Christian Methodist Episcopal
Southern Presbyterian
Christian Churches (Disciples)
Significant in this body was the inclusion of blacks. By 1968 the Consultation's annual discussions reached a point that it appointed a commission to draw up a plan of union which could be the guide for the creation of a mega-church for Protestants. The ambitions of the Consultation suffered a fatal set back in 1972 when the United Presbyterian Church withdrew from further participation in the Consultation's discussions and plans. Paul Crow, Jr., secretary for the Consultation, noted the heavy opposition to merger and the ecumenical movement among the laity. On the local level resistance seemed to center in the sense of power and threat to that power via organizational merger. One cannot avoid speculation on the roles which diminishing funds, inflation, and civil rights played in the resistance of local congre-

PROPOSED MERGER	NEW NAME	Proposed Date	Adopted Date
Presbyterian Church in the USA United Presbyterian Church of North America	United Presbyterian Church the USA	1955	1958
American Lutheran Church Evangelical Lutheran Church United Evangelical Lutheran Church	The American Lutheran Church	1954	1960
American Unitarian Association Universalist Church of America	Unitarian-Universalist Association	1955	1961
Evangelical United Brethren Church Methodist Church	United Methodist Church	1958	1968

gations to talks of merger and union. The extent to which these factors contributed to the resistance cannot be measured, but they must be acknowledged as part of the total picture which affected developments in American religious experience. Although no new organization among Protestants came of Blake's proposal, nor of the discussions in the Consultation on Church Union, a positive benefit emerged, and was operative through the remaining fifteen years. This benefit was the open expression of commonalities among Protestant groups, some sense of open discussion, an apparent appreciation for the contributions of diversity in heritage, a renewed appreciation for the liturgical dynamics of worship, a reemphasis on the centrality of Scripture, and greater openness among individual congregations to cross denominational lines for the accomplishment of a common goal within a community. These accomplishments accentuated the potentials of unity without union, thereby recognizing common religious concerns, but not forming a monolithic Protestant church.

While Protestants seemed to be exploring the question of a mega-church structure, the Roman Catholic Church was simultaneously experiencing a removal of the veil from its traditional monolithic image. This public change came with the election of Guiseppi Roncalli to the chair of St. Peter in 1958. John XXIII, as he chose to be called, was anticipated to be an interim pope. He chose to be an active, energetic, change effecting pontif, not bound by some of the strictures and traditions of papal form. To achieve one of his primary goals John XXIII announced early in 1959 (January 25) plans for a world council of the church. The last general council was 1869/70. This council promulgated the doctrine of papal primacy and infallibility, two traditional doctrines thereby raised to dogma. In announcing Vatican II, which met in four sessions—October 11 to December 8, 1962; September 29 to December 4, 1963; September 14 to November 21, 1964; and, September 14 to December 8, 1965—John XXIII hoped to provide the opportunity for the church openly to explore itself and its role in the modern world.

One of the first acts of Paul VI on his election to the papacy following the death of John XXIII June 3, 1963, was to declare his intention to continue the Council. He had the option not to continue it. Actions of the Council were lengthily debated, but four constitutions which emerged from the debate set the ideological basis for all other actions of the Council. They were the Constitutions on the Church, Divine Revelation, Sacred Liturgy, and the Church in the Modern World. Two of these were dogmatic constitutions and two were pastoral. The other actions of the Council were in the form of decrees or declarations. The actions which have received greatest visibility to date were those on the liturgy, the church, the church in the world, ecumenism, renewal of religious life, life and ministry of priests, and the lay apostolate.

Some of the immediate effects of Conciliar action were experienced in modifications to worship, which have been discussed earlier. Other dynamics of the impact of the Council have continued to be implemented through the decade since its close. One significant impact has been the greater visibility of the inner workings of the decision making processes within the whole church. To attempt to summarize the actions and implications of the Council is outside the scope of this writing, but mention must be made of some items which have been a force of renewal for both Roman Catholics and other religious groups.

Of greatest interest in terms of ecumenism was the Decree of Ecumenism, November 21, 1964. John XXIII's announcement that he was convening an Ecumenical Council was made January 25, 1959. This was the last day of the traditional annual season of prayers among Roman Catholics that Protestants would return to the one true church, and that the schism with the Orthodox since 1054 would be healed. The intention of the Pope was "to invite the separated Communities to seek again that unity for which so many souls are longing in these days throughout the world." To accomplish that purpose he asked that observers be sent from Orthodox and Protestant churches. In the meetings of the Council he had them seated across the aisle from the cardinals, and he established a Secretariat for Promoting Christian Unity to be at the service of the observers, providing that it should have equal status with Council commissions. To head the new Secretariat he appointed Augustin Cardinal Bea, a recognized Biblical scholar whose contacts with Protestants in Biblical studies had been unusually amicable. From the beginning the choice of terms describing non-Catholics was fortuitous. "Separated brethren" as applied to non-Catholics became a reality, not simply the diplomatic overtures in so large an undertaking.

Before his death John XXIII read the first drafts of the Decree on Ecumenism released by the Commission. On April 22, 1963, he instructed that the document be released to the bishops for study and recommendations. Five chapters of the original document involved the principles and practices of ecumenism and relations with Protestant and Orthodox churches. The fourth, relations with Jews, was ultimately deleted from the Decree on Ecumenism, but received separate treatment in the Declaration on the Relationship of the Church to Non-Christian Religions, October 28, 1965. The fifth chapter, dealing with religious freedom, was also removed and later issued as the Declaration on Religious Freedom, December 7, 1965.

The progress of the Decree on Ecumenism as it passed through the Council provided insight into the struggles within the church. On November 21, 1963, the Moderators asked the Council if they would accept the first three chapters as a basis for discussion. This was overwhelmingly accepted. After receiving more than one thousand proposals for change the Council accepted the modified document offered by the Secretariat in the third session of the Council. The Council closed the debate on the decree, scheduling a vote on November 20, 1964. On November 19, Paul VI made nineteen changes in the text, at a time when the Council could not consider them without rejecting the Decree. The Council approved the Decree, with the papal changes on November 20, and the formal, ceremonial vote was taken. By his action Paul VI was interpreting his prerogative of papal authority.

The Decree acknowledged that separation in the church was the result of sin on both sides, thereby acknowledging the responsibility which the church had in perpetuating divisions. The Decree asserted that those who believe in Christ are reborn, are brothers, and that God uses their worship to sanctify and save them. For generations of Protestants who had been called heretic, the Decree was a remarkable evidence of a change of heart. The Decree, while demonstrating a new openness, providing for prayers together on special occasions, and presenting a view of the centrality of Scripture for common ground, did not back off from the church's view of its primacy, its authority for teaching, nor from warning about the dangers of a falsely conciliatory approach.

In the decade since the Decree there has been a lessening of the tensions among Protestants and Roman Catholics. Through open dialog they have come to know and appreciate each other's traditions. Greater cooperation among clergy, particularly in America at weddings and funerals, has developed. Dialog with the Anglican Church has produced a common catechism, eucharistic interchange, and other mutually beneficial movements.

The Declaration on the Relationship of the Church to Non-Christian Religions was a special concern of Cardinal Bea. He had been specifically instructed by John XXIII of his desire that the Council speak on Jewish relationships. The world wide political relationship of the church was involved in the development of this statement, especially the tensions between Jews and Arabs which erupted in June 1967 and still was raging in 1975. The strength of the Declaration lay in its denial that the Jews were a "deicide" people. Rather than acknowledging Christian guilt for wrongs committed against Jews, this document, like the World Council statement from New Dehli in 1961, provided an absolution for Jewish guilt. The document is clear in its assertion that there is no ground or Christian sanction for discrimination against or persecution of Jews. Bishops from the more populated areas of the world had different concerns than bishops in areas of heavy Jewish populations. The former raised the issues which they encountered with world religions. The church affirmed for them that all the peoples of the world form one community and respect is due the spiritual, moral, and cultural values of Hinduism, Buddhism, and Islam. The declaration is unusual in the annals of Roman Catholic attitudes toward any who do not fall within the realm of allegiance to Rome.

The Council provided for greater direct authority of councils of regional bishops, a step toward the collegial concept. At the same time the traditional authority of the papacy was maintained. In the Constitution on the Church this was clearly spelled out in terms that the bishops' authority exists only in proper relationship to and at the pleasure of the pope. The bishops were specifically empowered in the Constitution on the Sacred Liturgy to make the necessary decisions concerning regional modifications to accomodate the liturgy to their geographical areas of jurisdiction. In other matters the bishops were bound to the authority of the papal office, and this was demonstrated for United States bishops in the question on birth control, 1968. The pope refused to accept any unnatural modes of contraception. On a practical basis there was some evidence that both bishops and people have ignored the teachings of the holy office. In 1971 *Newsweek* reported a special Gallup poll indicating that 58% of the Roman Catholics surveyed felt that "a good Catholic" could ignore the Pope's condemnation of artificial birth control, while 31% felt that this was not possible, and 11% responded that they did not know. At the same time the same poll revealed that 92% of the respondents could not name any decision of the National Conference of Catholic Bishops that had been important for their lives.

John XXIII sought to open the windows of the church and allow a cleansing breeze to blow through. Some declared it a tornado. The effects of Vatican II did provide for a sense of openness and moves toward reconciliation. Paul VI made an important move toward reconciliation when he met Athanagoras, Patriarch of Constantinople, in Jerusalem in December 1965. East and West had not spoken officially to each other amicably since 1054. Rome entered the ecumenical arena, but world problems eclipsed continued and concerted efforts. In the last quarter of the twentieth century there is still hope for the continued conversations and gains among all who affirm the Lordship of Christ.

Mobility and Denominations

In the previous chapter mention was made of indications of the decreasing influence of religion on the lives of Americans. Between 1962 and 1970 a 35% change was noted among those who evaluated religion as losing its influence, with a notation in 1969 that 85% younger adults felt this compared with 67% older adults. The reality of these figures is staggering to some who approach them. There may have been a sense of the lessening of influence, but it was awesome to be confronted with the realization that 75% of the populace affirmed this lessening of influence. Factors which contributed to this phenomenon have not been definitivly approached, but some speculation may be appropriate.

One of the first factors to receive attention was the increased mobility of American culture in the years since 1955. One has only to refer to the history of the development of the inter-state highway system to be aware of the levels of increased mobility. Post war and cold war affluence were also factors which contributed to the mobility of Americans. Affluence contributed to the development of a larger middle class with many of the concomitant problems of nouveau riche without noblesse oblige. Education became big business, and with federal subsidy in the sixties it became an expansive big business built on soft money. Urban life spread from the cities to the suburban communities. Even in traditionally agrarian belts middle class farm families had the activities and resources of surburban life. The whole American culture appeared to take on a complexity of relationships that gradually removed the effective influence of the church in the daily lives of the citizenry.

The picture of life lived by "average Americans" in the past two decades contrasted sharply with the nostalgic pictures of the simpler, more communal life styles of preceding decades. The comparisons may have in them the natural errors of faulty memory. But, the memories were those which were often voiced.

In West Central Alabama is a small community which has an agrarian base to its economy. The community is composed of approximately seventy-five families, some of whom have been on the land for a century or more. Others have come more recently, but their acceptance in the community has been conditional with their ability as farmers. In the community are four Protestant churches, each part-time, the last of which gave up having an evening service in 1975. The central grammar school for the people was closed in 1967, resulting in children being transported forty miles round trip. The school building is now a club house for the people, consistent with the wills of those who provided it as a school. Tennis courts and a swimming pool are also a part of the club house/community center. The swimming pool is an independent, membership organization, with members sharing maintenance responsibility. With the development of private schools in the surrounding communities, less than a dozen of the fifty-plus children were in public school in 1975. School loyalties and activities decimate the development of activities locally attractive and viable for youth. Gradually, during the course of two decades the loyalties and activities of the people have shifted from the interactions among themselves around the churches and school. Their energies seem dissipated by the time spent "with their foot in the road." The evidences of urbanization seem subtle until they are lined out as above. The commuter is not just an urban phenomenon. In the pace of life which these people lead their commitment to their religious institutions has taken the same toll that the same energy expenditures have claimed in larger, classically urban centers of life.

In another instance, which microcosmically may illustrate the dynamics of mobility and the effect which it has on denominational loyalties, the case of Ralph may be approached. In college during the mid-fifties Ralph was an active member of a Baptist congregation. He played the piano skillfully, and one of his collegiate activities was on a youth revival team for the Baptist Student Union at his college. This activity carried him and two other collegians to a variety of churches within a reasonable radius of his college community several times a month. The "love offering" from the churches provided a modicum of income for his college expenses. In college he met a girl with a Methodist background. Following their marriage, he joined the Methodist church because of her objection to the Baptist insistence on her immersion. Military service followed marriage, with stations in New York and California. Ralph earned two master's degrees, worked in several academic libraries, and returned to a major Southern university for his doctoral work. In California he and his wife joined a Presbyterian church because of the quality of the sermons, compatibility with social views of the congregation, and the quality of music and friends they found through the choir. At thirty-eight, he finds himself the director of a library in an urban university. In his recent move to this job he indicated that his church preference would probably be Presbyterian, since for the past five to seven years he and his wife had been comfortable with that denomination. Significantly he was not making the decision on the basis of theological or social issues, but on the basis of personal comfort. As an articulate and introspective person whose perception of some life events had a sacramental quality, he apparently does not stand alone in 1975. From many perspectives his pilgrimage has been an every-man phenomenon.

Another way of viewing the church orientation of Americans has been through polls conducted over the ten year period 1964-1973. The Gallup study indicated that church attendance among Protestants held steadily during the decade, at 37, 38, or 39 per cent, with the last three years of the survey reflecting the low figure. Among Roman Catholics, however, the change was remarkable with a drop of sixteen percentage points (71-55%) in the same period. In the last three years of the survey the figure showed a less significant drop. The findings of the poll also indicated that the drop came among the young adult group, 18-29 years old. Attendance by Jews showed a two per cent decline in the same decade (19-17%). Gallup surveys over a nineteen year period (1955-1973) verified a seasonal picture providing credence for barbs about "Easter and Christmas Christians." Attendance was shown to be higher during the Lenten months, and peaked in December. The nineteen year average showed a probability of 45% adult Americans attending church at least once in a given week. Comparing the first and last years of this survey, however, showed a decline of nine percentage points (49-40%). Other studies among Roman Catholics have indicated that the Archdiocese of New York experienced a 23% decline in attendance at mass between 1955-1970. Another study over the 1960-1970 period showed an 11% decline, with the greatest change being among the 20-30 year old group.

Attitudes of clergy toward the question of church attendance was reported in April 1971 by Gallup. To the question, "Do you think a person can be a good Catholic/ Protestant/Jew and not attend church/temple regularly?" several interesting patterns emerged. Rabbis reflected almost two to one that attendance at temple was not requisite. Among Protestants regular attendance was considered imperative by 74% of those under 39 years old, and 81% of those forty and over. Among Roman Catholic priests, those 39 years old or younger indicated a 51% response which expected church attendance, and a 74% response among those forty and over. The 23% spread among priests may account for the decline among Roman Catholics during the sixties.

Developing inferences and conclusions from the figures used above must remain cautionary. Those familiar with the lack of standards for collecting data about religious attitudes in America will have already read the figures with skeptical caution. Those unfamiliar with the problems can easily speculate on the difficulty of developing data which is truly representative. The best that can be said is that over a two decade period the figures assist in viewing a trend, but they contribute little to a clear understanding of the dynamics which produce trends. Thus, one is left with speculation, or to use the more scientific term, extrapolation, on the basis of observation. Keen social scientists are wary of conclusions reached on the basis of subjective observation.

One final observation, however, should be offered. Will Herberg's *Protestant-Catholic-Jew* was referred to in the section on civil religion. With the diminution of denominational demarcations and the reality of the strength of the American way of life, what are the distinctives among denominations in a culture which has reached a certain level of religious homogeneity? Obviously there are no concrete answers to the question, but does this absolve conscientious churchmen from the responsibility of entertaining the question?

Common Concerns

Bricks, baptisms, and budgets were a standard mode for evaluating the effectiveness of a congregation and its leadership. One of the clerical games of upmanship has been reviewing rival "since I came" reports on anniversary or resignation reports. In each of the criteria statistical information was clearly attainable, and increases or decreases were openly evidenced through the use of simple arithmetic.

In the heady days of the mid-fifties to the early sixties, with the feelings of comfort and affluence which came on the heels of military superiority, building booms among churches began. New church buildings had to be constructed for the growing suburbs. Older buildings needed renovation, or in some instances razing and replacement. In other situations, the "down town" churches decided to move its facilities to a suburban location, thereby abandoning to parking lots and office buildings their former sites.

Growth measured through developing membership also met the pragmatic evaluators of church development. To report a large number of baptisms among Roman Catholics was not unusual. To report this among some Protestants testified to energy, enthusiasm, aggressiveness, friendliness, and productive relationships. In the mid-and late fifties baptism statistics rose, as a part of the growth phenomenon related to the sense of revival then being experienced.

Budgets, of course, relate to buildings and to baptisms. The more baptisms the greater the potential and actual budget which may be projected. To see the increases in the budget reports from central offices among denominations was to see an ever rising line on a graph.

By the late sixties the boom had ended for many of the growth evaluators who gauged by bricks, baptisms, and budgets. Two factors may have contributed to the declining income levels of the churches. In some instances personal and localized dissatis-faction with policies of national denominational boards and/or committees caused credibility problems which resulted in les-sening income sources. The black power movement, and reflec-tions that some denominations had provided funds for the movement, created visible levels of displeasure. At the base of this dissatisfaction may have been a reflection of growing sus-piciousness of centralized authority. The church was among the last institutions of the culture in which individuals felt a sense of personal control.

The second factor may have been the persistent effect of infla-tion, both on individual purses and on institutional purses. This effect was seen in most national offices of American denomina-tions after 1968. The organizational functioning of the churches struggled with increased costs to provide services to which its constituency had become accustomed, yet facing lessened in-come from its constituency.

In this same period the "Madison Avenue" identity within American churches became more and more evident. National offices of denominations adopted the most current business procedures. Business consultants were used to evaluate the op-erational effectiveness of the national offices, in some instances to the cost benefit of the institutions. A realization that denomi-national life was big business became evident. Reported annual budgets in the multi-millions only reflected a small percentage of the total incomes of churches, since national offices received small percentages from each congregation. The business mind-set which was observed among the churches also had a negative effect on income levels. This came when it was recognized that tithing had been deemphasized, and younger churchmen were responding to church budgets on the basis of evidence of need and percentages of increase. They were treating the church like any other business or investment, holding it accountable, yet accepting the reality that it was an institution which would generally show no profit. From the view of taxes, it was a write-off item.

The bricks, baptisms, and budgets criteria for evaluating the effective ministry of a congregation or a denomination reflected the growing concern in American culture with the ability to quantify all of life. Occasionally a voice was heard crying in the wilderness of quantification. That voice said numbers have meaning, only if you read them with compassion. Some hearing of the wilderness voice made attempts to modify the straight jacket views based only on statistical reports. Those who responded to the voice made attempts to refocus the direction of the churches toward ministry in human situations.

New forms of ministry were a common concern in American religious experience in these two decades. In some instances the new forms of ministry were a redressing or restructuring of ministries the church had been performing for some time. For instance, the church's social ministries had been on an informal, need recognized basis. As the nation's awareness of social issues was increased, some congregations developed specific programs of ministry to deal with social issues. These programs ranged from development of head start, community action, senior citizen, and youth services programs. Occasionally individual churches cooperated with federal agencies, and in some cases the response was strictly on a congregational support level.

At the same time the institutions supported by churches—schools, hospitals, geriatric facilities, orphanages and children's homes—continued to require increasing levels of support. The traditional charitable institutions had accustomed themselves to the status of hand-to-mouth existence through long years of function on faith and friends. These institutions experienced spiraling inflation in the latter sixties. Their diminished support, coupled with inflation, partially dictated the results which came when some of them closed, especially small church supported colleges. Others terminated relationships which would restrict their receipt of government funds, and in some instances "went public" as private investments. By the mid-seventies with the decreases in federal funding and decreases in denominational funding, many institutions of social and educational service were finding their future to be bleak.

Sometimes cultural changes required adjustments for service institutions. Until 1960 adoption and personal care centers for illegitimate children were provided by churches as well as private foundations. The demographic impact of oral contraceptives caused a decrease in the demands for the services these institutions provided. Legalization of abortion created a definite crisis. Some of the facilities closed, but others were capable of adapting to the needs of the culture which in the late sixties and early seventies was dealing with drugs, run-away adolescents, and an increasing need for temporary domicile care for juvenile offenders or products of "the broken home."

Another area of common concern among the major religious groups of America was the domain of vocation, particularly the priestly vocation. The problems associated with the ministry as a vocation began to surface in the mid-sixties. One of the ways in which it surfaced was the declining enrollments in divinity schools and seminaries. Enrollment decline was not unique, it was a Protestant-Catholic-Jew problem. Responses to declining enrollments varied from a sense of relief that the post war enrollment booms of fox hole called clerics had been educated and were functioning, to a growing sense of malaise that something was seriously wrong since young men were not responding to the clerical call. In some instances, as the action of the Episcopal Church in America showed, closing seminaries was the only alternative. Even with that action, by 1975 the remaining seminaries were reported to be producing more priests than could be absorbed by the dioceses.

Roman Catholic problems were not only the decrease in candidates, but in some instances the number of priests leaving their offices and relinquishing their orders became alarming. To add to the alarm the reaction of some American priests to Paul VI's 1968 encyclical on birth control further confirmed the severity of the gap evident in the hierarchical authority of the church. At first it was novel for the announcement to be made that a priest had forsaken or had obtained release from his ordination. Then it became common, or at least common enough that the priest had to be otherwise newsworthy to merit mention. In 1969 when Charles Davis "left" his ordination, it was noteworthy because he was a leading Jesuit scholar, and was a "name" who was doing what only less well known priests had done. The Daniel Berrigan release from orders caused little ripple because Berrigan's political behavior had been an embarrassment to some of the church. When McLaughlin, resident priest in Nixon's White House staff announced he was forsaking his orders, few took note. Those media sources which noted the occurrence made no comment, carrying only a small announcement because the subject was of former national news prominence. To be a former priest or nun seemed to lose the stigma which had been associated with this status in former generations.

Declining numbers of religious vocations, however, plagued the church. In some instances media advertising was used as a means of attracting the attention of viable candidates. When an advertisement for a monastic community appeared in *Playboy*, some reaction was rather strong. Defenders and attackers of the notice seemed to miss the point of whether this was an action motivated by a perception of the desperate plight of the religious vocation, or was it a clever and appropriate means of communicating with a basically healthy group of young men. Either way, it was attempting to deal with the reality of decreased numbers of candidates.

From the other end of the spectrum, some of it already noted, was the problem of professional drop out in middle years. When this phenomenon was observed after 1970, only a few studies were being done. Preliminary reports indicated financial, personal, familial, and professional pressures seemed to be the main reasons for apparently successful Protestant ministers changing vocations. In 1975 concern for this problem was being voiced not only for the professionally religious, but for the then recognizable phenomenon of middle aged career switch. Industrial models of career switch were related to technology. Non-industrial, articulate professionals related their motivation in seeking a less cluttered, more personally controllable and satisfying life style. Recognition began to develop that clergy live under unusual pressure, some of it self imposed, some of it from those whom they serve. Inability to respond to continual pressure seemed to be the basis for many decisions of middle aged clerics to seek a less pressured vocation and life style.

Finally, a common concern among religious groups in America was the struggle and challenge to find new ways of meeting the religious needs of a changing culture. Between 1955-1975 American culture became more mobile than any time in the prior experience of the country. Mobility, one in five families moved annually, created problems not previously encountered in a more stable culture. Urbanization, not only in terms of developing cities, but in the attitudes of agrarian based communities presented challenges of overcoming isolation, creating dependable relationships, providing crisis assistance, and developing a new concept of community. Future shock became reality, and as religious institutions took seriously their responsibilty to minister to human need, their common concerns were seen in overlapping areas of man's life experiences. But, mobility also created problems for denominational identity, as previously noted.

American Judaism

Failure to consider the Jewish community in a review of American religious experience has been cited in the reviews of many works in this area. How to include Judaism has been a problem for every writer about American religious experience. Judaism, however, has been a factor in the religious history of this country from the very beginning. This factor must be recognized in two ways. First, the dominant symbols and images used in the colonial period, referring to the destiny of the continent, have their origin in the expression of the Old Testament. Exodus, wilderness, promised land, and other key symbols are the common property of the Judao-Christian tradition. Second, as part of the earliest settlers of America, and as a definite ethnically identified group which grew through the various periods of immigration, Judaism has contributed leadership to the fields of medicine, education, entertainment, social service, business, and government. Some of the sociological studies on Judaism have tended to verify the "rags to riches" stories, and the push to professionalism among second and third generation Jews in America. An attempt must be made, however, to approach the phenomenon of Judaism in the mid-twentieth century.

One of the first items to be noted concerning Judaism in the twentieth century would be a sense of openness and a sense of being distinctly a part of the religious scene in America. This can be illustrated best by noting that a synagogue in Birmingham, Alabama, has for the past five years provided a notable Jewish scholar as speaker for a forum to which all Christian ministers in the city and area were invited. The forum has been held during February's observations of brotherhood. The other evidence for the standing of Judaism must come only by referring the reader to Will Herberg's *Protestant-Catholic-Jew*. As the third religious force in the American way, Judaism stands alongside Christianity, not separate from it, in molding the American ethos. But, these two illustrations do not provide much to help understand Judaism in American life, 1955-1975.

One of the first items for consideration is recognizing the impact of the formation of Israel as a state. The accomplishment of this goal presented a unique problem for Jews, because this produced a subtle shift in the foundation of twentieth century

Judaism. Until 1948 Jews were an exiled national body, dispersed. In the reality of nationhood in Israel, exile terminated and the responsibility of world citizenship was experienced on a new level. Israelite statehood also provided a glaring visibility to Judaism culturally and religiously. The glare became constant after 1967 when the Arab-Israeli conflict intensified into a seven day war, skirmishes from which continued to the present. Statehood and international responsibility were new experiences in Judaism.

They raised another issue, race verses religion. Traditionally violating the precise meaning of race, and using it to describe a distinct ethnic identity, many people have used the term "Jewish race." The designation was sufficiently common, as well as descriptive, to become acceptable. The question was raised by younger Jews during the mid-twentieth century whether they constituted a "race," or whether Judaism was only a religious identity. Their response tended to be that their distinctly Jewish identity or heritage had little influence on their development or accomplishment. This has been interpreted in ways which reflect that Judaism in America, except for some unique groups like the Hasidic community, had allowed its most talented to exercise leadership outside the confines of Judaism. Thus, a leadership crisis within Judaism was projected.

American Judaism, composed mainly of three distinct groups, is organized differently from Judaism in other parts of the world. Orthodox, Conservative, and Reformed are the three major groups, with a type of confederated structure. Conservative and Reformed Judaism were distinctly American creations. European organization of Judaism was community based, and the governing body in the community set up synagogues and schools and provided personnel for them. In America Judaism organized on a congregational pattern, following the cultural and legal models of Protestantism which was the controlling and molding entity in American experience. With a synagogue, i.e., congregational, base to organization, local diversity was facilitated in American Judaism. The three dominant movements were attempts to provide some national structures, but in each instance their confederated status was always primary. Among American Judaism, then, was a spectrum as broad as synagogues which reflected the thought of nineteenth century humanistic associations and Unitarianism, and the rigidity of Hasidic Jewish communities in New York City.

In order to meet the needs of Jews in American culture synagogues have experimented with Sunday morning services, but favored Friday evening for worship. In some instances Sunday school has provided a convenient time for pre-confirmation instruction. The prayer books have been translated for worship, since Hebrew became less well known by second and third generations of American Jews. At the same time some congregations have stressed learning Hebrew as a modern language.

Joseph L. Blau in the mid-sixties interpreted American Judaism as a healthily diverse force, both in American culture generally and in Judaism specifically. To him the diversity within Judaism was a sign of strength, vitality, interest, and concern. Unification among the Jewish segments of American society would be deadly for the future of American Judaism. He also pointed to a direct threat to American Judaism in the growth of the "unsynagogued." These individuals remained culturally and ethnically Jews, but were forsaking the traditional religious identities of Judaism. In this instance the differentiation was voiced over the substitution of "Jewishness" for "Judaism." One could be a Jew without being a practitioner of Judaism.

Blau challenged Judaism, and Christianity when he pointed out that the "synagogued" (read also, "churched") must find ways of relating to and servicing society as non-synagogue related organizations through which individuals met religious dedication in service. To be able to meet religious or spiritual needs through social welfare, ethical activities, cultural creativity, and even political participation outside the synagogue threatened it through loss of membership, leadership, and income. Blau expressed the problem within Judaism during the late sixties and early seventies, but he also expressed the problem among Christian churches.

Judaism in America has experienced the same general problems, faced some of the same changes, and experienced the same challenges of Protestantism and Roman Catholicism. Each group is a microcosm of the total cultural experience.

Touch the kaleidescope, and you may see the same thing from a different angle.

7

Epilog: From Adolescence to Middlescence

Reading, reflecting, and writing about American religious experience between 1955-1975 has been unique. Part of the experience has been a trip of nostalgia, knowing the past cannot be fully recaptured. Part of it has been a level of frustration, knowing that much which is of importance cannot be included with any sense of detail, aware that some omission will reflect both ignorance and provincialism. But, part of the experience has been joy.

There was a joy in being eighteen years old in 1955. The future looked bright. There was no draft, and the civilian enticement to military service had been terminated. Veterans' educational benefits ended in March 1955, and were not resumed until the mid-sixties. What lay ahead for many American youth was four years of college, marriage, job, a new family, five or six moves up the ladder of the organization, and a stable future. Life looked good then. You could plan your life, and work your plan.

Looking back on twenty years and the forces which have molded your culture, makes you aware that your experience has been of value. You feel a sense of identity, a sense of understanding of some of the forces that are now history. Especially, when you recall that next year's freshmen will be a group that were not even born in 1955, and only a few of the seniors will already be 21, you know that your sense of heritage is stronger than theirs.

There is something unique in knowing that Jaroslav Pelikan's *The Secret of Roman Catholicism* presented the best apology for Protestant understanding that had been done in this century. There is something even more unique in having the veil lifted on Rome by Vatican II, and knowing that Pelikan's volume reflected pre-conciliar Romanism, but that postconciliar Romanism is still developing. Change—no more meatless Fridays—had come. Challenge came, too.

If you followed certain normal patterns for an eighteen year old in 1955, you have been married approximately 15-17 years, and you have two or three children, teenagers. You have changed jobs three times, you are living in your third house, and you have two cars, wondering how you will make out with four drivers. Your wife may work, at least part time, and you feel fortunate you have not divorced. Then, again, some normal patterns are that you and your wife are former divorcees, and you find your-selves struggling with the responsibilities you have assumed, especially when your kids and her kids are in the same weekend.

Being eighteen in 1955 also made you eligible for welfare on a separate check. You were black, or Puerto Rican, or Mexican, and you had always been poor. Life among the poor was miserable in 1955. It was still miserable in 1975, even with the billions in federal and state assistance programs. Few middle class people know what it is to be poor all your life, to see your kids hungry. You know you should not have had the last two kids, broke your health, but you couldn't get the pills. No money, and your state didn't provide them for welfare. You talked to your social worker 'bout that operation, but she said, no money. At least the gov-ernment check increased a little each month with the birth of each of the last two children. Now I can stay home to raise 'em decent. But still, no money.

Being eighteen in 1955 you could remember the first time you saw TV. It was still new then. Billy Graham was the preacher. "The Bible says..." and he would tell you what the Bible said about sex, drinking, marriage, divorce, and almost any other subject. Seldom said a word about loving the blacks or Asians, except at a distance. His brand of religion was pretty personal. Just you and Jesus. TV was new. The programs had little violence in them.

In 1965 you were glad you were too old for the draft. After all, this wasn't really our war. Where'n hell was Viet Nam, anyway? Besides, if I went, it surely would mess things up here. I'm just getting started and we're feeling comfortable. And now that the kids are in school, we can begin to look forward to a little extra. Wife has gone back to teaching. Having the kids twenty months apart was pretty rough then, but now, well, we don't have to worry.

Try to remember—
Autherine Lucy
Marilyn Monroe
Babe Ruth
Bishop Pike
Rap Brown
Jessee Jackson
Lee Harvey Oswald
Chicago Seven
Daniel Berrigan
Elizabeth O'Connor
Joseph Feltcher
Thomas Altizer
Maharaji Mahesh Yogi
John XXIII
Oral Roberts
Carl McIntyre
Cynthia Wedel
Alison Cheek

Sometimes the struggle to remember who they were and what they represented is difficult. They were in the news—but was it before 1970, or after? Oh, well, if I really need to know, I guess I can find it in the encyclopedia. Besides I have a bridge game to concentrate on.

Sunday is important. That's the day we go to church. I need church. Somehow being there restores my faith. All the violence and war news on TV these days is enough to drive you mad. And then, the young people. I know I'm just over thirty, but I don't really understand them. Did you see them on TV last week at the convention? Police should be commended for being so careful with them. Let me tell you if that new preacher don't get off this social gospel bit, he's gonna find himself looking for a new pulpit. I want my kids to be taught right from wrong, respect for authority, and to love Jesus. In a couple years they'll be on their own and they need what they get in Sunday school. Sunday is important. It's a family day. We go to church.

He was so young. That's what the doctor said. Thirtyseven. A heart attack. A little unusual, but becoming more common. The pressure at work has been terrific, and we both felt it. The kids have been doing okay, I think. Now I'm alone. Thank God, I've got a job.

1955-1975. A lot of Americans moved from adolescence to middlescence. Where have they touched, or been touched by the religious groups and institutions in this county?

Touch the kaleidescope. See a reflection.

Suggested Reading

Abbott, Walter M., ed., *Documents of Vatican II:* with notes and comments by Catholic, Protestant, and Orthodox Authorities. New York: Associated Press, 1964.

Augenstein, Leroy. *Come, Let Us Play God.* New York: Harper & Row, 1969.

Barth, Karl. *Church Dogmatics.* 13 parts. Allenson, 1936-1969.

Bellah, Robert N. *The Broken Covenant: American Civil Religion in Time of Trial.* Philadelphia: Seabury, 1975. cf. McLoughlin.

Berne, Eric. *Games People Play: The Psychology of Human Relationships.* New York: Grove, 1964.

Blau, Joseph L. cf. McLoughlin.

Bloomfield, Harold H., et. al. *TM: Discovering Inner Energy and Overcoming Stress.* New York: Delacorte, 1975.

Bonhoeffer, Dietrich. *Letters and Papers from Prison* rev. ed. New York: Macmillan, 1967.

Brunner, Emil. *I Believe in the Living God, Sermons on the Apostles' Creed.* Holden, John, tr. Philadelphia: Westminster, 1959.

Buber, Martin. *For the Sake of Heaven.* Ludwig, Lewisohn, tr. Greenwood, 1953. *I and Thou.* Kaufman, Walter, tr. New York: Scribner, 1970. *Two Types of Faith: The Interpretation of Judaism and Christianity.* New York: Harper & Row, nd.

Bultmann, Rudolf. *Jesus and the Word.* Smith, Louise Pettibone

141

and Lanterr, Erminie Huntress, trs. New York: Scribner, 1958.

Buttrick, Arthur, ed. *The Interpreter's Bible.* 12 vols. Nashville: Abingdon. *The Interpreter's Dictionary.* 4 vols. Abingdon, 1960.

Barth, Karl. *Epistle to the Romans.* Hoskyns, Edwyn C., tr. Oxford, 1933.

Calvin, John. *Institutes of the Christian Religion.* 2 vols. Ed. John T. McNeill. Library of Christian Classics. Vol 20-21. Westminster, 1960.

Cone, James. *Black Theology and Black Power.* Philadelphia: Seabury, 1969.

Cox, Harvey. *The Secular City.* rev. ed. Macmillan, 1966.

Culbertson, Judi and Bard, Patti. *Games Christians Play, an Irreverent Guide to Religion Without Tears.* New York: Harper & Row, 1967.

Enroth, Ronald M. et al. *The Jesus People: Old Time Religion in the Age of Aquarius.* Grand Rapids: Eerdmans, 1972.

Ellwood, Robert. *One Way: The Jesus Movement and Its Meaning* Englewood Cliffs, N.J. Prentice Hall, 1973. *Religious Groups and Spiritual Groups in Modern America.* Englewood Cliffs, N.J.: Prentice Hall, 1972.

Fletcher, Joseph. *Situation Ethics: The New Morality.* Philadelphia: Westminster, 1966.

Foy, Felician A., ed. *Catholic Almanac 1976.* Our Sunday Visitor: Huntington Ind., 1975.

Frazier, E. Franklin. *The Negro Church in America.* New York: Shocken, 1963.

Friedan, Betty. *The Feminine Mystique.* New York: Norton, 1963.

Gallup, George H. *The Gallup Poll; Public Opinion, 1935-1971.* 3 vols. New York: Random House, 1972.

Guyer, Alan and Peerman Dean, eds. *Theological Crossings.* Grand Rapids: Eerdmans, 1971.

Harkness, Georgia. *Women in Church and Society.* Nashville: Abingdon, 1972.

Heschel, Abraham Joshua. *God in Search of Man: A Philosophy of Judaism.* New York: Holt, 1955. Octagon (1972 reprint). *Man is*

Not Alone: A Philosophy of Religion. Holt, 1955. Octagon, 1972 reprint.

Herberg, Will. *Protestant-Catholic-Jew: An Essay in Religious Sociology.* New York: Doubleday, 1955.

Hoge, Dean R. *Commitment on Campus: Changes in Religion and Values Over Five Decades.* Philadelphia: Westminster, 1974.

Johnson, James Weldon. *God's Trombones.* Viking, nd.

Kean, Samuel. *To a Dancing God.* New York: Harper & Row, 1970.

Kelley, Dean M. *Why Conservative Churches are Growing.* New York: Harper, 1972.

Liebman, Joshua Loth. *Peace of Mind.* New York: Simon & Schuster, 1947.

Lindbergh, Ann Morrow. *Gift From the Sea.* New York: Random, 1955.

McCall, Emmanuel, comp. *The Black Religious Experience.* Nashville: Broadman, 1972.

McLoughlin, William G. and Bellah, Robert N. *Religion in America.* New York: Houghton-Mifflin, 1967.

Merton, Thomas. *The Seven Storey Mountain.* New York: Doubleday, 1948.

Mitchell, Henry H. cf. McCall.

Moltmann, Jurgen. *Theology of Hope.* Harper & Row, 1967.

Neale, Robert E. *In Praise of Play: Toward a Psychology of Religion.* Harper, 1969.

The New Abingdon Bible Commentary. Abingdon, 1975.

Niebuhr, Reinhold. *Leaves From the Notebook of a Tamed Cynic.* New York: Meridan, =1929= 1957. *The Nature and Destiny of Man.* 2 vols. New York: Scribner, 1949.

Peale, Norman Vincent. *Guide to Confident Living.* Englewood Cliffs, N.J. Prentice Hall, 1948. *The Power of Positive Thinking.* Prentice Hall, 1952.

Pelikan, Jaroslav. *The Search of Roman Catholicism.* Nashville: Abingdon, 1959.

Rauschenbusch, Walter. *Prayers for the Social Gospel.* New York: Pilgrim Press, 1910. *A Theology for the Social Gospel.* Nashville: Abingdon, =1917 Macmillan=.

Richey, Rusell E. and Jones, Donald. *American Civil Religion.* New York: Harper & Row, 1974.

Robinson, John. *Honest to God.* Westminster, 1963.

Rogers, Dale Evans. *Angel Unaware.* Old Tappan, N.J. Revel, nd.

Ramm, Bernard. *The Evangelical Heritage.* Waco: Word, 1973.

Review and Expositor, "Women," LXXII, #1, Winter 1975. (Southern Baptist Theological Seminary, Louisville, Ky.)

Rosten, Leo. *Religions of America.* New York: Simon & Schuster, 1975.

Sklare, Marshall. *The Jew in American Society.* New York: Behrman House, Inc., 1974.

Sheldon, Charles M. *In His Steps.* Nashville: Broadman. *His Brother's Keeper.* Chicago: Advance Publ. Co., 1898.

Tillich, Paul. *The Eternal Now.* New York: Scribner, 1963. *The New Being.* New York: Scribner, 1955. *The Shaking of the Foundations.* New York: Scribner, 1948.

Visser't Hooft, W.A. *New Dehli Speaks about Christian Witness, Service, Unity.* New York: Association Press, 1962.

Washington, Joseph. *Black Religion.* Boston: Beacon Press, 1964.

White, James F. *New Forms of Worship.* Nashville: Abingdon, 1971.

Yankelovich, Daniel. *The New Morality: a Profile of American Youth in the 70's.* New York: McGraw-Hill, 1974.